The Emergency Medicine Trauma Handbook

T0201464

The Emergency Medicine Trauma Handbook

Edited by
Alex Koyfman
UT Southwestern Department of Emergency Medicine

Brit Long
SAUSHEC Department of Emergency Medicine

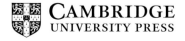

CAMBRIDGE
UNIVERSITY PRESS

University Printing House, Cambridge CB2 8BS, United Kingdom

One Liberty Plaza, 20th Floor, New York, NY 10006, USA

477 Williamstown Road, Port Melbourne, VIC 3207, Australia

314–321, 3rd Floor, Plot 3, Splendor Forum, Jasola District Centre, New Delhi – 110025, India

79 Anson Road, #06–04/06, Singapore 079906

Cambridge University Press is part of the University of Cambridge.

It furthers the University's mission by disseminating knowledge in the pursuit of education, learning, and research at the highest international levels of excellence.

www.cambridge.org
Information on this title: www.cambridge.org/9781108450287
DOI: 10.1017/9781108647397

© Cambridge University Press 2020

First published 2020

Printed in Singapore by Markono Print Media Pte Ltd

A catalogue record for this publication is available from the British Library.

Library of Congress Cataloging-in-Publication Data
Names: Koyfman, Alex, editor. | Long, Brit, 1986- editor.
Title: The emergency medicine trauma handbook / edited by Alex Koyfman, Brit Long.
Description: Cambridge, United Kingdom ; New York, NY : Cambridge University Press, 2020. | Includes bibliographical references and index.
Identifiers: LCCN 2019004817 | ISBN 9781108450287 (pbk. : alk. paper)
Subjects: | MESH: Emergency Treatment–methods | Wounds and Injuries–therapy | Emergencies
Classification: LCC RD93 | NLM WB 105 | DDC 617.1–dc23
LC record available at https://lccn.loc.gov/2019004817

ISBN 978-1-108-45028-7 Paperback

Contents

Contributors

Michael K. Abraham, MD, MS
Department of Emergency Medicine, University of Maryland School of Medicine, Baltimore, MD

Michael D. April, MD, DPhil, MSc
SAUSHEC Department of Emergency Medicine, Fort Sam Houston, TX

Ashley Brady, MD
Department of Emergency Medicine at the University of Texas Southwestern Medical Center, Dallas, TX

Christopher B. Colwell, MD
Zuckerberg San Francisco General Hospital and Trauma Center, and Department of Emergency Medicine, UCSF School of Medicine, San Francisco, CA

R. Erik Connor, MD
SAUSHEC Department of Emergency Medicine, Fort Sam Houston, TX

Katja Goldflam, MD
Department of Emergency Medicine, Yale School of Medicine, New Haven, CT

Michael Gottlieb, MD, RDMS
Department of Emergency Medicine, Rush University Medical Center, Chicago, IL

Matthew Greer, MD
Department of Anesthesia, Washington University in Saint Louis, School of Medicine, Saint Louis, MO

Jeffery Hill, MD, Med
Department of Emergency Medicine, University of Cincinnati, Cincinnati, OH

Timothy Horeczko, MD
Department of Emergency Medicine and Pediatric Medicine, Harbor-UCLA Medical Center, Torrance, CA

Mike Jackson, DO, LCDR
Department of Emergency Medicine, Naval Medical Center Portsmouth, Portsmouth, VA

Colin Kaide, MD
Department of Emergency Medicine, Wexner Medical Center at the Ohio State University, Columbus, OH

Norah Kairys, MD
Emergency Medicine, Temple University Hospital, Philadelphia, PA

Kristen Kann, MD
SAUSHEC Department of Emergency Medicine, Fort Sam Houston, TX

Dennis Kim, MD, FACS
Division of Surgery/Critical Care, Harbor-UCLA Medical Center, Torrance, CA

Andrew King, MD
Wexner Medical Center at the Ohio State University, Columbus, OH

Ryan LaFollette, MD
Department of Emergency Medicine, University of Cincinnati, Cincinnati, OH

Matthew R. Levine, MD
Department of Emergency Medicine, Northwestern Memorial Hospital, Chicago, IL

E. Liang Liu, MD
Department of Emergency Medicine at the University of Texas Southwestern Medical Center, Dallas, TX

Brit Long, MD
SAUSHEC Department of Emergency Medicine, Fort Sam Houston, TX

Brandon Morshedi, MD, DPT
Department of Emergency Medicine at the
University of Texas Southwestern Medical
Center, Dallas, TX

R. Grant Morshedi, MD
Little Rock Eye Clinic, Little Rock, AR

Jason F. Naylor, DSc, PA-C
US Army Institute of Surgical Research,
Department of Emergency Medicine, JBSA
Fort Sam Houston, TX

Ryan O'Halloran, MD, MS
Emergency Medicine Residency, Icahn
School of Medicine at Mount Sinai, New
York, NY

John D. Pemberton, DO, MBA
Oculoplastics, Harvey and Bernice Jones
Eye Institute, University of Arkansas
College of Medicine,
Little Rock, AR

Zachary Repanshek, MD
Emergency Medicine, Lewis Katz School of
Medicine at Temple University,
Philadelphia, PA

Steven G. Schauer, DO, MS
US Army Institute of Surgical Research,
JBSA Fort Sam Houston, TX

Kaushal Shah, MD
Education Emergency Department, Mount
Sinai Hospital, Icahn School of Medicine,
New York, NY

Manpreet Singh, MD
Department of Emergency Medicine,
Harbor-UCLA Medical Center,
Torrance, CA

Richard Slama, MD, LT
Department of Emergency Medicine, Naval
Medical Center Portsmouth,
Portsmouth, VA

Terren Trott, MD
Emergency Medicine, Critical Care
Medicine Cooper Health/Rowan School of
Medicine, University of Kentucky,
Lexington, KY

Brian T. Wessman, MD, FACEP, FCCM
Washington University in Saint Louis,
School of Medicine, Saint Louis, MO

Preface

Student, you do not study to pass the test. You
study to prepare for the day when you are the
only thing between a patient and the grave.
– *Mark Reid*

Next to creating a life, the finest thing a man
can do is save one.
– *Abraham Lincoln*

The best way to find yourself is to lose
yourself in the service of others.
– *Mahatma Gandhi*

One of the major causes of death worldwide is trauma. Many of these patients are managed
in the emergency department (ED). Emergency clinicians are masters of evaluating and
managing life-threatening diseases in the chaotic setting of the ED. From the first contact of
the injured patient, emergency clinicians play a vital role in their assessment and treatment.

Though trauma is often considered "the bread and butter" of emergency medicine,
several conditions associated with trauma can be challenging, as patients can be at death's
door upon initial presentation. If patients do not receive timely, quality care, they may die.
Knowledge of these conditions is imperative to ensuring we optimally care for trauma
patients, whether they arrive by emergency medical services with "lights and sirens," they
are dropped off at the door, or they simply walk in to the ED.

This text, *The Emergency Medicine Trauma Handbook*, presents a focused breakdown of
topics in trauma, with the goal to provide emergency physicians, residents, medical
students, nurses, and other healthcare workers vital information for the evaluation and
management of the patient with trauma, whether minor or life-threatening.

We thank all of the authors involved in the construction of this book, and we greatly
appreciate the assistance of the staff at Cambridge University Press. We also extend our
gratitude to our families for their amazing support and patience during the writing and
editing phases. We hope this book improves your clinical knowledge and practice, and
thank you for reading!

Disclaimer

This book and the content within does not reflect the views or opinions of the US government, Department of Defense, Brooke Army Medical Center, US Army, US Air Force, or SAUSHEC EM Residency Program.

Chapter 1

General Approach to Traumatic Injuries

Ryan O'Halloran and Kaushal Shah

Introduction

Trauma is the fourth leading cause of death overall in the United States and the number one cause of death for ages 1 to 44 – second only to heart disease and cancer in those older than 45 (CDC).[1] As the disease burden from infectious diseases declines and secondary prevention of chronic conditions improves, the relative importance of the practice of trauma care becomes even more apparent. Though safety engineering has improved across many industries (one need only consider examples such as crosswalk and bike lane planning, football helmet technology, and motor vehicle computerized improvements), trauma remains a significant threat to life and limb in emergency medicine.

The Trauma Team

The American College of Surgeons, the governing body for credentialing trauma centers, has provided guidelines for optimal resources necessary for a coordinated response to a critically injured trauma patient. Box 1.1 demonstrates the players suggested for an optimal response.

While response teams may vary, several principles are key to the functioning of a good, interdisciplinary team. These include clearly establishing roles for members of the team, following policy and protocols established in advance, briefing prior to the arrival of the patient, and debriefing after the event, whether immediately after the event or through quality case review. Successful team dynamics include the ability to be fluid, adaptable, and communicative.

Team leaders must focus on the big picture: overall physiologic status of the patient, triage of resources available in the trauma room, assigning tasks to individuals or groups of

---

Box 1.1   Human Resource Response to Trauma Activations

- Emergency Physician
- Emergency/Trauma Nurses
- Trauma Surgeon
- Anesthesiologist
- Radiology Tech (and radiologist)
- Blood Bank, Laboratory Support Staff
- Respiratory Therapist
- Social Worker
- Security

Table 1.1 Adapted in part from ALiEM article by Arlene Chung, an effective team debriefing checklist[2]

✓ Set ground rules (purpose, safe environment) and time expectations (5–10 minutes)	
✓ Present facts of the case (avoid excessive detail)	*Can you give us an overview about what happened from your viewpoint?*
✓ Elicit thoughts	*What was your first thought or most prominent thought?*
✓ Discuss reactions (emotions)	*How did that go? What were you feeling?*
✓ Discuss the facts of the case, medicine, and teamwork	*What was the worst? What was the best?*
✓ Teaching and learning	*What could have gone better?*
✓ Re-entry and closure (validate emotions, highlight learning points)	

Box 1.2   Trauma Teams That Are Successful at Helping Patients Work Together Well

- Institutionally organized policy and plans for interdepartmental cooperation
- Designated team leader
- "Pre-briefing" prior to arrival of trauma patients
- Debriefing and/or quality clinical reviews, of trauma resuscitations
- Closed-loop, concise, out-loud communication
- Systematic, reproducible approach to every trauma patient
- Ability to be fluid, adaptable, and communicative

---

individuals, and planning for the next series of actions for the patient and team. A systematic approach to the patient is important (discussed in Box 1.2), as is a systematic approach to directing the team. Critical actions, while they may be pre-designated to a member of the team by policy, must be verbalized and confirmed. Intravenous access, for example, is crucial for a sick trauma patient. Direct, closed-loop communication among team members is essential in trauma management. This call-and-response principle can be extrapolated to all critical tasks in the trauma room.

Trauma team members are often exposed to high stress, highly emotional situations. Team debriefing is critical for emotional well-being, education, and resolution of deficiencies, demonstrated in Table 1.1. It is ideal that a formal debriefing, even if only a few minutes, be completed after every trauma team activation. These meetings may be delayed based on the circumstances of the patient (e.g., going immediately to the operating room), but should be attempted as often as is practical, with as many of the team members as possible.

Emergency Medical Services (EMS)

The first step in the series of steps that can optimize outcome in trauma is accurate triage (with overtriage preferred over undertriage), rapid care that addresses immediate life

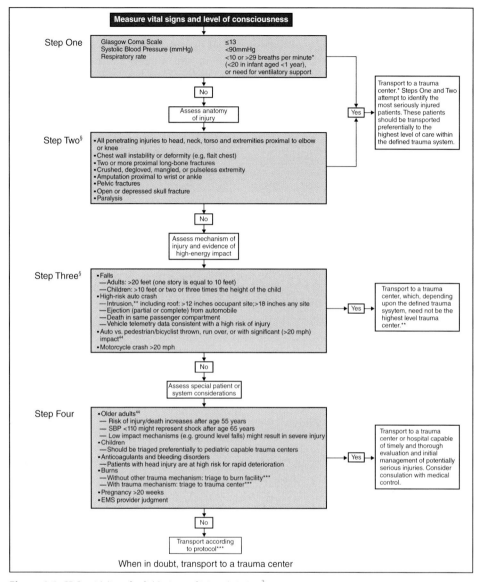

Measure vital signs and level of consciousness

Step One
Glasgow Coma Scale — ≤13
Systolic Blood Pressure (mmHg) — <90mmHg
Respiratory rate — <10 or >29 breaths per minute* (<20 in infant aged <1 year), or need for ventilatory support

No → Assess anatomy of injury

Yes → Transport to a trauma center.* Steps One and Two attempt to identify the most seriously injured patients. These patients should be transported preferentially to the highest level of care within the defined trauma system.

Step Two§
- All penetrating injuries to head, neck, torso and extremities proximal to elbow or knee
- Chest wall instability or deformity (e.g. flail chest)
- Two or more proximal long-bone fractures
- Crushed, degloved, mangled, or pulseless extremity
- Amputation proximal to wrist or ankle
- Pelvic fractures
- Open or depressed skull fracture
- Paralysis

No → Assess mechanism of injury and evidence of high-energy impact

Step Three§
- Falls
  — Adults: >20 feet (one story is equal to 10 feet)
  — Children: >10 feet or two or three times the height of the child
- High-risk auto crash
  — Intrusion,** including roof: >12 inches occupant site; >18 inches any site
  — Ejection (partial or complete) from automobile
  — Death in same passenger compartment
  — Vehicle telemetry data consistent with a high risk of injury
- Auto vs. pedestrian/bicyclist thrown, run over, or with significant (>20 mph) impact††
- Motorcycle crash >20 mph

Yes → Transport to a trauma center, which, depending upon the defined trauma sysytem, need not be the highest level trauma center.**

No → Assess special patient or system considerations

Step Four
- Older adults††
  — Risk of injury/death increases after age 55 years
  — SBP <110 might represent shock after age 65 years
  — Low impact mechanisms (e.g. ground level falls) might result in severe injury
- Children
  — Should be triaged preferentially to pediatric capable trauma centers
- Anticoagulants and bleeding disorders
  — Patients with head injury are at high risk for rapid deterioration
- Burns
  — Without other trauma mechanism: triage to burn facility***
  — With trauma mechanism: triage to trauma center***
- Pregnancy >20 weeks
- EMS provider judgment

Yes → Transport to a trauma center or hospital capable of timely and thorough evaluation and initial management of potentially serious injuries. Consider consulation with medical control.

No → Transport according to protocol***

When in doubt, transport to a trauma center

Figure 1.1 CDC guidelines for field triage of injured victims[3] (courtesy of the Centers for Disease Control, USA)

threats, and prompt transport to the appropriate level trauma center (see CDC guidelines chart, Figure 1.1) by EMS personnel.[3]

EMS professionals perform an abridged version of the hospital team's primary and secondary surveys. Many EMS systems rely on basic-level Emergency Medical Technicians (EMTs) to respond to calls for traumatic injuries. Modern EMT-staffed Basic Life Support ambulances carry equipment more advanced than simple standard first aid, such as tourniquets and hemostatic dressings for severe hemorrhage, and supraglottic airway devices. Paramedics, the highest trained pre-hospital providers, are capable of intubation, needle decompression, and IV and IO access. Regardless of the level of skill, or equipment available, rapid transport to the appropriate hospital is key to survival. Some controversial studies have suggested that police officers ought not to wait for EMS to transport victims – inferring that speed, rather than care provided in the interim of transport, is most important.[4-9]

EMS notification to the receiving hospital allows for the trauma team to assemble, prepare equipment, and "pre-brief," as described earlier, in anticipation of their arrival. In some urban systems this may be a quick "heads-up" that the ambulance is around the corner. In rural settings, the patient may be coming by air or ground from hours away. In extreme circumstances, notification may provide time for the calling-in backup personnel (such as in multiple or mass casualty incidents) or setup of decontamination equipment.

Upon entering the trauma room, the team leader ought to obtain a brief history from EMS about the mechanism of injury, vital signs, interventions started, and IV or IO access already obtained. This information, while easily ignored in haste to begin assessment and treatment, may be invaluable. A brief period of time should be set aside (30–60 seconds) where the EMS personnel can convey the critical data points or "bullet" to the team leader, discussed in Table 1.2.

Primary Survey

The primary survey is a rapid (less than two minutes), focused, and requisitely thorough process of identifying immediate threats to life, shown in Table 1.3. It should be completed

Table 1.2 Critical information to obtain from EMS during transition of care

EMS Bullet Information	
Critical Information	**Additional Information (if possible to obtain)**
Mechanism of Injury	Details of the mechanism (e.g., size of knife, type of gun, passenger
Latest Vital Signs (and trends)	space intrusion)
	Number of additional anticipated victims
Mental Status (and trend)	Past medical or surgical history, medications, allergies
IV/IO Access (if already obtained)	
Interventions	

Table 1.3 Immediately life-threatening conditions that must be identified during the primary survey

A – Airway	B – Breathing	C – Circulation	D – Disability	E – Exposure
• Swelling	• Pneumothorax	• Uncontrolled bleeding	• Herniation	• Any hiding injury
• Excessive fluid	• Hemothorax	• Hypotension	• Neurologic deficit suggestive of SCI	
• Burns	• Hypoxia			
• Tracheal injury	• Respiratory failure			

by a physician at the head-of-the-bed and start with a brief introduction: "my name is Dr. Smith, focus on me and my voice; lots of people are here to help and will be doing lots of things around you."

In the era of terrorism, high-power gunfire on city streets, and improvised explosive devices, it is important to immediately consider significant, life-threatening bleeding. Major uncontrolled external bleeding should be addressed before proceeding with the traditional "ABCDE" primary assessment; first with direct pressure, then consideration given to applying a tourniquet to the proximal extremity (or the "CABCDE" assessment).

At the end of the primary survey, while there is still more work to be done, the team leader has enough information to start considering the anticipated next steps, for example, the CT scanner, the intensive care unit, the operating room, or an operating room alternative such as interventional radiology.

A – Airway (Key Question: Do We Need to Take Control of the Airway Right Now?)

In many patients, a thorough assessment of the airway can be completed by asking one question: "what is your name?" A speaking patient, answering a question directly, typically has a patent and self-maintained airway. Changes in voice, gurgling, stridor, or the inability to speak in full sentences should be noted as clues to impending airway problems. Ultimately the decision must be made if it is necessary to immediately take control of the airway. Box 1.3 lists the most important things to consider when deciding to intubate a trauma patient.[10,11]

If the patient must be intubated, it is critical to mentally and physically prepare for an anatomically and physiologically difficult airway. Anatomy may be severely distorted by the trauma or simply difficult to visualize due to a cervical collar in place, swelling, or bleeding. The need for a backup plan should always be anticipated; before intubating, have a gum elastic bougie, supraglottic airway, video laryngoscope, and/or scalpel for cricothyrotomy available. As with any other anticipated difficult airway, a verbalized plan for front-of-the-neck access should be in place should a cricothyrotomy be required.

The already-physiologically-stressed trauma patient may respond profoundly to induction and paralytic agents – as many are already reliant on a sympathetic surge to maintain their cardiac output. Consider medication selection in the context of the patient's physiology. For example, ketamine[12–18] or etomidate[19–23] are better choices for induction in the context of hypotension, as they are less likely to cause a drop in blood pressure. Relative contraindications for paralytic agents should also be considered.[24–26] Likewise, consider

---

Box 1.3 Indications For Early or Immediate Intubation in the Trauma Room[10,11]
- Severe head injury, with significantly decreased mental status (GCS <8, mGCS <6)
- Penetrating neck trauma (such as gunshot wounds, or poorly visualized stab wounds)
- Severe burns (especially involving inhalation injury to the airway)
- Significant blunt or penetrating chest trauma impairing breathing efforts
- Severely intoxicated or agitated patients prohibiting assessment of life-threatening injuries
- Anticipated course (such as transport to another facility, or immediate surgery)
- Severely ill, unresponsive, or otherwise in extremis

adjusting the dosages of medications for hypotension; lower doses of sedatives and higher doses of paralytics may be required.[27] Attention should be given to beginning pre-oxygenation and optimization of the patient's physiology (mean arterial pressure, oxygen saturations, etc.). If the mental status allows, insert a supraglottic airway, place a nasal cannula, apply a bag valve mask, and/or utilize noninvasive ventilation to pre-oxygenate as would be expected with any non-trauma patient.

B – Breathing (Key Questions: Are Chest Tubes Required? Is There Bleeding in the Chest?)

Assessment of breathing is a look (ensure equal chest rise, quantify the respiratory rate, check for wounds), listen (auscultate bilaterally), and feel (press on the chest wall to assess for crepitus or flail rib segments) process. Glance at the monitor and note the oxygen saturation. Pneumothorax can be more subtle than anticipated. Careful attention to asymmetric breath sounds (as referred sounds from one side of the chest could be heard on the collapsed-lung side), neck veins, and tracheal deviation could be crucial to picking up a pneumothorax or hemothorax before it develops tension physiology.

If there is concern for pneumothorax or hemothorax in a hemodynamically unstable patient, needle decompression of the chest or placement of a chest tube should be completed immediately. This is both a diagnostic and therapeutic procedure in critically ill trauma patients, especially those with penetrating trauma to the chest.

C – Circulation (Key Question: Where Are They Bleeding and Do They Need Blood?)

Coagulopathy, acidosis, and hypothermia – the trauma triad of death –all primarily stem from shock in trauma. Finding and promptly methodically stopping major hemorrhage is paramount. The trauma adage is that blood can be found in six major places: the chest, the abdomen, the pelvis, the retroperitoneum, the thighs (or areas around other long bones), and the street.

External hemorrhage may be obvious or discovered when exposing the patient. Internal hemorrhage may be more subtle and requires considering the patient's heart rate, blood pressure, and appearance. Obtain a complete set of vital signs and assess peripheral circulation. Weak pulses and cool extremities imply a shock state, as does a more objective rise in the shock index (heart rate divided by systolic blood pressure). While cutoffs for tachycardia and blood pressure are more poorly defined in the literature, a shock index <0.7 or >1.3 is correlated with poorer outcomes,[28] and a shock index >0.95 is correlated with the need for massive transfusion.[29]

Ensure that good intravenous access has been obtained – at least two large-bore (i.e., at least 18-gauge) IVs in most trauma patients. While short, 18-gauge peripheral IVs are excellent methods for volume resuscitation, consideration should be given to placement of an intraosseous or central venous line if peripheral access is limited or difficult. While obtaining IV access, lab work should be sent, including a typical trauma panel of labs: complete blood count, venous blood gas (serum lactate), basic chemistry, coagulation studies, and type-and-screen for potential transfusion. Additional labs may be obtained, but they usually do not guide initial management. Initial hemoglobin and hematocrit levels may be falsely reassuring, as it takes time for blood concentrations of heme to equilibrate to rapid blood loss. Patients known to be on anticoagulants, or with elevated coagulation times, ought to be reversed in the context of active hemorrhage.

Hypotension/Shock

Classically taught "classes of shock" based on various vital sign cutoffs is important to appreciate; however, the literature demonstrates that they are not entirely reliable and often insensitive predictors of shock.[30,31] Normotensive elderly patients might be in shock. Children and healthy adults might compensate very well, leading to deceptively normal vital signs. The trajectory in tachycardia, mean arterial pressure, and mental status must be considered in any trauma patient with the potential for active bleeding.

If the patient is hypotensive, blood loss must be at the top of the differential for the cause, but also consider non-bleeding causes of hypotension in trauma; namely, tension pneumothorax, cardiac tamponade, spinal cord injury, myocardial dysfunction (from contusion, underlying heart disease, arrhythmia, or infarction), and toxic ingestions. Box 1.4 discusses causes of hypotension in trauma.

External bleeding should be stopped with direct pressure. Consider that holes in the skin are not always lined up with where blood originates. Attempts to apply pressure at potentially retracted vascular structures, or over proximal pressure points, may be reasonable additional measures. If blood loss from an extremity cannot be stopped with direct pressure, consider placing hemostatic stitches (e.g., a figure-of-eight or whip stitch) or staples if the wound is small enough. If bleeding cannot be controlled from a larger wound, such as an amputation, utilize a tourniquet (preferably a commercially available product or manual blood pressure cuff).

Blood loss from the pelvis is often associated with pelvic fractures, which may be stabilized with binding (either with a commercially available device or properly placed and secured bedsheet). While there are various types of pelvic fractures – some of which do not benefit from binding – a hypotensive patient with suspected active bleeding in the pelvis might benefit from empiric binding as a temporary measure.

Box 1.4   Differential for Hypotension in the Trauma Patient

Hemorrhagic Shock
- Bleeding (chest, abdomen, pelvis, retroperitoneum, long bones, street)

Obstructive Shock
- Tension pneumothorax
- Cardiac tamponade

Neurogenic Shock
- Spinal cord injury

Cardiogenic Shock
- Myocardial dysfunction (contusion, underlying heart disease, arrhythmia, infarction)

Distributive Shock (or other mechanisms)
- Toxic ingestion (poisoning, substance use)

Whether suffering from internal or external bleeding, a hemodynamically unstable patient needs to have replaced what has been lost: whole blood. Transfusion with packed red blood cells alone may not be adequate. Consider initiating a massive transfusion protocol. Protocols vary by institution but should include a mix of products containing packed fresh frozen plasma (FFP), platelets, and red blood cells (PRBC). The PROPPR and PROMMTT trials have demonstrated that overall transfusion in a ratio of 1:1:1 of FFP: Platelets:PRBCs is optimal.[32,33] Prothrombin Complex Concentrate (PCC) can be considered as an alternative to FFP, as it does not require thawing and is often more readily available. Consider supplemental calcium, as citrate in blood products can chelate body stores of calcium, potentiating hypotension. The CRASH-2 trial also demonstrated the efficacy of tranexamic acid (TXA), if given within the first three hours, to improve mortality in patients in hemorrhagic shock from trauma.[34] While IV fluids can temporarily elevate the circulating blood volume, they dilute clotting factors and perhaps unnecessarily increase the mean arterial pressure affecting hemostasis. They should be used sparingly and only as a bridge to blood products. Vasopressors have no role in hemorrhagic shock from trauma. Target resuscitation to a MAP of 65 mm Hg typically – and increase this goal to 80 mm Hg in any patient suspected of head injury or spinal cord injury.[35–37] This strategy of allowing penetrating trauma patients to remain slightly hypotensive is sometimes referred to as "permissive hypotension," and, although it has been demonstrated to be effective in one randomized trial, subsequent human trials have not been able to validate the benefit; therefore, the strategy remains controversial.[38]

Lastly, consideration may be given to more invasive hemostasis options such as a resuscitative thoracotomy[39–41] or placement of a Resuscitative Endovascular Balloon Occlusion of the Aorta (REBOA),[42–44] in select patients nearing death.

D – Disability (Key Question: Is There a Major Neurologic Deficit?)

During the primary survey the neurological assessment should include Glasgow Coma Scale (GCS),[45] pupillary exam, and gross motor/sensory assessment of all four extremities. Mental status is a key assessment in the overall status of the trauma patient. GCS can help assess the trajectory of the patient over time. Studies have indicated that simply assessing the motor component of the GCS can be a simplified, binary assessment (can the patient follow simple commands?) and is equally predictive of the need for airway management and mortality, discussed in Table 1.4.[46] Localized neurologic (or vascular) deficits in the context

Table 1.4 Glasgow Coma Scale GCS score[45] is used to stratify mental status in trauma patients[46]

Eye		Verbal		Motor	
4	Spontaneous opening	5	Oriented	6	Obeys commands
3	Opens to voice	4	Confused	5	Localizes pain
2	Opens to pain	3	Inappropriate	4	Withdraws from pain
1	No eye opening	2	Incomprehensible	3	Flexes to pain
		1	No verbal response	2	Extends to pain
				1	No motor response

Table 1.5 Key questions to consider in each portion of the primary survey

Airway	*Do we need to take control of the airway right now?*
Breathing	*Are chest tubes required? Is there bleeding in the chest?*
Circulation	*Where are they bleeding and do they need blood?*
Disability	*Is there a major neurologic deficit?*
Exposure	*What injuries haven't been found yet?*

of a mangled or deformed extremity may prompt a rapid bone or joint reduction and improve the likelihood of limb salvage.

All trauma patients with a significant mechanism of injury should be placed in a cervical collar until it is demonstrated they do not have an injury to the cervical spine, whether by clinical decision rules (in highly assessable patients, such as NEXUS or the Canadian C-Spine Rule) or by imaging and exam.[47,48]

If using induction or paralytic agents for intubation, the next possible neurologic exam will likely be significantly delayed. Consider performing a thorough baseline exam, if possible, prior to intubation.

If there is clinical evidence of brain herniation from head trauma, hyperosmolar therapy should be started to partially abate rises in intracerebral pressure (and subsequent losses in cerebral perfusion pressure).[49-56] Any intubation performed in this context should be completed by an experienced provider, as first-pass success minimizes hypotension and hypoxia.[55,57,58] Definitive therapy will require neurosurgical intervention.

E – Expose (Key Question: What Injuries Haven't Been Found Yet?)

Norman McSwain, a trauma surgeon and developer of the initial Advanced Trauma Life Support (ATLS) program, noted that "paranoia prevents disasters: the most severe injury is under the unremoved clothes." Every trauma patient should be exposed from head-to-toe in order to be examined thoroughly for injuries. Careful attention must be paid to areas that hide injuries, such as the axilla, skin folds, and the perineum. All patients must be rolled to examine the back. Key questions to consider in the primary survey are listed in Table 1.5.

Secondary Survey

As a continuation of the exposure portion of the primary survey, start from the head and work inferiorly, visualizing every square inch of the trauma patient. Descriptions of wounds ought to be as objective as possible and documented either with drawings of the body or precise anatomical locations. For example, "exit wound on the right flank" may be better stated as "1 cm ballistic wound in the R flank at the level of T5, 4 cm to the right of the midline." Excess qualifiers ("exit wound") serve to define the mechanism of injury in ways not typically known to the trauma team and do not provide additional, useful medical information. Remember these statements in the medical record may have criminal or legal implications for the patient or assailant.

A complete head-to-toe secondary survey, including rolling the patient and checking the posterior anatomy, should take no more than three to four minutes. Decisions should be

Table 1.6 General overview of the process of the trauma assessment

Primary Survey	Secondary Survey
• Massive Bleeding/Circulation	• Head-to-toe exam, including the back
• Airway	• Medications and allergies
• Breathing	• Past medical and surgical history
• Circulation	• Last oral intake
• Disability	• Discuss events leading to the trauma
• Expose	• Consider imaging

made at this point about what imaging needs to be completed in the trauma bay, i.e. what imaging is pivotal to deciding the next steps for the patient. While rolling the patient, consider placing plain film radiology plates underneath the patient's chest and pelvis.

Lastly, the secondary survey includes asking about the patient's past medical and surgical history, current medications (paying special attention to those immediately relevant to the trauma resuscitation, such as anticoagulant or antiplatelet agents), allergies, last oral intake, tetanus status, and any other details of the incident that led to the trauma in the first place. The general overview of the trauma assessment is listed in Table 1.6.

Imaging

Trauma Bay Imaging

A chest x-ray has long been the tradition for the trauma bay imaging of choice to evaluate for pneumothorax. In reality, a chest x-ray is poor at identifying this pathology, with sensitivity of 28–75%, especially if performed supine. The alternative is the eFAST (Extended Focused Assessment with Sonography in Trauma). This ultrasound exam is more sensitive (86–98%) than chest x-ray, and equally specific. It can be performed faster (no pun intended), and synergize better with the next steps.[59] If the patient is unstable with traumatic mechanism and there is clinical evidence to suggest pneumothorax (especially tension pneumothorax), a chest tube should be placed empirically without waiting for imaging.

The eFAST is a six-part study that assesses for abdominal free fluid, pericardial effusion, and pneumothorax. The prominent role for this procedure was largely designed to replace the need for diagnostic peritoneal lavage (DPL) to rule-out or rule-in abdominal sources of bleeding in blunt trauma patients with unstable vital signs, primarily as a means to guide operative therapy. In practice, the eFAST exam is also performed routinely on stable trauma patients, looking to identify the same abdominal and pericardial pathology early, and to identify pneumothoraces without the need for a chest x-ray. Positioning of the patient is key to enhancing the sensitivity of the exam. Brief periods in Trendelenburg (for the right and left upper quadrant views), reverse-Trendelenburg (for the suprapubic view), and supine (for the subxiphoid and lung views) will help position organ tissue, fluid, and air to improve diagnostics. Serial eFAST exams are not unreasonable in a stable patient, or one in whom the clinical picture has changed (sudden hypoxia or hypotension). Ultrasound has been

Ryan O'Halloran and Kaushal Shah

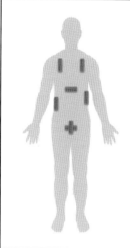

Extended Focused Assessment with Sonography in Trauma (eFAST) Views

1. Right upper quadrant view
2. Left upper quadrant view
3. Suprapubic view (two axes)
4. Subxiphoid view
5. Lung views (bilaterally)

Figure 1.2 The eFAST assesses six locations, looking for intraperitoneal fluid, pericardial fluid, and pneumothorax. Extended Focused Assessment with Sonography in Trauma (eFAST) views: (1) Right upper quadrant view; (2) Left upper quadrant view; (3) Suprapubic view (two axes); (4) Subxiphoid view; and (5) Lung views (bilaterally)

noted to be as high as 100% sensitive for identifying the need for laparotomy in unstable patients, though only 75% sensitive (and 98% specific) for identifying free fluid in stable and unstable trauma patients cohorted together.[60–65] Figure 1.2 describes ultrasound views.

If the mechanism or primary and secondary survey suggest a possible pelvic fracture, a portable film of the pelvis should be completed as well. As mentioned above, any unstable patient where a pelvic source of bleeding is suspected should empirically have the pelvis placed in a binding device. Suspected pelvic fracture is an indication for portable pelvis x-ray in the trauma bay, but this may be omitted to pursue more expedient definitive CT imaging in the hemodynamically stable patient.

CT Scans

Given the limitations of chest x-ray, pelvic x-ray, and the eFAST exam, more advanced imaging is often required to completely assess injuries. CT scans should be completed for areas where potentially clinically relevant injury has occurred. Priority should be given to scans identifying immediate life threats (such as intracranial hemorrhage in an obtunded fall victim with clinical evidence of herniation) over operative planning scans (such as three-dimensional reconstruction images of a trimalleolar ankle fracture) that do not immediately impact the next steps in management or disposition of the patient.

Some decision rules may aid in ruling-out clinically relevant injury, such as the NEXUS,[47] Canadian Head CT,[66] and C-spine[48] rules, though clinical judgment will dictate when most CT imaging is ordered. Some strategies involve major trauma patients routinely receiving whole-body or "pan-scan" CT imaging; others advocate for more selective imaging based on mechanism and exam. Whole Body CT (WBCT) typically includes non-contrast studies of the head and c-spine, as well as IV contrast enhanced studies of the chest, abdomen, and pelvis. In the era of multi-detector CT scanners, a trauma "pan-scan" typically delivers approximately 20 mSv of radiation (a 0.35% increased risk of cancer in one's lifetime, compared to the population's lifetime inherent risk of death from cancer of approximately 25%).[67] Proponents of whole-body scans argue that diagnoses are less likely to be missed and are identified faster. Advocates for the selective scanning highlight the unnecessary radiation exposure and increased incidental, clinically irrelevant findings that lead to further unnecessary – or at worst potentially harmful – testing and treatment. Little prospective evidence exists on the matter. Most recently, the REACT-2 trial, a prospective, multicenter study with intention-to-treat analysis of major trauma patients, found no difference in mortality (24-hour, 30-day, or overall) for WBCT vs. selective imaging. While the evidence is scant, WBCT may be a better option in patients who are not easily assessed (intoxicated, severely injured, altered mental status with unreliable exam, etc.).[68]

Disposition and Ongoing Care

Final disposition of the trauma patient is based on the dynamic assessment of hemodynamic status and findings on evaluation. Due to improved CT imaging, many trauma patients can be discharged home more rapidly and, similarly, many patients who might have been taken for exploratory laparotomy can now be observed for progression of injuries.

Unstable patients with active bleeding, internally or externally, require source control, and are often taken to the operating room or interventional radiology suite. Efficient use of resources (personnel, imaging, and multidisciplinary brain power) in the trauma bay, as explained in this chapter, will get the patient what they need, when they need it, and as methodically as possible.

Key Points

- Trauma systems are complex and expensive, but regionalized, systemized, tiered care saves lives of the sickest injured patients.
- The team dynamic is critical to success in trauma; having the right people, empowered to do their jobs, who communicate well, is necessary for the best outcomes.
- EMS has valuable information; be sure to ask about details of the mechanism of injury, interventions already completed, and trends in vital signs or mental status.
- The primary survey (airway, breathing, circulation, disability, exposure) is designed to identify immediate threats to life. The secondary survey is designed to identify every injury, complete a thorough evaluation, and guide imaging.
- The eFAST exam is sensitive for bleeding (most strongly in unstable patients) and more sensitive than chest x-ray for pneumothorax. CT scans make critical diagnoses and should not be delayed, even in the stable trauma patient.

References

1. Kochanek K, Murphy S, Xu J, Tejada-Vera B. National vital statistics reports deaths: final data for 2014. Centers for Disease Control. www.cdc.gov. 2016.

2. Chung A. Wellness and resiliency during residency: debriefing critical incidents and podcast. *Academic Life in Emergency Medicine*. Online blog entry. www.aliem.com/2017/01/wellness-resiliency-debriefing-critical-incidents/. 2017.

3. McCoy CE, Chakravarthy B, Lotfipour S. Guidelines for field triage of injured patients: In conjunction with the morbidity and mortality weekly report published by the center for disease control and prevention. *West J Emerg Med.* 2013;14 (1):69–76.

4. Gonzalez RP, Cummings GR, Phelan HA, Mulekar MS, Rodning CB. Does increased emergency medical services prehospital time affect patient mortality in rural motor vehicle crashes? A statewide analysis. *Am J Surg.* 2009;197(1):30–34.

5. McCoy CE, Menchine M, Sampson S, Anderson C, Kahn C. Emergency medical services out-of-hospital scene and transport times and their association with mortality in trauma patients presenting to an urban level I trauma center. *Ann Emerg Med.* 2013;61(2):167–74.

6. Seamon MJ, Fisher CA, Gaughan J, et al. Prehospital procedures before emergency department thoracotomy: "scoop and run" saves lives. *J Trauma.* 2007;63(1):113–20.

7. Branas CC, Sing RF, Davidson SJ. Urban trauma transport of assaulted patients using nonmedical personnel. *Acad Emerg Med.* 1995;2(6):486–93.

8. Demetriades D, Chan L, Cornwell E, et al. Paramedic vs private transportation of trauma patients: effect on outcome. *Arch Surg.* 1996;131(2):133–38.

9. Band RA, Salhi RA, Holena DN, et al. Severity-adjusted mortality in trauma patients transported by police. *Ann Emerg Med.* 2014;63(5):614.e3.

10. Shah K, Lee J, Medlej K, Weingart SD, eds. *Practical Emergency Resuscitation and Critical Care.* Cambridge: Cambridge University Press; 2013.

11. Strayer R. Reasons to intubate. Emergency Medicine Updates Web Site. http://emupdates.com/2016/12/29/reasons-to-intubate/. Updated 2016. Accessed October 5, 2017.

12. Price B, Arthur AO, Brunko M, et al. Hemodynamic consequences of ketamine vs etomidate for endotracheal intubation in the air medical setting. *Am J Emerg Med.* 2013;31(7):1124–32.

13. Heffner AC, Swords D, Kline JA, Jones AE. The frequency and significance of postintubation hypotension during emergency airway management. *J Crit Care.* 2012;27(4):417.13.

14. Fields AM, Rosbolt MB, Cohn SM. Induction agents for intubation of the trauma patient. *J Trauma.* 2009;67 (4):867–69.

15. Weingart SD, Trueger NS, Wong N, et al. Delayed sequence intubation: a prospective observational study. *Ann Emerg Med.* 2015;65(4):349–55.

16. Dewhirst E, Frazier WJ, Leder M, Fraser DD, Tobias JD. Cardiac arrest following ketamine administration for rapid sequence intubation. *J Intensive Care Med.* 2013;28(6):375–79.

17. Morris C, Perris A, Klein J, Mahoney P. Anaesthesia in haemodynamically compromised emergency patients: does ketamine represent the best choice of induction agent? *Anaesthesia.* 2009;64 (5):532–39.

18. Miller M, Kruit N, Heldreich C, et al. Hemodynamic response after rapid sequence induction with ketamine in out-of-hospital patients at risk of shock as defined by the shock index. *Ann Emerg Med.* 2016;68(2):188.e2.

19. Oglesby AJ. Should etomidate be the induction agent of choice for rapid sequence intubation in the emergency department? *Emerg Med J.* 2004;21 (6):655–59.

20. Zed PJ, Abu-Laban RB, Harrison DW. Intubating conditions and hemodynamic effects of etomidate for rapid sequence intubation in the emergency department: an observational cohort study. *Acad Emerg Med.* 2006;13(4):378–83.

21. Sokolove PE, Price DD, Okada P. The safety of etomidate for emergency rapid sequence intubation of pediatric patients. *Pediatr Emerg Care.* 2000;16(1):18–21.

22. Jellish WS, Riche H, Salord F, Ravussin P, Tempelhoff R. Etomidate and thiopental-based anesthetic induction: comparisons between different titrated levels of electrophysiologic cortical depression and

response to laryngoscopy. *J Clin Anesth.* 1997;9(1):36–41.

23. Guldner G, Schultz J, Sexton P, Fortner C, Richmond M. Etomidate for rapid-sequence intubation in young children: hemodynamic effects and adverse events. *Acad Emerg Med.* 2003;10(2):134–39.

24. Taha SK, El-Khatib MF, Baraka AS, et al. Effect of suxamethonium vs rocuronium on onset of oxygen desaturation during apnoea following rapid sequence induction. *Anaesthesia.* 2010;65(4):358–61.

25. Curley GF. Rapid sequence induction with rocuronium – a challenge to the gold standard. *Crit Care.* 2011;15(5):190.

26. Heier T, Caldwell JE. Rapid tracheal intubation with large-dose rocuronium: a probability-based approach. *Anesth Analg.* 2000;90(1):175–79.

27. Reich DL, Hossain S, Krol M, et al. Predictors of hypotension after induction of general anesthesia. *Anesth Analg.* 2005;101(3):8, table of contents.

28. Singh A, Ali S, Agarwal A, Srivastava RN. Correlation of shock index and modified shock index with the outcome of adult trauma patients: a prospective study of 9860 patients. *N Am J Med Sci.* 2014;6(9):450–52.

29. Rau C, Wu S, Kuo SCH, et al. Prediction of massive transfusion in trauma patients with shock index, modified shock index, and age shock index. *Int J Environ Res Public Health.* 2016;13(7):683.

30. Thomas I, Dixon J. Bradycardia in acute haemorrhage. *BMJ.* 2004;328(7437):451–53.

31. Guly HR, Bouamra O, Little R, et al. Testing the validity of the ATLS classification of hypovolaemic shock. *Resuscitation.* 2010;81(9):1142–47.

32. Holcomb JB, Tilley BC, Baraniuk S, et al. Transfusion of plasma, platelets, and red blood cells in a 1:1:1 vs a 1:1:2 ratio and mortality in patients with severe trauma: the PROPPR randomized clinical trial. *JAMA.* 2015;313(5):471–82.

33. Holcomb JB, Fox EE, Wade CE, PROMMTT Study Group. The PRospective Observational Multicenter Major Trauma Transfusion (PROMMTT) study. *J Trauma Acute Care Surg.* 2013;75(1 Suppl 1):1.

34. Roberts I, Shakur H, Coats T, et al. The CRASH-2 trial: a randomised controlled trial and economic evaluation of the effects of tranexamic acid on death, vascular occlusive events and transfusion requirement in bleeding trauma patients. *Health Technol Assess.* 2013;17(10):1–79.

35. Wiles MD. Blood pressure management in trauma: from feast to famine? *Anaesthesia.* 2013;68(5):445–49.

36. Berry C, Ley EJ, Bukur M, et al. Redefining hypotension in traumatic brain injury. *Injury.* 2012;43(11):1833–37.

37. Maas AI, Dearden M, Teasdale GM, et al. EBIC-guidelines for management of severe head injury in adults. European brain injury consortium. *Acta Neurochir (Wien).* 1997;139(4):286–94.

38. Bickell WH, Wall MJ, Jr, Pepe PE, et al. Immediate versus delayed fluid resuscitation for hypotensive patients with penetrating torso injuries. *N Engl J Med.* 1994;331(17):1105–09.

39. Moore EE, Knudson MM, Burlew CC, et al. Defining the limits of resuscitative emergency department thoracotomy: a contemporary Western trauma association perspective. *J Trauma.* 2011;70(2):334–39.

40. Hunt PA, Greaves I, Owens WA. Emergency thoracotomy in thoracic trauma – a review. *Injury.* 2006;37(1):1–19.

41. Seamon MJ, Haut ER, Van Arendonk K, et al. An evidence-based approach to patient selection for emergency department thoracotomy: a practice management guideline from the Eastern Association for the Surgery of Trauma. *J Trauma Acute Care Surg.* 2015;79(1):159–73.

42. Brenner M, Hoehn M, Teeter W, Stein D, Scalea T. Trading scalpels for sheaths: catheter-based treatment of vascular injury can be effectively performed by acute care surgeons trained in endovascular techniques. *J Trauma Acute Care Surg.* 2016;80(5):783–86.

43. Biffl WL, Fox CJ, Moore EE. The role of REBOA in the control of exsanguinating

torso hemorrhage. *J Trauma Acute Care Surg.* 2015;78(5):1054–58.

44. Stannard A, Eliason JL, Rasmussen TE. Resuscitative endovascular balloon occlusion of the aorta (REBOA) as an adjunct for hemorrhagic shock. *J Trauma.* 2011;71(6):1869–72.

45. Teasdale G, Jennett B. Assessment of coma and impaired consciousness. A practical scale. *Lancet.* 1974;2(7872):81–84.

46. Chou R, Totten AM, Carney N, et al. Predictive utility of the total Glasgow coma scale versus the motor component of the Glasgow coma scale for identification of patients with serious traumatic injuries. *Ann Emerg Med.* 2017;70(2):157.e6.

47. Hoffman JR, Wolfson AB, Todd K, Mower WR. Selective cervical spine radiography in blunt trauma: methodology of the national emergency X-radiography utilization study (NEXUS). *Ann Emerg Med.* 1998;32 (4):461–69.

48. Stiell IG, Wells GA, Vandemheen KL, et al. The Canadian C-spine rule for radiography in alert and stable trauma patients. *JAMA.* 2001;286(15):1841–48.

49. Battison C, Andrews PJ, Graham C, Petty T. Randomized, controlled trial on the effect of a 20% mannitol solution and a 7.5% saline/6% dextran solution on increased intracranial pressure after brain injury. *Crit Care Med.* 2005;33(1):8.

50. Ware ML, Nemani VM, Meeker M, et al. Effects of 23.4% sodium chloride solution in reducing intracranial pressure in patients with traumatic brain injury: a preliminary study. *Neurosurgery.* 2005;57 (4):36.

51. Shackford SR, Bourguignon PR, Wald SL, et al. Hypertonic saline resuscitation of patients with head injury: a prospective, randomized clinical trial. *J Trauma.* 1998;44(1):50–58.

52. Sakowitz OW, Stover JF, Sarrafzadeh AS, Unterberg AW, Kiening KL. Effects of mannitol bolus administration on intracranial pressure, cerebral extracellular metabolites, and tissue oxygenation in severely head-injured patients. *J Trauma.* 2007;62(2):292–98.

53. McGraw CP, Howard G. Effect of mannitol on increased intracranial pressure. *Neurosurgery.* 1983;13(3):269–71.

54. James HE. Methodology for the control of intracranial pressure with hypertonic mannitol. *Acta Neurochir (Wien).* 1980;51 (3–4):161–72.

55. Brain Trauma Foundation, American Association of Neurological Surgeons, Congress of Neurological Surgeons, et al. Guidelines for the management of severe traumatic brain injury. II. hyperosmolar therapy. *J Neurotrauma.* 2007;24(Suppl 1):14.

56. Hinson HE, Stein D, Sheth KN. Hypertonic saline and mannitol therapy in critical care neurology. *J Intensive Care Med.* 2013;28 (1):3–11.

57. Jaeger M, Dengl M, Meixensberger J, Schuhmann MU. Effects of cerebrovascular pressure reactivity-guided optimization of cerebral perfusion pressure on brain tissue oxygenation after traumatic brain injury. *Crit Care Med.* 2010;38(5):1343–47.

58. Elf K, Nilsson P, Ronne-Engstrom E, Howells T, Enblad P. Cerebral perfusion pressure between 50 and 60 mm hg may be beneficial in head-injured patients: a computerized secondary insult monitoring study. *Neurosurgery.* 2005;56(5):71.

59. Wilkerson RG, Stone MB. Sensitivity of bedside ultrasound and supine anteroposterior chest radiographs for the identification of pneumothorax after blunt trauma. *Acad Emerg Med.* 2010;17(1):11–17.

60. Stengel D, Rademacher G, Ekkernkamp A, Guthoff C, Mutze S. Emergency ultrasound-based algorithms for diagnosing blunt abdominal trauma. *Cochrane Database Syst Rev.* 2015;(9): CD004446.

61. Quinn AC, Sinert R. What is the utility of the focused assessment with sonography in trauma (FAST) exam in penetrating torso trauma? *Injury.* 2011;42(5):482–87.

62. Wherrett LJ, Boulanger BR, McLellan BA, et al. Hypotension after blunt abdominal trauma: the role of emergent abdominal sonography in surgical triage. *J Trauma.* 1996;41(5):815–20.

63. Rozycki GS, Ballard RB, Feliciano DV, Schmidt JA, Pennington SD. Surgeon-performed ultrasound for the assessment of truncal injuries: lessons learned from 1540 patients. *Ann Surg.* 1998;228(4):557–67.

64. McKenney M, Lentz K, Nunez D, et al. Can ultrasound replace diagnostic peritoneal lavage in the assessment of blunt trauma? *J Trauma.* 1994;37(3):439–41.

65. Ng A. The FAST examination how good is FAST. Trauma.org Web site. www.trauma.org/archive/radiology/FASThowgood.html. Updated 2001. Accessed October 5, 2017.

66. Stiell IG, Wells GA, Vandemheen K, et al. The Canadian CT head rule for patients with minor head injury. *Lancet.* 2001;357 (9266):1391–96.

67. Brenner DJ, Elliston CD. Estimated radiation risks potentially associated with full-body CT screening. *Radiology.* 2004;232(3):735–38.

68. Sierink JC, Treskes K, Edwards MJ, et al. Immediate total-body CT scanning versus conventional imaging and selective CT scanning in patients with severe trauma (REACT-2): a randomised controlled trial. *Lancet.* 2016;388(10045):673–83.

Trauma Airway

Colin Kaide and Andrew King

Airway management is of paramount importance in trauma resuscitations; in fact, virtually all management algorithms begin with the assessment and protection of the airway. Trauma airways are often compromised and among the most difficult to manage due to hemodynamic instability from multi-organ dysfunction, cervical trauma, or direct trauma to airway structures.

Important Considerations for Airway Management in Trauma Patients

Airway management in the trauma patient can pose many challenges, even for the most experienced clinicians. These factors can occur independently or collectively to complicate the care of the trauma patient. There are a few specific, unique aspects of trauma airway management that require special preparation and caution (Box 2.1).

Consider Pre-existing Difficult Airway

A fundamental rule of airway management is to ensure caution when considering the paralysis of a patient who is expected to be a difficult or impossible intubation, unless the clinician has a specific plan to address a failed airway. Further, the ability to adequately mask ventilate should be considered when determining the type and method of airway intervention.

Trauma Immobilization

The physical process of trauma immobilization with a cervical collar and backboard can significantly limit access to the airway and the anterior neck. A properly placed collar limits mouth opening and intentionally prevents repositioning of the head and neck. If time

---

Box 2.1 Complicating Factors in the Trauma Airway

- Pre-existing difficult airway (anterior larynx, short neck, poor jaw mobility, etc.)
- Physical constraints of trauma immobilization
- Potential or actual injuries to the cervical spine
- Mechanical distortion of the airway anatomy from direct trauma to oral, pharyngeal, or laryngeal structures
- Mechanical distortion of the airway from injuries to contiguous structures (lower neck, thorax, or trachea)
- Other non-airway factors such as hypotension, brain injury, or pneumothorax which compete with the urgency to control the airway
- Hypoxia from underlying lung injury, such as pulmonary contusion

allows, patients should be log rolled off a backboard, and providers should remove the cervical collar and utilize inline stabilization during intubation attempts.

Mechanical Distortion of the Airway and Contiguous Structures

Direct trauma; previous surgery; or cancers to the face, larynx, or thorax can alter the normal anatomical relationships of the airway structures and can significantly increase the difficulty of the intubation.

Indications for Airway Intervention

The decision to intubate a trauma patient is among the most important and definitive steps in the management algorithm. The primary goals of airway management are to improve gas exchange, relieve respiratory distress by decreasing the work of breathing, and protection against aspiration (Box 2.2). Secondary goals range from the control of the agitated patient to the delivery of heated, humidified oxygen to facilitate core rewarming.[1]

Traumatic Injuries with Associated Difficult Airways

Closed Head Injury

- Changes in hemodynamics, oxygenation, and ventilation should be minimized in an attempt to maintain adequate cerebral perfusion pressure (CPP).
- CPP = MAP – ICP, where ICP is intracranial pressure and MAP is mean arterial pressure.
- Laryngoscopy causes an increase in ICP secondary to its resultant hypertension.
- The goal during intubation is to minimize the two main contributors to increased ICP – patient position and hypoventilation (Box 2.3).
- Obtain a focused neurologic examination prior to intubation and the administration of sedatives and paralytics in an effort to guide further care.
- Opiates, such as Fentanyl, may be given two-to-three minutes prior to intubation in an effort to blunt the sympathetic response.
- Ketamine, etomidate, or propofol can be used as an induction agent.

Box 2.2 Intubation Considerations

Indications for Intubation
- Oxygenation Failure: PO_2 <60 on FiO_2 >40%
- Ventilation Failure: pH of <7.3 associated with hypoventilation or pCO_2 >55 with previously normal pCO_2 or rise in pCO_2 by 10 acutely in COPD
- Intentional Hyperventilation
- Profound Shock: Reduces energy expenditure used during rapid breathing
- Intentional Paralysis: To accomplish necessary procedures in a non-compliant patient
- Aspiration Protection
- Mechanical Obstruction
- Core rewarming

Box 2.3 Airway Management Pearls in Closed Head Injury
- Preparation: Ensure proper positioning, pre-oxygenation, and use apneic oxygenation with nasal cannula
- Elevate the head of the bed to improve cerebral perfusion pressure and decrease aspiration risk
- Premedication regimens are controversial. Fentanyl or esmolol may decrease catecholamine surge and control the hemodynamic response to intubation
- Ketamine and etomidate are the best induction agents – with the least hemodynamic effects
- Propofol has neuroprotective effects, but hypotension and decreased CPP can result
- Post-intubation analgesia and sedation are essential – drips should be prepared prior to intubation to minimize the effects of agitation on ICP

- Ketamine increases cerebral blood flow and counters systemic hypotension. Evidence suggests that it does not elevate ICP.
- Although propofol can be used, it should be used with caution and with reduced doses in patients who are hemodynamically unstable.

Maxillofacial Trauma
- Facial trauma can significantly distort normal anatomy, and injuries can range in severity from minimal to severe.
- In cases where airway obstruction is either present or imminent, immediate decisive action is required. Alternatively, some patients initially present with minor respiratory difficulty, but pose a significant risk of rapid deterioration.
- A few moments should be taken to plan an effective strategy to safely intervene without resulting in further harm.
- Expectant management or delayed decision-making may force a cricothyrotomy.
- Preparation including arrangements for back up plans significantly increases the chances of successfully securing the airway.
- The patient's neck should immediately be prepped for a surgical airway in the event of a likely difficult airway or failed intubation.
- There is an associated cervical spine injury in up to 5% of patients with maxillofacial trauma and neurologic injury in up to 36%.[2,3]
- If there is no concern for C-spine injury, place the patient in an upright position to allow blood and secretions to drain. Check the oropharyngeal anatomy and ensure jaw mobility.
- RSI is the initial method of choice – if not possible or contraindicated then a surgical airway should be performed (Box 2.4).

Direct Airway Trauma
- Important signs or symptoms of airway involvement include dyspnea, cyanosis, subcutaneous emphysema, hoarseness, and air bubbling through the wound site (Box 2.5).
- Penetrating trauma has a high degree of morbidity and mortality; in fact, the overall mortality is as high as 11%,[4] with up to 40% of patients requiring emergent intubation.[5,6]

Box 2.4 Airway Management Pearls in Maxillofacial Trauma
- Preparation: Examine oropharyngeal anatomy and ensure jaw mobility. Rapidly devise a specific strategy
- Can rapidly deteriorate – delayed decision-making may result in cricothyrotomy
- Associated cervical spine and neurologic injuries can occur
- RSI initial method of choice – if not possible or contraindicated then cricothyrotomy

Box 2.5 Airway Management Pearls in Direct Airway Trauma
- Important signs or symptoms of airway involvement include dyspnea, cyanosis, subcutaneous emphysema, hoarseness, and air bubbling through the wound site
- Indications for intubation in penetrating trauma include acute respiratory distress, airway compromise from blood or secretions, extensive subcutaneous emphysema, tracheal shift, or altered mental status
- GSW to the anterior neck is an indication for early intubation due to expanding hematoma; stab wounds need intubation only if there is evidence of airway or vascular trauma
- Awake airway evaluation or intubation can be performed with sedation (Ketamine) and topical anesthesia
- Blunt neck trauma has a high incidence of associated cervical spine injury

- Zone I – between the clavicles and cricoid cartilage – is the least common neck injury, but the most likely to require emergent airway management due to the close proximity of major pulmonary and vascular structures.[5]
- Tracheobronchial injury occurs in approximately 10–20% of patients with penetrating trauma to the neck.[7–10]
- Indications for intubation in the setting of penetrating trauma include acute respiratory distress, airway compromise from blood or secretions, extensive subcutaneous emphysema, tracheal shift, or altered mental status.[11]
- Gunshot wound to the anterior neck is also an indication for early intubation in order to prevent obstruction from an expanding hematoma.[12]
- A stab wound to the anterior neck is an indication for early intubation only if there is evidence of vascular or direct airway trauma.[13]
- Orotracheal intubation with RSI is the technique of choice in penetrating neck trauma[12]; however, administration of paralytics may result in an obstructed airway due to the relaxation of a damaged airway segment.
- An awake airway evaluation or an awake intubation can be performed under sedation and topical anesthesia. Ketamine has been suggested as a good induction agent to use in this setting without paralytics.[14]
- Occasionally the entrance wound provides a direct communication between the anterior neck and the trachea – in this case, it may be easier to intubate directly through the wound.
- Blunt trauma to the neck is frequently more complicated as it is associated with a high incidence of C-spine injuries. Specifically, up to 50% of blunt airway trauma patients have concurrent C-spine injuries.[15]

- In terms of securing the airway in patients with blunt neck trauma, there are essentially three initial methods of choice: RSI, awake intubation, and awake fiberoptic intubation. The exception occurs in a laryngeal fracture, in which emergent tracheostomy is the best first maneuver.

Cervical Spine Injury

- All trauma patients who present with cervical spine precautions should be assumed to have a cervical spine injury until proven otherwise (Box 2.6).
- The two initial methods of choice for securing the airway are oral intubation with RSI or awake fiberoptic intubation.
- When performing RSI, the anterior portion of the collar should be removed to allow for manual in-line axial head and neck stabilization (MILS).
- MILS has been shown to immobilize the c-spine better in the setting of endotracheal intubation than the c-collar alone.[16]
- However, MILS can make intubation attempts difficult, and it may not reduce the risk of cervical spine movment.[17,18]
- Consider airway adjuncts such as using video assisted laryngoscopy to improve the chance of success while maintaining MILS.

Thoracic Trauma

- Thoracic trauma may present difficulties when it causes a distortion of the trachea from its normal midline position (Box 2.7).
- Occasionally a large pneumothorax can cause significant subcutaneous emphysema tracking into the neck, which can interfere with the ability to identify the trachea and/or cricothyroid membrane.
- Pneumothorax, hemothorax, or significant trauma to the lung (pulmonary contusion) can inhibit the ability to adequately pre-oxygenate the patient prior to the intubation.
- A pneumothorax should be treated prior to intubation if possible.

Box 2.6 Airway Management Pearls Cervical Spine Injury
- All trauma patients should be assumed to have a C-spine injury until proven otherwise
- RSI or awake fiberoptic intubation are the preferred methods
- When performing RSI, the anterior portion of the cervical collar should be removed to allow for manual in-line stabilization
- Consider airway adjuncts to improve chances of success while maintaining manual in-line stabilization

Box 2.7 Airway Management Pearls Thoracic Trauma
- Thoracic trauma can displace the trachea from the normal midline position or distort the normal anatomy and landmarks
- RSI or awake fiberoptic intubation are the preferred methods
- Thoracic injuries can inhibit pre-oxygenation
- Treat pneumothorax prior to intubation if able

> **Box 2.8** Airway Management Pearls in Burns
>
> - Upper airway edema is progressive over hours – advisable to secure an airway early, but reasonable to consult with burn specialist in many circumstances
> - Liberal use of nasopharyngoscopy can help with the decision to intubate or manage expectantly
> - If prolonged transport is needed to a burn center, consider a secure airway prior to transfer
> - RSI is the method of choice, but could also consider awake intubation or fiberoptic intubation
> - Indications for intubation:
>   - Stridor or hoarseness
>   - Known inhalation of toxic fumes
>   - Increased work of breathing
>   - Burn or edema to airway structures
>   - Carbonaceous sputum or soot in nares or mouth

Burns

- Upper airway edema is progressive over 24–36 hours after the burn; therefore, it is advisable to secure an airway earlier rather than later (Box 2.8).
- Because burn injuries develop over hours, it is often is reasonable to consult a burn specialist prior to securing an airway when appropriate.
- If transport is needed to a burn center, particularly a prolonged transport, consider a secure airway with intubation prior to transfer.
- Indications for intubation include: Stridor or hoarseness, known inhalation of toxic fumes, and increased work of breathing. Nasopharyngoscopy by the treating clinician or an ENT consultant can help to look for evidence of burns or edema of the posterior pharyngeal or glottis structures. If no burns to these structures are discovered and the patient remains stable, intubation can be withheld. Remember, however, that this is a dynamic situation. Any change with respect to the patient's work of breathing or stridor should prompt another nasopharyngoscopic evaluation or definitive airway management with intubation.
- Standard oral endotracheal intubation with RSI is the initial method of choice to secure the airway when no obvious obstruction is visualized.
- If concerned about obstruction, "an awake look" should be performed under sedation and topical anesthetics.
- Because of the incidence of upper airway edema, there should be a low threshold for moving to fiberoptic intubation or cricothyrotomy.

Rapid-Sequence Intubation (RSI)

RSI is currently considered the method of choice for emergent airway control in the trauma patient, unless specific contraindications are present (Box 2.9).[19–21]

Rapid Sequence Intubation (RSI): The Technique

A teaching tool to describe the steps of RSI was developed by Walls.[21] The "P's" of RSI are described below in a modified form that reflects emphasis on some new considerations.

Box 2.9 RSI Contraindications

- Absolute Contraindications:
    . Total upper airway obstruction requiring surgical airway
    . Loss of facial/oropharyngeal landmarks requiring surgical airway

- Relative Contraindications:
    . Anticipated difficult airway scenario where endotracheal intubation may not be successful, relying on bag-valve-mask
    . Crash airway scenario with the patient in a cardiac arrest situation, unconscious, and apneic, which requires immediate intervention with no medications

P – Plan B

The first P in this series refers to the predetermined plan for dealing with a difficult or failed orotracheal intubation. A complicated situation can rapidly become a disaster if no pre-implemented plan is in place to mitigate unanticipated difficulty. An emergency airway cart, containing difficult intubation equipment, can keep all needed tools readily available. See Box 2.10 for an example emergency airway cart.

P – Predict a Difficult Intubation

A thorough evaluation of the patient prior to attempts at laryngoscopy can help to predict a difficult intubation. The LEMON law can be used as a tool for airway evaluation. The description below adds "S" for saturation.

By discussing out loud your primary plan, your plan B, and the conditions which will mandate an emergent cricothyrotomy, it will make it easier to move to cricothyrotomy if indicated.

L – Look Externally

External anatomical features that can predict difficult intubation are short muscular neck, protruding upper incisors, high-arched palate, receding mandible, and severe facial trauma.

E – Evaluate Internally: The 3-3-2 Rule

The rule describes the ideal external dimensions of the airway.

3 – the opening of the jaw should be far enough to accommodate three fingers (3–4 cm).
3 – the distance from the mentum to the hyoid bone should be at least three fingerbreadths.
2 – the distance from the floor of the mouth to the thyroid cartilage should be at least two fingerbreadths.

M – Mallampati

The Mallampati classification was developed to correlate a simple visual inspection of the patient's pharynx with the ability to obtain direct visualization of the larynx. Airways are designated as Class I, II, III, or IV. Mallampati classes roughly correlate with the Cormack and Lehane direct laryngoscopic views, graded as 1, 2, 3, and 4 (Figure 2.1).

Box 2.10   Airway Management Supplies

Emergency Airway Supplies (example)

- A complete set of RSI drugs

  - Induction/Sedation agents: Etomidate, ketamine
  - Paralytic agents: Succinylcholine, rocuronium, vecuronium
  - Adjunctive medications: Atropine, lidocaine

- Various ET tube sizes and types: Pediatric and adult

  - Oropharyngeal and nasopharyngeal airways

- Additional laryngoscope parts

  - Miller and Macintosh blades
  - Standard laryngoscope handle
  - Pediatric laryngoscope handle

- Video laryngoscopy tools

  - GlideScope
  - C-Mac
  - Airtraq

- Airway Adjuncts

  - Tracheal Introducer (Bougie)
  - LMA – laryngeal mask airway
  - ILMA – intubating LMA
  - King LT
  - Retrograde intubation sets

- Surgical Airway Tools

  - Percutaneous and open cricothyrotomy kits
  - Scalpels (#10, #11, #15 blades)
  - Extra instruments

- Various size needles and syringes

O – Obstruction

Blood in the upper airway, foreign body, expanding hematoma, abscess, swelling of intraoral structures, or laryngeal edema.

N – Neck mobility

Inability to flex or extend the neck (c-collar, arthritis, etc.), Cervical spine injury.

S – Saturation

An oxygen saturation <85% portends an impending desaturation that can occur very rapidly. This does not allow much time to perform the intubation and may result in cardiac arrest due to hypoxemia.

- Mallampati Class I: No difficulty: Soft palate, uvula, fauces, pillars visible
- Mallampati Class II: No difficulty: Soft palate, uvula, fauces visible
- Mallampati Class III: Moderate difficulty: Soft palate, base of uvula visible
- Mallampati Class IV: Major difficulty: Hard palate only visible

By Jmarchn (Own work) reproduced under CC BY-SA 3.0 (https://creativecommons.org/licenses/by-sa/3.0)

Figure 2.1 Mallampati classification

- Mallampati Class I: No difficulty: Soft palate, uvula, fauces, pillars visible
- Mallampati Class II: No difficulty: Soft palate, uvula, fauces visible
- Mallampati Class III: Moderate difficulty: Soft palate, base of uvula visible
- Mallampati Class IV: Major difficulty: Hard palate only visible

(by Jmarchn (Own work), reproduced under CC BY-SA 3.0; https://creativecommons.org/licenses/by-sa/3.0)

P – Prepare

Preparation includes the following:

- Remove dentures.
- Bring the difficult airway cart to the bedside.
- Have the chosen intubation method set up.
- Verify the integrity of the balloon on the ET tube.
- Have suction ready at the bedside. When preparing suction, it is useful to have two suction options available. A standard Yankauer tip works well for loose secretions but does not adequately aspirate larger food pieces.
- Verify the integrity of IV access.
- Have color-change capnography and/or end-tidal CO_2 device ready.

P – Preoxygenate

As early as possible the patient should be placed on high flow oxygen, as close to 100% FiO_2 as possible (Figure 2.2). A typical NRB mask with oxygen reservoir can only provide an FiO_2 in the mid 60% range. The FiO_2 can be substantially raised by placing a nasal cannula set at 15 LPM on the patient during the preoxygenation period. A full 15 LPM can be effectively delivered via a standard cannula.[22] A non-rebreather mask with a reservoir is then added over the nasal cannula and set at the absolute maximum possible setting. This means that the oxygen flow knob will be turned until it will not turn any further. During the intubation procedure, the mask is removed, but the nasal cannula is left in place during intubation. Passive oxygenation, also known as apneic oxygenation, provides real oxygen delivery to the patient and can help maintain saturations above 90% for an extended period of time.[22,23] Patients should be positioned sitting up during pre-oxygenation, as patients will have less ventilation/perfusion mismatch compared to lying flat.

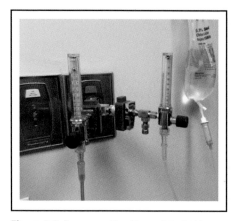
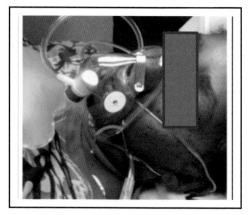

Figure 2.2 Preoxygenation (Photos: Colin Kaide)

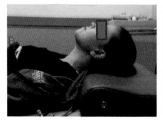
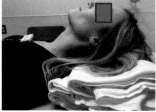
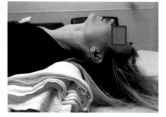

Proper positioning with earlobe in line with sternal notch and face parallel to the floor. Used with permission courtesy of Colin Kaide.

Proper positioning with earlobe in line with sternal notch and face parallel to the floor using multiple blankets.

Incorrect positioning with earlobe not in line with sternal notch and neck hyperextended. Used with permission courtesy of Colin Kaide.

Figure 2.3 Positioning (Photos: Colin Kaide)
Proper positioning with earlobe in line with sternal notch and face parallel to the floor (used with permission, courtesy of Colin Kaide)
Proper positioning with earlobe in line with sternal notch and face parallel to the floor using multiple blankets
Incorrect positioning with earlobe not in line with sternal notch and neck hyperextended (used with permission, courtesy of Colin Kaide)

P – Position

Many trauma patients present in a c-collar (Figure 2.3). After collar removal, the c-spine should be maintained with manual in-line stabilization. If the patient's c-spine can be cleared, the patient should be placed such that the head is elevated off the bed by a few inches (approximately four inches). The head is subsequently extended on the neck so that the face is parallel to the ceiling, while the earlobe is aligned with the sternal notch.[22] This maximizes the alignment of the oral axis, pharyngeal axis, and the glottis axis. Except in the pediatric patient, placing the pillow or towel roll beneath the shoulders to force hyperextension of the neck without elevating the head is not helpful, and should be avoided.

P – Put to Sleep

- Induction agents are given simultaneously to or in rapid succession with paralytic agents (Table 2.1).
- Cricoid pressure (Sellick's Maneuver) is no longer recommended routinely. It has no proven benefits and can potentially make intubation more difficult.[24]

Table 2.1 Sedation agents

	Etomidate	Ketamine	Propofol
Dosage	IV 0.3 mg/kg IV 0.15 mg/kg in hypotensive patients	IV push 1–2 mg/kg, with decreased doses in hypotension	Adult and Children: 2–2.5 mg/kg IV slowly over 30 sec; with decreased doses in hypotension
Pregnancy Category	C	Unknown, but likely safe	B
Preparation	2 mg/mL	100, 50, and 10 mg/mL	10 mg/mL
Description	Non-barbiturate, sedative hypnotic with anesthetic and amnestic properties (no analgesia)	Dissociative anesthetic; PCP derivative. May act at multiple receptor sites including opioid and cholinergic *Ketamine is the only single agent with anesthetic, amnestic, and analgesic properties*	Non-barbiturate, sedative-hypnotic with anesthetic and amnestic properties
Onset & Duration	<60 sec; 6–10 min	IV 30–60 sec; 10–15 min	<60 sec; 5–10 min
Reversal Agent	None	None proven; naloxone and physostigmine may have some theoretical effect	None
Ideal Patient	• Need for rapid induction • Excellent for older patients or those with tenuous cardiovascular status • Induction in a hypotensive patient, but at reduced doses	• Induction in a hypotensive patient, but at reduced doses • The need for induction in a patient with bronchospasm	• Induction of anesthesia in hemodynamically stable patients
Contraindications	• Allergy to etomidate • In Addison's Disease, must supplement corticosteroids	• Ischemic Heart Disease • Age <3 mo	• Allergy to albumin or egg whites • Compromised cardiac function • Caution in elderly patients (exaggerated hypotension)

Table 2.1 (cont.)

	Etomidate	Ketamine	Propofol
Major Side-Effects	• Apnea-related to dose and rate of administration is rare and only minor respiratory depression is seen. • Pain on injection common • Decreased ICP and cerebral perfusion pressure • Spontaneous myoclonus (not seizure) is seen in up to 30% of patients • Transient ACTH-resistant/ hydrocortisone-responsive decrease in the production of cortisol • Vomiting and hiccups are possible during and post-procedure	• Transient 20–30% increase in BP and heart rate • Nystagmus • Nausea – vomiting is rare and usually occurs late after emergence • Excess salivation – use atropine/ glycopyrrolate • Hallucinations on awakening (rare in children <13) – hallucinations are much less frequent than previously reported in adults and are virtually eliminated by the addition of 2 mg of midazolam • Transient apnea is very rare and seen only with rapid-push of high doses • Laryngospasm in patients with recent URI or history of severe asthma (not a significant concern when used with a paralytic agent) • *Side-effects rarely outweigh the potential benefits of ketamine as an induction agent in the hypotensive patient*	• Transient hypotension and apnea are related to dose and rate of administration • Pain on injection (10%) • Decreased ICP and cerebral perfusion pressure

- Avoid ventilating the patient until reoxygenation is required, as indicated by oxygen saturation falling below 90%.

P – Paralyze

- Depolarizing agents such as succinylcholine act at the ACh receptor and act to initially cause depolarization of the motor endplate and induce contraction, manifesting clinically as fasciculations (Table 2.2).
- Subsequently, the receptor is blocked by the succinylcholine, preventing ACh from binding and producing further contraction. The paralysis lasts until succinylcholine is degraded by acetylcholinesterase.
- Non-depolarizing agents such as vecuronium and rocuronium competitively inhibit the ACh receptor, occupying it and then exiting the site. These agents are removed

Table 2.2 Paralytic agents

	Succinylcholine	Rocuronium
Dosage	1.5–2 mg/kg IV rapid push	0.6–1.2 mg/kg IV rapid push. 1 mg/kg is preferred dose
Pregnancy Category	C	B
Preparation	20 mq/mL	10 mg/mL
Description	Depolarizing neuromuscular blocking agent	Non-depolarizing neuromuscular blocking agent
Onset	30–60 sec	45–90 sec
Duration	6–12 min	15–40 min
Reversal Agents	None	Neostigmine, Sugammadex
Ideal Patient	First-line paralytic agent in RSI	• May be used as 1st or 2nd line agent for RSI • Rapid onset (slower than SUX) but long duration of action
Contraindications	• Burn or spinal cord injury patients >48 h post-injury • Neuromuscular diseases • CVA less than 6 months out • Open-globe ocular injury • Use can cause bradycardia unless pretreatment with anticholinergic • Known hyperkalemia	• Hypersensitivity to rocuronium • Hypersensitivity to bromides
Major Side-Effects	• Muscular fasciculation • Transient hyperkalemia • Increased ICP and intraocular pressure	• Tachycardia • Transient hypo/hypertension

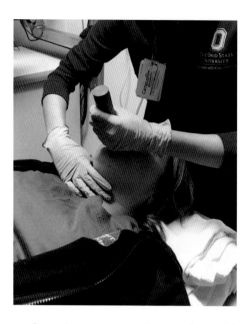

Figure 2.4 External laryngeal manipulation (Photo: Colin Kaide)

from the neuromuscular junction and broken down in the liver. Their duration and onset of action are generally longer than succinylcholine. Vecuronium is not ideal for RSI and is best used for ongoing paralysis.

P – Pass the Tube

One technique which has been described to facilitate direct visualization of an anterior larynx is called "BURP" (Backward-Upward-Rightward-Pressure).[25,26] The assistant applies pressure to the thyroid cartilage, first backward (toward the table), then upward (toward the head), and finally rightward. The adult larynx should be displaced backward so as to abut the vertebrae, 0.5–2 cm to the right and about 2 cm cephalad. Meanwhile, the intubator attempts direct visualization of the larynx.

External Laryngeal Manipulation (ELM) achieves the same backward, upward, and rightward airway repositioning as does "BURP," however the pressure is applied by the intubator with his or her right hand.[27,28] This allows the intubator to visualize the effects of the manipulations and adjust the pressure accordingly. The final position of the larynx can be held by the assistant, freeing the intubator's right hand to complete the procedure (Figure 2.4).

Video Laryngoscopy

The introduction of video laryngoscopy has virtually made most other airway devices obsolete. This device uses a fiberoptic lens attached to the laryngoscope blade or at the end of a stylet to transmit a picture of the cords to a portable LCD screen. Direct visualization of the tube passing through the cords can be obtained.

The GlideScope

- Unlike with a conventional laryngoscope, the GlideScope blade is inserted in the middle of the tongue without a sweeping motion.

- Owing to the steep curvature of the blade, the cords can be easily seen, even in an anterior airway.
- Occasionally, the cords and tube can be seen, but difficulty arises in trying to pass the tube through the opening. Passage of the tube can be made easier by using the rigid GlideScope stylet.

The C-MAC

- Conceptually similar to the GlideScope, but the C-MAC uses a blade configured much like a conventional Macintosh blade, whereas the glidescope blade has a more hyperacute angle.
- The CMAC can be used to perform DL, with the back-up of having a video view of the cords.
- One study suggested that the C-MAC and GlideScope both provided good views of the cords, however use of the C-MAC resulted in faster times to passage of the tube successfully through the cords.[29]

P – Prove Placement

The final step is to verify the correct placement of the ETT into the trachea. After the tube is passed and the cuff is inflated, the chest should be auscultated for breath sounds. Physical exam alone is not sufficient to definitively confirm ETT placement into the trachea, with a sensitivity of 94% and specificity of 83%.[30] The American College of Emergency Physicians policy statement states that additional modalities should be used in conjunction with examination.[31]

The detection of end-tidal carbon dioxide (ETCO$_2$) is the most accurate way to evaluate ETT position with sensitivities approaching 100% in patients who are adequately perfusing.[30] The sensitivity drops off significantly in patients in cardiac arrest or with severe disturbances in perfusion as the lack of lung perfusion can lead to the absence of CO$_2$ and a lack of detection, despite the correct placement of the ETT in the trachea. There are two main methods of detecting ETCO$_2$: Continuous quantitative waveform capnography and colorimetric devices (Figures 2.5 and 2.6).

- The preferred method uses detection and quantitation of CO$_2$ as displayed in a continuous waveform. Continuous capnography can not only detect correct ETT placement, but also can help with assessing the degree of resuscitation and monitoring of ETT position during transport or procedures.

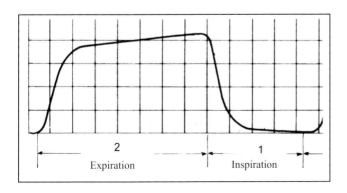

Figure 2.5 Capnography waveform (from Rschiedon at Dutch Wikipedia, reproduced under CC-BY-SA-3.0; http://creativecommons.org/licenses/by-sa/3.0/)

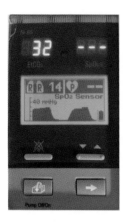

Figure 2.6 Hand held capnography device showing a good CO_2 waveform
(Photo: Colin Kaide)

- The use of inexpensive color-change CO_2 detectors represents a practical alternative. The detection of CO_2, indicated by a purple to yellow color change, is 100% specific for tracheal placement of the ETT, whereas the failure to detect color change strongly suggests esophageal intubation.[32]

P – Post-Intubation Management

There are three important issues to address after successful intubation: Ventilator settings, sedation/analgesia, and continued paralysis.

Ventilator Settings

A detailed discussion of ventilator management is beyond the scope of this article, but a few basic points should be highlighted. A study in the *Annals of Emergency Medicine* looked at the effects of implementing early lung-protective ventilation and found it was associated with "significant improvements in the delivery of safe mechanical ventilation and clinical outcome."[33] The following summarizes this lung-protective ventilation strategy.

Post-Intubation Ventilator Settings

- Tidal Volume (TV): The minimum TV that can keep the patient oxygenated and ventilated should be used. TV should be calculated using ideal body weight, as determined by the patient's height. 6–8 mL/kg should be used.
  - Males: Ideal body weight = 50 kg + 2.3 kg for each inch over 5 feet.
  - Females: Ideal body weight = 45.5 kg + 2.3 kg for each inch over 5 feet.

- Respiratory Rate: 20–30 breaths per minute.
- PEEP: Start with an initial PEEP of ≥5 mm Hg. PEEP can be increased if there is a need for increasing FiO_2.
  - BMI >30 set PEEP to 8 mm Hg.
  - BMI >40 set PEEP to 10 mm Hg.

- FiO_2: Begin to rapidly titrate the FiO_2 down to less than 60%, with a goal of decreasing it to 30–40% while keeping the O_2 sat between 90–95% or a PaO_2 of 55–60 mm Hg.
- Plateau Pressures: Try to limit plateau pressures to <30 mm Hg.
- Head of Bed: Unless contraindicated, the head of the bed should be raised to >30 degrees.

Post-Intubation Sedation/Analgesia

- Post-intubation sedation/analgesia should be initiated as soon as possible after intubation. The duration of paralysis, particularly when using rocuronium, is much longer than the duration of the induction agent, leaving the patient potentially awake and fully paralyzed.
- The overall conclusion suggested by the literature is that post-intubation should maximize pain control early using opioids and add light sedation and titrate to the patient's response. Sedative and amnestic agents should be given during any period of chemical paralysis. One should avoid prolonged heavy sedation by adequately controlling the patient's pain.

Post-Intubation Paralysis

Appropriate use of paralytics might include:

- The need to rapidly obtain imaging studies that require a patient to remain still.
- The patient who remains physically agitated despite pain control and sedation when the excessive physical activity may harm the patient or the treatment process.
- Excessive fighting of the ventilator, leading to breath stacking and elevated airway pressures.

The overall goal is to minimize the time the patient remains paralyzed and work to transition to adequate pain control and appropriate sedation. Table 2.3 discusses medications for sedation.

Table 2.3 Post intubation sedation

Agent	Action	Onset	Clinical Duration*	Bolus Dose	Infusion Rate
Propofol	Sedative/Amnestic	1–2 min	5–15 min	1–2 mg/kg	5–50 mcg/kg/min
Midazolam	Sedative/Amnestic	2–5 min	15–20 min	5–10 mg	0.02–0.1 mg/kg/h
Lorazepam	Sedative/Amnestic	15–20 min		1–2 mg	0.01–0.1 mg/kg/h
Dexmedetomidine	Sedative/Amnestic	5–10 min	–	1 mcg/kg†	0.2–0.7 mcg/kg/h
Ketamine	Sedative/Amnestic/ Analgesic	1 min	15–20 min	1–2 mg/kg	0.05–0.4 mg/kg/h
Fentanyl	Analgesic	1–2 min	1 h	1–2 mcg/kg	0.7–10 mcg/kg/h
Morphine	Analgesic	5–10 min	1–2 h	0.15 mg/kg	2–30 mg/h
Hydromorphone	Analgesic	5–15 min		1–2 mg	0.5–3 mg/h
Rocuronium	Non-Depolarizing Paralytic	1–1.5 min	45–80 min	0.6–1.2 mg/kg	
Vecuronium	Non-Depolarizing Paralytic	1.5–3 min	45–90 min	0.1–0.3 mg/kg	

* Clinical duration of action after a bolus dose. †Bolus over 10 minutes, followed by infusion

P – Problem Solving

It is important to be able to troubleshoot problems that can arise after intubation. One of the most concerning problems that can arise is sudden, progressive problems with ventilating the patient. An easy way to remember problems post-intubation is "DOPES."

- D – Dislodged ETT: During the process of securing the tube or moving the patient, the tube may come out of the trachea. Check end-tidal CO_2 using a color change device or preferably a continuous capnographic waveform to assure endotracheal placement of the ETT. Revisualizing that the tube is still going through the cords may also be helpful.
- O – Obstruction: Placing a suction catheter down the ETT and suctioning secretions can help assure the tube is not blocked.
- P – Pneumothorax: Does the patient have a pneumothorax? Chest x-ray or real-time visualization of lung sliding on bedside ultrasound can quickly answer the question.
- E – Equipment Failure: Take the patient off the ventilator and bag the patient with a BVM on 100% FiO_2. This will eliminate the ventilator as the cause of the problem. Check for cuff leak.
- S – Stacked Breaths: Breath stacking creates autopeep. This happens in patients with asthma and COPD who do not completely exhale after each breath because of air trapping. Take the patient off the ventilator or BVM and allow the patient to fully exhale. They can be assisted by slowly compressing the chest, helping to force exhalation.

Difficult Intubation

This section deals with the potentially disastrous situation in which the patient's airway either presents a substantial challenge or has proved unintubatable by standard methods. In general, up to 10% of patients will be difficult to intubate with direct laryngeal visualization.[34]

As discussed above, the primary intubation technique in the trauma patient is oral endotracheal with RSI. In some circumstances, however, this is either not possible or contraindicated (e.g. closed tracheal disruption). It is also important to have back-up methods of securing the airway. There are many alternative intubation techniques and airway adjuncts.

Devices That Facilitate Intubation

Endotracheal Tube Introducer

The endotracheal tube introducer, commonly known as a Bougie, is designed to enter the trachea blindly and allow an ETT to be guided into position. In studies with patients with simulated cervical spine injuries and a Mallampati score of 3 or less, successful first attempt intubations are reported at 96–100%, compared to significantly lower rates with a traditional stylet.[35]

- While the jaw and tongue are lifted by a laryngoscope, the device is placed blindly into the pharynx with the introducer aligned in the midline and the angled tip pointed upward. The angle of the tip facilitates placement under the epiglottis and through the cords. When tracheal placement is achieved, the tip of the introducer is advanced over the tracheal rings, creating a "washboard" sensation.

- When it is fully inserted, the tip should impact on the carina and provide resistance to further insertion. An ETT can then be placed over the introducer and guided into the trachea, with subsequent removal of the device through the ETT. This device may have significant utility in trauma patients for whom limited neck mobility is expected.

Flexible Fiberoptic Bronchoscope (FFB)

Although the fiberoptic bronchoscope provides excellent visualization of the upper airway anatomy during intubation, it is rarely used by emergency physicians in the management of the trauma airway, as many emergency physicians have limited experience with this instrument. There are certain well-defined indications for fiberoptic bronchoscopy in airway management. Examples include:

- The awake patient with a known difficult airway.
- The patient with an unstable cervical spine injury.
- The patient with upper airway burns.
- The patient with an expanding neck hematoma.

Because intubation over a fiberoptic bronchoscope requires more time and technical skill than conventional laryngoscopy, it is not recommended in the setting of penetrating neck trauma.[36]

The AirTraq® is a fully integrated high definition optical device with a magnified wide-angle (panoramic) view, with no need for an external monitor (Figure 2.7). There is a guide channel on the side into which the ETT is pre-loaded. When the cords are visualized, the ETT is advanced directly through the cords.

- It has been shown to improve intubation success rates when compared with the Macintosh blade, with decreased time to intubation, decreased failed attempts, and decreased cardiovascular effects seen during intubation.[37]
- The device is single use, so there is no risk of cross-contamination.
- They have an anti-fog system in place.
- It is particularly useful in difficult airway situations, including traumatic neck injuries (no need for extension of the neck), obese patients, and semi-seated intubations.

The King Vision is conceptually similar to the AirTraq®, but utilizes a small LCD screen instead of a physical lens.

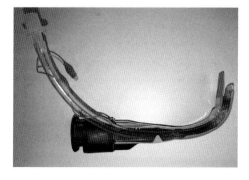

Figure 2.7 AirTraq® with endotracheal tube in place in the track (Photo: Colin Kaide. Used with manufacturer's permission)

Devices That Temporarily Substitute for Endotracheal Intubation

Supraglottic Airways

Laryngeal Mask Airway (LMA), the Intubating Laryngeal Mask Airway (ILMA), and the i-Gel

The laryngeal mask airway (LMA) is an endotracheal tube with an attached silicone rubber collar which covers the supraglottic area, thereby enclosing the larynx. Two forms of LMA are in widespread use: the classic LMA and the intubating LMA (ILMA). Both are relatively easy to use and serve as quick rescue devices for patients who cannot be intubated by conventional means.

- The classic LMA comes in sizes #3 for adolescents and small adults and sizes #4 and #5 for average size and large adults (Figure 2.8).
- Before inserting the LMA, apply water-soluble lubricant to the sides of the collar. When inserting the LMA, place the tip of the cuff against the patient's hard palate and advance it along the natural curve of the hypopharynx until resistance is met. The cuff is then inflated with the size appropriate amount of air (20 cc #3, 30 cc #4, 40 cc #5).

The ILMA is designed to allow for the placement of an ETT through the device and into the trachea.

- Success rates of intubation with the ILMA were comparable to those achieved with a fiberoptic scope in patients with anticipated difficult intubation.[38] The ILMA only comes in adult sizes, equivalent to sizes 3, 4, and 5 found in the classic LMA, based on the patient's weight (Figure 2.9).[39,40]

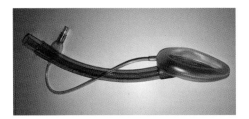

Figure 2.8 Laryngeal mask airway (Photo: Colin Kaide)

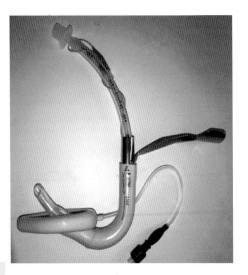

Figure 2.9 Fastrach® intubating laryngeal mask airway with endotracheal tube inserted (Photo: Colin Kaide. Used with manufacturer's permission)

- The ILMA is inserted in the same manner as the classic LMA, but with the assistance of the handle (Figure 2.9). Once in place with the cuff inflated, the ETT (up to size 8.0) is placed into the metal tube of the ILMA and advanced into the trachea. The ILMA can then either be left in place or withdrawn over the ETT.

Another variation of the LMA is a product called the i-Gel. It is similar in function to an LMA, except that the cuff that covers the glottic opening is made of a soft and pliable gel-like thermoplastic elastomer. It is placed in a similar fashion to an LMA, but does not require inflation.

The Failed Airway

There are many definitions of a failed airway. The one that is favored in the National Airway Course occurs when any of three scenarios develop[34]:

1. Orotracheal intubation is unsuccessful after three attempts by an experienced physician, even if adequate oxygenation is maintained.

    This is the "**can't** Intubate, **can** oxygenate" scenario.
2. A failed attempt at orotracheal intubation with the inability to maintain adequate oxygenation (>85%) "during or after one or more failed laryngoscopic attempts." This is the "**can't** Intubate, **can't** oxygenate" scenario.
3. One failed "best attempt" in the situation where the physician is "forced to act" (because of rapid deterioration, etc.) despite a predicted difficult intubation can also be considered a failed airway.

If the "can't intubate, can't oxygenate" scenario arises, a surgical airway is clearly indicated. If supraglottic devices are available, they can be used as a temporizing measure in preparation for a more definitive airway. Since these adjuncts do not place a cuffed endotracheal tube into the trachea, they do not substitute for definitive management.

Remember: The quickest way to kill a patient is to keep trying the same failing technique over and over again. *Failure to STOP doing an ineffective strategy and START cutting a hole in the neck means almost certain death in a patient whose oxygen saturation continues to fall!*

Surgical Airway

With all of the advances in adjunctive airway techniques, cricothyrotomy is performed infrequently. The National Emergency Airway Registry II reported a 1.7% ED cricothyrotomy rate in trauma patients and 1% over all ED intubations.[41] Due to the infrequent need for surgical airways, physicians may lack the experience and skill needed to practice this technique safely and efficiently.[42] For this reason, it is essential for the emergency physician to be familiar with the anatomy of the neck and the steps required to perform the procedure (Figure 2.10).

- There are several indications for cricothyrotomy, the most common of which is the inability to intubate the trachea in a patient who cannot be oxygenated or ventilated. Another significant indication includes trauma to the face severe enough to significantly distort airway anatomy.
- Cricothyrotomy is contraindicated in cases of laryngeal fracture and in the setting of complete laryngotracheal separation, as the skin may be the only tissue holding the proximal trachea in the neck.[43,44]

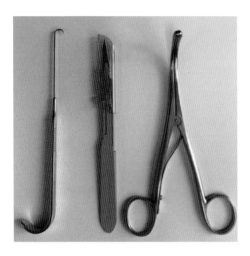

Figure 2.10 Tools for performing a 4-step cricothyrotomy. Trach hook, scalpel and a Trousseau dilator (Photo: Colin Kaide)

- Owing to the small size of the cricothyroid membrane, the procedure is also contraindicated in children less than 8 years of age, in whom a needle cricothyrotomy is the preferred technique.

Holmes et al.[45] designed the rapid 4-step technique in an effort to simplify the procedure and decrease the time involved.

- In this technique, the cricothyroid membrane is identified by palpation.
- A horizontal stab incision is then made through both the skin and cricothyroid membrane with a number 20 scalpel blade.
- The larynx is stabilized with a tracheal hook pulling caudal traction on the inferior aspect of the cricoid cartilage.
- A Shiley tracheal tube is introduced into the trachea.

This technique has been shown to be much faster than the standard method in a cadaver study.[46]

The wire-guided technique using a percutaneous cricothyrotomy set is not recommended for the failed airway, as it often takes longer to perform than an open cricothyrotomy. Common equipment utilized for cricothyrotomy is demonstrated in Figure 2.10.

Conclusion

At the core of airway management in all patients is a good understanding of when and how to intervene and provide definitive airway control. Although the setting and injury patterns can be dramatic, management of the trauma airway involves the same basic skills required for any other difficult airway. The well-prepared physician should possess sound, basic intubation skills and be intimately familiar with the various induction and paralytic agents. He or she should have a working knowledge of some of the common airway adjuncts and the requisite skills to create a surgical airway. Finally, the physician should be aware of, and have a plan to deal with, the potential pitfalls and disasters which can occur while taking control of a patient's vital functions.

Key Points
- **All** trauma airways should be considered difficult airways. Manual in-line stabilization is effective in maintaining cervical spine immobilization but can make airways difficult.
- Develop a personal trauma airway algorithm that can be applied to all trauma cases. Ensure familiarity with all airway adjuncts and their proper use and indications.
- The need to perform a cricothyrotomy does not represent a failed airway. Some trauma conditions necessitate a surgical airway.
- Rapid Sequence Intubation (RSI) is the preferred method to follow, when possible, for endotracheal intubation. Know the doses for both induction agents and paralytics.
- Ensure appropriate post-intubation sedation is administered promptly after the airway has been secured. Watch for intubation associated hypotension.

References
1. Kaide C. Invasive and non-invasive ventilation. In: Hoekstra JW, ed. *Handbook of Cardiovascular Emergencies*, 2nd ed. Philadelphia, PA: Lippincott, Williams & Wilkins; 2001.

2. Conforti PJ, Haug RH, Likavec M. Management of closed head injury in the patient with maxillofacial trauma. *J Oral Maxillofac Surg*. 1993;51:298.

3. Hills MW, Eeane SA. Head injury and facial injury: is there an increased risk of cervical spine injury? *J Trauma*. 1993;34:549.

4. Asensio JA, Valenziano CP, Falcone RE, et al. Management of penetrating neck injuries: the controversy surrounding zone II injuries. *Surg Clin North Am*. 1991;71:267–96.

5. Cicala RS. The traumatized airway. In: Benumof JL, ed. *Airway Management: Principles and Practice*. St. Louis: Mosby-Year Book; 1996, pp. 736–59.

6. Angood PB, Attia EL, Brown RA, et al. Extrinsic civilian trauma to the larynx and cervical trachea: important predictors of long-term morbidity. *J Trauma*. 1986;26:869.

7. Gussack GS, Jurkovich GJ, Luterman A. Laryngotracheal trauma: a protocol approach to a rare injury. *Laryngoscope*. 1986;96:660–65.

8. McConnell DB, Trunkey DD. Management of penetrating trauma to the neck. *Adv Surg*. 1994;27:97–127.

9. Thompson JN, Strausbaugh PL, Koufman JA, et al. Penetrating injuries of the larynx. *South Med J*. 1984;77:41–45.

10. Eggen JT, Jorden RC. Airway management, penetrating neck trauma. *J Emerg Med*. 1993;11:381–85.

11. Walls RM. Contemporary issues in trauma: management of the difficult airway in the trauma patient. *Emerg Med Clin North Am*. 1998;16:45–62.

12. Walls RM, Wolfe R, Rosen P. Fools rush in? Airway management in penetrating neck trauma [editorial]. *J Emerg Med*. 1993;11:479–82.

13. Capan LM, Miller SM, Turndorf H. Management of neck injuries. In: Caplan LM, Miller SM, Turndorf H, eds. *Trauma Anesthesia and Intensive Care*. Philadelphia: JB Lippincott; 1991, pp. 415–18.

14. Sinclair D, Schwartz M, Gruss J, et al. A retrospective review of the relationship between facial fractures, head injuries, and cervical spine injuries. *J Emerg Med*. 1988;6:109–12.

15. American Society of Anesthesiology. Practice guidelines for management of the difficult airway. A report by the American Society of Anesthesiologists Task Force on Management of the Difficult Airway. *Anesthesiology*. 1993;78:597–602.

16. Abrams KJ, Desai N, Datsnelson T. Bullard laryngoscopy for trauma airway management in suspected cervical spine injuries. *Anesth Analg*. 1992;74:619–23.

17. Thiboutot, F, Nicole PC, Trépanier CA, Turgeon AF, Lessard MR. Effect of manual in-line stabilization of the C-spine on the rate of difficult orotracheal intubation by direct laryngoscopy; a randomized controlled trial. *Can J Anaesth.* 2009;56 (6):412–18.

18. Manoach, S, Paladino L. Manual in-line stabilization for acute airway management of suspected cervical spine injury: historical review and current questions. *Ann Emerg Med.* 2007;50(3):236–45.

19. Tobias JD. Airway management for pediatric emergencies. *Pediatr Ann.* 1996;25(6):317–28.

20. Walls RM. Management of the difficult airway in the trauma patient. *Emerg Med Clin N Am-Contemp Issues Trauma.* 1998;16(1):45–61.

21. Walls RM. Rapid sequence intubation in head trauma. *Ann Emerg Med.* 1993;22:1008–13.

22. Weingart SD, Richard M, Levitan RM. Preoxygenation and prevention of desaturation during emergency airway management. *Ann Emerg Med.* 2012;59 (3):165–75e1.

23. Wong DT, Yee AJ, Leong SM, Chung F. The effectiveness of apneic oxygenation during tracheal intubation in various clinical settings: a narrative review. *Can J Anaesth.* 2017;64(4): 416–27.

24. Algie CM, Mahar RK, Tan HB, et al. Effectiveness and risks of cricoid pressure during rapid sequence induction for endotracheal intubation. *Cochrane Database of Syst Rev.* 2015;(11): CD011656.

25. Knill RL. Difficult laryngoscopy made easy with a "BURP." *Can J Anaesth.* 1993;40 (3):279–82.

26. Takahata O, Kubota M, Mamiya K, et al. The efficacy of the "BURP" maneuver during a difficult laryngoscopy. *Anesth Analg.* 1997;84(2):419.

27. Knopp RK. External laryngeal manipulation: a simple intervention for difficult intubations. *Ann Emerg Med.* 2002;40:38–40.

28. Levitan RM, Mickler T, Hollander JE. Bimanual laryngoscopy: a videographic study of external laryngeal manipulation by novice intubators. *Ann Emerg Med.* 2002;40:30–37.

29. Healy DW, Picton P, Morris M, Turner C. Comparison of the glidescope, CMAC, Storz DCI with the Macintosh laryngoscope during simulated difficult laryngoscopy: a manikin study BMC. *Anesthesiol.* 2012;12:11.

30. Grmec S. Comparison of three different methods to confirm tracheal tube placement in emergency intubation. *Intensive Care Med.* 2002;28:701–4.

31. ACEP Policy. Verification of endotracheal tube placement. *Ann Emerg Med.* 2009;54:141–42.

32. Reardon RF, Carleton SC. Direct laryngoscopy. In: Brown III CA, Sakles JC, Wick MW, eds. *The Walls Manual of Emergency Airway Management*, 5th ed. Alphen aan den Rijn, Netherlands: Wolters Kluwer, 2017.

33. Fuller BM, Ferguson IT, Mohr NM. Lung-protective ventilation initiated in the emergency department (LOV-ED): a quasi-experimental, before-after trial. *Ann Emerg Med.* 2017;70(3):406–18.

34. Brown III CA, Walls RM. Identification of the difficult and failed airway. In: Brown III CA, Sakles JC, Wick MW, eds. *The Walls Manual of Emergency Airway Management*, 5th ed. Philadelphia, PA: Wolters Kluwer, 2017.

35. Green DW. Gum elastic bougie and simulated difficult intubation. *Anaesthesia.* 2003;58(4):391–92.

36. Angood PB, Attia EL, Brown RA, et al. Extrinsic civilian trauma to the larynx and cervical trachea: important predictors of long-term morbidity. *J Trauma.* 1986;26:869.

37. Koh JC, Lee JS, Lee YW, et al. Comparison of the laryngeal view during intubation using Airtraq and Macintosh laryngoscopes in patients with cervical spine immobilization and mouth opening limitation. *Korean J Anesthesiol.* 2010;59(5):314–18.

38. Langeron O, Semjen F, Bourgain JL, Marsac A, Cros AM. Comparison of the intubating laryngeal mask airway with the fiberoptic intubation in anticipated difficult airway management. *Anesthesiology*. 2001;94:968–72.

39. Brain AI, Berghese C, Addy EV, et al. The intubating laryngeal mask: II. A preliminary clinical report of a new means for intubating the trachea. *Br J Anaesth*. 1997;79:704–9.

40. Kapila A, Addy EV, Berghese C, et al. The intubating laryngeal mask airway: an initial assessment of performance. *Br J Anaesth*. 1997;79:710–13.

41. Walls RM, Brown CA III, Bair AE, et al. Emergency airway management: a multi-center report of 8937 emergency department intubations. *J Emerg Med*. 2011;41(4):347–54.

42. Chang RS, Hamilton RJ, Carter WA. Declining rate of cricothyrotomy in trauma patients with an emergency medicine residency: implications for skill training. *Acad Emerg Med*. 1998;5: 247–51.

43. Bent JP, Silver JR, Porubsky ES. Acute laryngeal trauma: a review of 77 patients. *Otolaryngol Head Neck Surg*. 1993;109:441–49.

44. Einarsson O, Rochester CC, Rosenbaum S. Airway management in respiratory emergencies. *Clin Chest Med*. 1984;15:13–34.

45. Holmes JF, Panacek EA, Sackles JC, Brofeld BT. Comparison of 2 cricothyrotomy techniques: standard methods verses rapid 4-step technique. *Ann Emerg Med*. 1998;32:442–46.

46. Davis DP, Bramwell KJ, Vilke GM, et al. Cricothyrotomy technique: standard verses rapid 4-step technique. *J Emerg Med*. 1999;17(1):17–21.

Chapter 3

Transfusion in Trauma

Brit Long

Introduction

Hemorrhage is a leading cause of death in trauma, following head injury. Shock is defined by inadequate tissue perfusion with hemodynamic instability and organ dysfunction.[1-10] In trauma, the most common cause of shock is due to acute hemorrhage. Advanced Trauma Life Support (ATLS) describes four classes of hemorrhage,[1] but these are not relevant to real world practice, due to different injury types (blunt vs. penetrating), age (due to blunted physiologic responses in the elderly), comorbidities, and medication use (beta blockade reduces the chance of tachycardia in response to decreased blood pressure).[6-14] Bradycardia may also be seen in hemorrhage, due to several causes including vagal stimulation and failure to mount a tachycardic response.[13,14]

Management of hemorrhage in trauma requires: (1) hemorrhage control, (2) restoring intravascular volume, (3) delivering adequate oxygen, and (4) maintaining functional blood composition. This chapter will focus on restoring intravascular volume, specifically transfusion. Balanced resuscitation and massive transfusion protocol (MTP) are also key resuscitation components.[3-8]

Blood Products

A variety of blood products may be provided (Table 3.1). There are several types of blood antigens.

- Three primary categories of blood antigens are A, B, and AB. Group O has no antigen type.
- Blood type O is the universal donor (due to lack of antigens), while AB+ is the universal recipient.
- The Rhesus (Rh) system contains over 50 antigens, with the D antigen the most important (usually specified as + or −).[3-8,15]

For non-emergent transfusions, blood is typically typed and crossed. In a massive transfusion protocol, this is not possible. Blood products set aside for a massive transfusion protocol should be checked before trauma.[15-18]

- For male trauma patients, type O+ blood can be provided if the patient's type is unknown, and for females, type O− blood should be given if the patient's blood type is unknown.

Negatives of Crystalloid Resuscitation

Traditional ATLS teaching is to provide 1–2 L of crystalloid solution, though more recent editions lean away from this.[1] Crystalloids in trauma can result in dilutional coagulopathy,

Table 3.1 Blood products[15–18]

Product	Contents	Considerations and Volume	Threshold	Potential Complications
Packed red blood cells (pRBCs)	Red blood cells improve oxygen-carrying capacity	• 1 unit = 450 mL, increases Hgb by 1 g/dL • Infuse with normal saline, not lactated ringers • Provide O− for females, O+ for males, in MTP • Citrate may result in hypocalcemia • Cell lysis can cause hyperkalemia, acidosis	• Provide in hemorrhagic shock with injury • TRICC trial showed Hgb level >7.0 g/dL is safe	Fluid overload, transfusion reaction, infection, fever, allergy
Fresh frozen plasma (FFP)	Contains all clotting factors	• Volume = 250 mL, with 400 mg fibrinogen • Can provide type AB or A for MTP; must be ABO compatible otherwise • Portion of blood formed when whole blood is centrifuged and RBCs removed	• Provides clotting factors necessary for traumatic coagulopathy • Hemorrhage in DIC, cirrhosis • Patients with anticoagulation needing reversal	Infection, inflammatory complications
Cryoprecipitate	Contains factor VIII, vWF, fibrinogen	• 250 mg of fibrinogen per unit • Cold insoluble fraction formed with thawing of FFB	• Smaller volume with delivery of clotting factor • Provide for fibrinogen levels <100–150	Infection, inflammatory complications
Platelets	Apheresis pack is equal to 6 units of non-apheresis packs	• Rh− patients need Rh− platelets • 1 pack apheresis platelets increases platelets by 40–60 • Thrombocytopenia may occur late in hemorrhage	• Provide in balanced resuscitation	May result in TRALI

43

impaired oxygen delivery to tissues due to dilutional anemia, hypothermia worsening metabolic acidosis if normal saline is utilized, and clot dislodgement.[4,9,10]

Trauma Coagulopathy and the Lethal Triad

Coagulopathy in severe trauma is associated with increased morbidity, higher transfusion, increased organ dysfunction, and increased mortality. The lethal triad of (1) hypothermia, (2) coagulopathy, and (3) acidosis is classically associated with worse outcomes in trauma (Figure 3.1, Table 3.2). These three factors cause and contribute to further bleeding and coagulopathy.[4–10]

- Coagulopathy occurs in close to 25% of trauma patients due to many causes including: depletion and consumption of clotting factors, platelet dysfunction, increased fibrinolysis, and loss of RBCs.
- Resuscitation should focus on restoring the coagulation system, clot strengthening, hemorrhage control, and replace volume with appropriate products.[4–10,19]

Blood product transfusion centers on several aspects. Packed RBCs provide oxygen and nutrients. Other aspects of hemostasis include clot initiation, amplification, and propagation.[3–10,15,19]

- Endothelial injury exposes prothrombogenic substances to platelets, forming a loose plug, which acts as a catalyst for coagulation proteins (the coagulation cascade).
- Thrombin activates other factors, amplifying thrombin production and activating factor XIII. This forms fibrin cross-links that stabilize the clot. Thrombin also activates a fibrinolytic process that prevents coagulation system overactivity.

Table 3.2 Treatments for components of the lethal triad

Lethal Triad Factor	Treatment
Hypothermia	Warmed fluids and blood products, forced air patient warming device/warm blankets, minimize exposure, increase ambient temperature, continuous monitoring
Acidosis	Correct underlying physiology by correcting hemodynamic status, balanced resuscitation, control source of hemorrhage
Coagulopathy	Balanced blood product resuscitation, correction of other factors in lethal triad

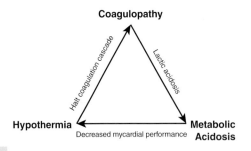

Figure 3.1 Lethal triad of trauma (from https://upload.wikimedia.org/wikipedia/commons/thumb/d/d4/Trauma_triad_of_death.svg/280px-Trauma_triad_of_death.svg.png under CC BY 3.0 license https://creativecommons.org/licenses/by/3.0/)

Box 3.1 DCR Components
- Hemorrhage control with compressive/hemostatic dressings/devices
- Permissive hypotension (otherwise minimal volume normotension)
- Early hemostatic resuscitation and managing lethal triad
- Use of TXA if <3 hours from time of injury
- Damage control surgery

- Massive hemorrhage is associated with an overwhelmed coagulation system, which is unable to balance between coagulation and fibrinolysis. Traumatic coagulopathy often presents early in resuscitation due to tissue injury, ischemia, clotting factor dilution, hypocalcemia, hypothermia, acidosis, inflammation, and fibrinolysis, independent of clotting factor deficiency.[3–7,19]

Damage Control Resuscitation

Damage control resuscitation (DCR) possesses several aspects (Box 3.1). DCR is a systematic approach to trauma management and severe injury, beginning in the ED, through the operating room (OR), and into the intensive care unit (ICU). It aims to maintain intravascular volume, control hemorrhage, and correct the lethal triad. Stages include (1) recognition (often pre-hospital), (2) hemostatic resuscitation, (3) rapid movement to the OR for damage control surgery, and (4) stabilization in the ICU, with reoperation in 24–26 hours.[3–10]

Damage control surgery focuses on management of the metabolic derangement of ongoing bleed, with abbreviated surgical operations that control hemorrhage and spillage from anatomical areas including the gastrointestinal system. Definitive operation is deferred until the patient is stabilized, targeting normothermia, the use of fewer products, and decreased coagulopathy.[3–10]

Permissive Hypotension

This is also known as hypotensive resuscitation. The focus is to maintain adequate perfusion while avoiding the disruption of an unstable clot at an injury site.[3–10]

- Penetrating trauma commonly includes a focal site of injury, and preventing clot disruption may improve bleeding control. Cyclic over-resuscitation may lead to rebleeding, worsening hypotension.
- Low blood pressure is not the target, as this can worsen organ perfusion. Rather, hemorrhage control is the goal. Once control is achieved, hemodynamic normalization is appropriate.
- Controversial: The strategy is largely based on animal studies, with one study being a non-blinded study in 1994.[20] There are several interpretations of permissive hypotension goals. Studies have not demonstrated worse outcomes for permissive hypotension in penetrating trauma. It has not demonstrated similar outcomes in blunt trauma, and, in head trauma, permissive hypotension is contraindicated due to the risk of hypotension aggravating secondary injury. This is also dangerous in prolonged transport/retrieval and in patients with chronically elevated hypertension.[3–10,20–22]

- Permissive hypotension, if followed, should be administered with care. Factors to consider include patient mental status, the likelihood of CNS injury, type of injury, and injury severity (such as ongoing hemorrhage). Delayed fluid resuscitation is likely more harmful unless rapid, emergent surgical exploration with rapid bleeding control is possible.[3–10]

Minimal Volume Normotension

A more optimal approach is minimal volume normotension, recently advocated in the literature.

- A target mean arterial pressure of 65 mm Hg is utilized with a good radial pulse and pulse oximetry waveform, as long as intracranial injury is not suspected and this level allows adequate perfusion. If perfusion is not adequate, a higher target can be used.[3–6]

Strategy:
- MAP <65 mm Hg → Provide balanced blood products
- MAP >65 mm Hg → Evaluate perfusion with pulses, lactate, mental status, capillary refill
  - If MAP >65 mm Hg with perfusion → no action required
  - If MAP >65 mm Hg with poor perfusion → provide analgesia with fentanyl (doses of 25 mcg IV), which will decrease catecholamine release and allow vasodilation. If MAP decreases <65 mm Hg, then provide balanced resuscitation

Balanced Resuscitation

Balanced resuscitation focuses on reversing traumatic coagulopathy early in resuscitation. This is completed though providing blood products in a close to equal ratio (1:1:1) of packed red blood cells (pRBCs), fresh frozen plasma (FFP), and platelets, avoiding dilution of coagulation factors, which begins in minutes.[23–27]

- Balanced resuscitation includes decreasing traumatic coagulopathy while maintaining or improving end-organ perfusion.
- FFP possesses properties and substances that can reduce endovascular leak.
- Massive transfusion protocols decrease the incidence of transfusion complications, reduce traumatic coagulopathy, and improve patient outcomes. Massive transfusion entails providing 1:1:1 (pRBCs:FFP:platelets) (Box 3.2).[23–27]
- Balanced resuscitation and MTP should target several parameters, most importantly patient hemodynamic status and hemorrhage control (Box 3.3).

Box 3.2 MTP Definition
- Total replacement of >1 blood volume in 24 hours, or
- >50% blood volume replacement in 4 hours, or
- In children, transfusion of >40 mL/kg

Box 3.3 Goal Parameters

- Improvement in hemodynamic status
- Hemorrhage control
- Temperature >35°C
- pH >7.2, base excess <−6, lactate <4 mmol/L
- Ionized Ca >0.9–1.1 mmol/L
- Hemoglobin: Do not use alone, but only in conjunction with hemodynamic status and other markers
- Platelets >50 × 10^9/L
- PT/APTT <1.5× of normal
- Fibrinogen >1.0 g/L

Primary Literature for MTP

PROMMTT

Demonstrated 1:1:1 vs. 1:1:2 was associated with improved 6-hour survival after admission.[26,27]

PROPPR

Demonstrated 1:1:1 vs. 1:1:2 was associated with no difference in mortality at 24 hours or 30 days, though more patients in the 1:1:1 group achieved hemostasis and experienced fewer deaths due to exsanguination by 24 hours.[23]

When Should Massive Transfusion Be Activated?

This strategy should be utilized in several circumstances, though a low threshold to activate is advised[23,28–30]:

(1) Clinical judgment in the setting of severe trauma with hemorrhage shock.
(2) Clinical scores may be utilized, such as the ABC score.[29,30] A score greater than 2 (points for systolic BP <90 mm Hg in the ED, HR >120 bpm, positive FAST exam, and penetrating mechanism of injury) or with physician judgment/concern for hemorrhage shock due to injury warrants activation of MTP.

Other factors warranting consideration for MTP include uncontrolled bleeding, SBP <110 mm Hg, HR >105 bpm, Hct <32%, pH <7.25, INR >1.4. However, clinical judgment is recommended over use of defined numbers.[3–10]

How to Run MTP

Multiple points of IV access are advised. pRBCs provide volume and oxygen carrying capacity and are often the first product provided. Platelets should be started at the same time through an additional IV, but platelets cannot be provided through a blood warmer. O− blood should be given for females, O+ blood for males. One pack of apheresis platelets is equivalent to six packs of platelets. These should not be cooled. For plasma, AB plasma is the universal donor. AB and A plasma can be used. Once the patient is hemodynamically stable or bleeding is controlled, massive transfusion can be deescalated.[3–10,31]

Cryoprecipitate contains Factor VIII, Von Willebrand factor, and fibrinogen. If the patient continues to bleed with resuscitation or if the massive transfusion is deescalated, check fibrinogen. If fibrinogen is less than 100–150 mg/dL, 10 units of cryoprecipitate should be provided, which raises the fibrinogen by approximately 100.[3–8,32] Calcium supplementation may also be required.

Other Products

Tranexamic Acid (TXA)

TXA is an anti-fibrinolytic that stabilizes the acute clot formed at the site of injury. Several studies, including the MATTERS and CRASH-2 studies, support its use.[33–36] Its use is recommended in patients with traumatic hemorrhage receiving blood products as 1 g IV over 15 minutes, followed by 1 g over 8 hours if the patient can receive it within 3 hours post injury. Past 3 hours, TXA may worsen outcomes.[33–36]

Calcium

Hypocalcemia is common in critically ill patients and trauma. Calcium functions as a cofactor in the coagulation cascade. Citrate, which is an anticoagulant used in blood components, can worsen hypocalcemia through calcium chelation. Ionized calcium less than 0.7 mmol/L can worsen coagulopathy. Calcium should be provided per ionized calcium level, targeting at least levels of 0.9 mmol/L, or with every four units of pRBCs provided.[3–10,37,38]

PCC

Prothrombin complex concentrate (PCC) is a concentrate of factors II, VII, IX, and X. This was initially developed for hemophilia; however, it is beneficial in reversal of warfarin and direct oral anticoagulants.[39,40] PCC can be used for coagulopathy correction in trauma, but it should be used after FFP. Other indications include intracerebral hemorrhage, where volume is limited. If a patient is on oral anticoagulation, PCC is recommended as first line therapy to reverse anticoagulation. Vitamin K with PCC is needed for reversal of vitamin K antagonsists such as warfarin. PCC use in conjunction with FFP to reverse traumatic coagulopathy in patients not on oral anticoagulation may improve reversal and reduce costs, but further study is required.[39,40]

Factor VII

Recombinant factor VIIa was developed for hemophilia and congenital factor deficiency. Factor VII functions as a principle trigger for clot formation. However, it should only be used in salvage therapy in hemorrhage shock with continued bleeding. Routine use is not advised, as the medication may worsen outcomes.[3–10,19,22,41]

Product Guided Resuscitation

Coagulation assessments including PT, INR, and aPTT/PTT may offer prognostic value, but are difficult to use in guiding transfusion. Another tool is thromboelastography (TEG) or rotational thromboelastometry (ROTEM), which can be used to guide product transfusion (Table 3.3 and Figure 3.2).[42–46]

Table 3.3 TEG properties[42–46]

Value	Description	Measures	Normal	Abnormal	Transfuse
TEG-ACT	Activated clotting time to initiation of fibrin formation	Intrinsic and extrinsic clotting factors	80–140 sec	>140 sec	FFP
R time	Reaction time to initial fibrin formation	Intrinsic clotting factors	5–10 min	>10 min	FFP
K time	Kinetic time to fibrin cross linkage	Fibrinogen and platelet number	1–3 min	>3 min	Cryoprecipitate
α angle	Angle from baseline to slope of tracing representing clot formation	Fibrinogen and platelet number	53–72°	<53°	Cryoprecipitate +/− platelets
MA	Maximum amplitude of tracing	Platelet number and function	50–70 mm	<50 mm	Platelets
G value	Calculated value of clot strength	Entire coagulation cascade	5.3–12.4 dynes/cm^2	–	–
LY 30	Clot lysis at 30 min following MA	Fibrinolysis	0–3%	>3%	Tranexamic acid

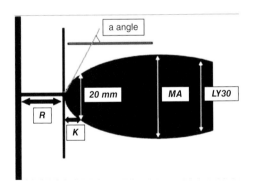

Figure 3.2 TEG representation (from da Luz et al.,[47] reproduced here under the CC BY 2.0 license; https://creativecommons.org/licenses/by/2.0/)

- This assessment evaluates whole blood coagulation, allowing targeted product transfusion.
- TEG evaluates clot initiation, clot maximum strength, and clot lysis in a real-time manner. The machine must be calibrated several times per day, and, after blood draw, the sample must be tested within several minutes.[42–46]

Resuscitation Goals

Blood pressure is commonly utilized in resuscitation as a marker of end organ perfusion. However, blood pressure can be falsely reassuring in trauma. Other goals include lactate <2 mmol/L, urinary output >0.5 mL/kg/h, normal base deficit, and normal hemoglobin/hematocrit. Examination markers such as normal mental status (if able to assess), normal capillary refill, and improved perfusion are also valuable to assess. Trends are also important, rather than absolute points in time.[3–10,20] As discussed, hemorrhage control is another goal.

Anticoagulants

The patient with active hemorrhage from trauma and on anticoagulation is challenging. Coumadin (warfarin) is the standard medication for thromboembolic disease and atrial fibrillation. It acts as an inhibitor of vitamin K epoxide reductase, decreasing the synthesis of factors II, VII, IX, and X, as well as anticoagulant proteins C and S. Effect is measured through PT and INR, and the duration of a single dose ranges from 2–5 days.[40,48–52]

- For the patient with active bleeding in trauma, vitamin K 10 mg IV slow infusion should be provided.
- For the patient with intravascular loss from bleeding, FFP should be provided at 10–15 mL/kg. One unit of FFP corrects clotting factors by 2.5–5%, and, to improve clotting status, factor levels must reach 10%.
- Four factor prothrombin complex concentrate (PCC) provides faster reversal of warfarin, with initial dosing 25–50 IU/kg. PCC can also be prepared and infused faster than FFP, with each 500 unit vial of PCC equivalent to 4 units FFP.[4,48–52]

Direct oral anticoagulants (DOAC) are potent inhibitors of coagulation used for venous thromboembolic disease and atrial fibrillation (in those without mechanical valve) (Table 3.4). With DOACs, reversal of anticoagulation is needed in intracranial hemorrhage, hemodynamic instability, and failure to control site of hemorrhage.[4,48–52]

- Standard coagulation tests such as PT, INR, and aPTT/PTT may be elevated but cannot be relied on to rule out DOAC effect.
- MTP should be activated, and, if the patient has taken DOAC outside of 12–14 hours, then the anticoagulant effects have likely worn off.
- Reversal requires PCC or several newer, investigational therapies (Table 3.4).

Table 3.4 Direct oral anticoagulant considerations[4]

Medication	Rivaroxaban (Xarelto®)	Apixaban (Eliquis®)	Edoxaban (Savaysa®)	Dabigatran (Pradaxa®)
Mechanism	Factor Xa inhibitor			Factor IIa inhibitor
Renal elimination	66%	25%	35%	80%
Reversal agent	• 4-factor PCC (Octaplex, Beriplex, Kcentra) at a dose of 50 IU/kg up to 2,000 units, with TXA 1 g IV and vitamin K 10 mg IV • Andexanet Alfa may be effective, but more study is required			• 4-factor PCC, vitamin K 10 mg IV, TXA 1 g IV • Idarucizumab (Praxbind) 5 g IV over 15 min

Transfusion Complications

Several complications may arise with transfusion, related to the products and immunomodulating effects (Table 3.5).[15,53–56] Complications of massive transfusion include hypothermia, as one unit of pRBCs can decrease the core temperature by 0.25°C. Acidosis, hyperkalemia, hypocalcemia, and hypothermia are others.[15,53–56]

Table 3.5 Transfusion reaction classification[15]

Reaction	Pathophysiology	Symptoms	Occurrence (Units Transfused)
Febrile non-hemolytic reaction	Recipient antibodies react with antigens in the product provided and increased cytokines in product	Fever, often low grade, which resolves with acetaminophen	Approximately 1 in 100–500 units transfused
Bacterial infection	Products can provide medium for bacterial growth. Risk highest with platelet products	High fever, chills, hypotension, rigor, nausea/vomiting	1 in 250,000 units transfused
Allergic	Exposure to foreign plasma proteins, often in patients with IgA deficiency	Urticaria, pruritis, hypotension, nausea/vomiting, which may meet criteria for anaphylaxis	1 in 333 units transfused. Anaphylactic reaction in 1 in 20,000 units
Acute hemolytic reaction	ABO incompatibility results in immune reaction and destruction of transfused cells	Symptoms of anaphylaxis with hypotension, tachycardia, confusion, arrhythmia, dyspnea, shock, cardiac arrest	1 per 250,000–600,000 units transfused
Transfusion associated acute lung injury (TRALI)	Transfused cytokines and interaction of patient WBC with antibodies in donor	Acute respiratory distress with fever, pulmonary edema, hypotension, with symptoms within 2–6 hours	1 in 5,000–150,000 units transfused
Transfusion associated circulatory overload (TACO)	Edema, dyspnea, orthopnea, hypertension	Volume overload seen in patients with impaired cardiac function	Approximately 1–8 in 100 units transfused, but varies with disease presence and comorbidities
Delayed hemolytic reaction	Fever, jaundice, darkened urine, but may have sub-clinical reaction	Patient antibodies to RBC antigens, often in patients with prior transfusion and shortened RBC survival	Unknown
Transfusion-associated graft-vs.-host disease (GVHD)	Range of presentations – anaphylaxis to tachycardia, fever, and hypotension. Often fatal	Immunologic attack of transfused cells against recipient, more common in immunosuppressed patients	1 in 100–1,000 units transfused in patients with cancer

Controversies – Whole Blood

Whole blood (WB) is currently in use by the military and is FDA approved for administration if collected, tested for transfusion-associated diseases, and stored properly. There are two types: fresh whole blood (FWB) and stored whole blood (SWB). FWB, or a walking blood bank, is stored up to 24 hours after collection at room temperature. If stored and refrigerated within 8 hours of collection, it is known as SWB.[57–60] SWB is approved for use in the civilian setting, but only FWB is used in the military. WB is the ultimate physiologic replacement for hemorrhage in trauma, as it contains platelets and is not as diluted as separated blood products.[58–61] WB must be ABO-identical if transfused, but low-titer group O WB can be used in emergencies.[57,62] Though WB simplifies transfusion and is likely ideal for resuscitation, further study is required. Future studies will likely result in regular use of SWB.

Key Points

- Hemorrhagic shock is the most common cause of death in trauma.
- A variety of blood products are available, most notably pRBCs, FFP, and apheresis platelets.
- The Lethal Triad consists of hypothermia, coagulopathy, and acidosis, with coagulopathy occurring in 25% of patients.
- Damage Control Resuscitation consists of minimal volume normotension (targeting MAP 65 mm Hg and hemorrhage control), hemostatic resuscitation, and damage control surgery.
- Permissive hypotension is controversial, and a better strategy is minimal volume normotension.
- Balanced resuscitation seeks to avoid coagulopathy with 1:1:1 of pRBCs:FFP:platelets.
- MTP should be activated based on clinical judgment or scoring.
- In MTP, 1:1:1 of pRBCs:FFP:platelets is recommended, with type O− blood for females or O+ for males and AB or A FFP.
- TXA 1g IV is essential. Calcium and PCC are adjuncts.
- Product guided resuscitation may be beneficial with TEG or ROTEM.
- Anticoagulants with hemorrhage provide significant challenges, and reversal includes Vitamin K, PCC/FFP, and several antidotes.
- There are multiple transfusion reactions, with careful consideration of transfusion reactions.
- Whole blood, especially stored whole blood, is the next frontier in transfusion.

References

1. ATLS Subcommittee; American College of Surgeons' Committee on Trauma; International ATLS working group. Advanced trauma life support (ATLS®): the ninth edition. *J Trauma Acute Care Surg.* 2013;74(5):1363–66.

2. Ball CG. Damage control resuscitation: history, theory and technique. *Can J Surg.* 2014;57(1):55–60.

3. Weingart S, Meyers CM. Thoughts on the resuscitation of the critically ill trauma patient. EmedHome.com. Available March, 2008.

4. Dutton RP. Damage control anesthesia. *Int TraumaCare.* 2005;(Fall):197–201.

5. Duchesne JC, McSwain NE Jr, Cotton BA, et al. Damage control resuscitation: the new face of damage control. *J Trauma-Inj Infect Crit Care.* 2010;69(4):976–90.

6. Kaafarani HM, Velmahos GC. Damage control resuscitation in trauma. *Scand J Surg.* 2014;103(2):81–88.

7. Giannoudi M, Harwood P. Damage control resuscitation: lessons learned. *Eur J Trauma Emerg Surg.* 2016 ;42:273–82.

8. Janson JO, Thomas R, Loudan MA, et al. Damage control resuscitation for patients with major trauma. *BMJ.* 2009;338:1436–40.

9. Cohen MJ, Kutcher M, Redick B, et al. Clinical and mechanistic drivers of acute traumatic coagulopathy. *J Trauma Acute Care Surg.* 2013;75(1 Suppl 1):S40–47.

10. Fox CJ, Bowman JN. Advances in resuscitation in the setting of vascular injury. *Perspect Vasc Surg Endovasc Ther.* 2011;23(2):112–16.

11. Deakin CD, Low JL. Accuracy of the advanced trauma life support guidelines for predicting systolic blood pressure using carotid, femoral, and radial pulses: observational study. *BMJ.* 2000;321 (7262):673–74.

12. Guly HR, Bouamra O, Little R, et al. Testing the validity of the ATLS classification of hypovolaemic shock. *Resuscitation.* 2010;81(9):1142–47.

13. Thompson D, Adams SL, Barrett J. Relative bradycardia in patients with isolated penetrating abdominal trauma and isolated extremity trauma. *Ann Emerg Med.* 1990;19 (3):268–75.

14. Thomas I, Dixon J. Bradycardia in acute haemorrhage. *BMJ.* 2004;328 (7437):451–53.

15. Long B, Koyfman A. Red blood cell transfusion in the emergency department. *J Emerg Med.* 2016;51(2):120–30.

16. Hebert PC, Wells G, Blajchman MA, et al. A multicenter, randomized, controlled clinical trial of transfusion requirements in critical care. Transfusion requirements in critical care investigators, Canadian Critical Care Trials Group. *N Engl J Med.* 1999;340:409–17.

17. Squires JE. Risks of transfusion. *South Med J.* 2011;104(11):762–69.

18. Sandler SG. Transfusion reactions. Medscape. Available at: http://emedicine.medscape.com/article/206885-overview. Published July, 2016. Accessed July, 2017.

19. Davenport R. Pathogenesis of acute traumatic coagulopathy. *Transfusion.* 2013;53(Suppl 1):23S–27S.

20. Bickel WH, Wall MJ Jr, Pepe PE, et al. Immediate versus delayed fluid resuscitation for hypotensive patients with penetrating torso injuries. *N Engl J Med.* 1994;331:1105–9.

21. Turner J, Nicholl J, Webber L, et al. A randomized controlled trial of prehospital intravenous fluid replacement therapy in serious trauma. *Health Technol Assess.* 2000;4:1–57.

22. Dutton RP, Mackenzie CF, Scalea TM. Hypotensive resuscitation during active haemorrhage: impact on in-hospital mortality. *J Trauma.* 2002;52:1141–46.

23. Holcomb JB, Tilley BC, Baraniuk S, et al. Transfusion of plasma, platelets, and red blood cells in a 1:1:1 vs a 1:1:2 ratio and mortality in patients with severe trauma: the PROPPR randomized clinical trial. *JAMA.* 2015;313(5):471–82.

24. Holcomb JB, Jenkins D, Rhee P, et al. Damage control resuscitation: directly addressing the early coagulopathy of trauma. *J Trauma.* 2007;62(2):307–10.

25. Holcomb JB, Pati S. Optimal trauma resuscitation with plasma as the primary resuscitative fluid: the surgeon's perspective. *Hematology Am Soc Hematol Educ Program.* 2013;2013:656–59.

26. Holcomb JB, del Junco DJ, Fox EE, et al. PROMMTT Study Group. The prospective, observational, multicenter, major trauma transfusion (PROMMTT) study: comparative effectiveness of a time-varying treatment with competing risks. *JAMA Surg.* 2013;148(2):127–36.

27. del Junco DJ, Holcomb JB, Fox EE, et al. PROMMTT study group. Resuscitate early with plasma and platelets or balance blood products gradually: findings

from the PROMMTT study. *J Trauma Acute Care Surg.* 2013;75(1 suppl 1):S24–30.

28. McLaughlin DF, Niles SE, Salinas J, et al. A predictive model for massive transfusion in combat casualty patients. *J Trauma.* 2008;64(2 Suppl):S57–63; discussion S63.

29. Nunez TC, Voskresensky IV, Dossett LA, et al. Early prediction of massive transfusion in trauma: simple as ABC (assessment of blood consumption)? *J Trauma.* 2009;66(2):346–52.

30. Cotton BA, Dossett LA, Haut ER, et al. Multicenter validation of a simplified score to predict massive transfusion in trauma. *J Trauma.* 2010;69(Suppl 1):S33–39.

31. Weingart S. Podcast 197 – The logistics of the administration of massive transfusion. Available at: https://emcrit.org/emcrit/logistics-administration-massive-transfusion/ Published April, 2017. Accessed July, 2017.

32. Cryoprecipitate. Medscape. Available at: http://reference.medscape.com/drug/cryo-cryoprecipitate-999498. Accessed July, 2017.

33. Cap AP, Baer DG, Orman JA, et al. Tranexamic acid for trauma patients: a critical review of the literature. *J Trauma.* 2011;71(1 Suppl):S9–14.

34. Crash-2 trial collaborators. Effects of tranexamic acid on death, vascular occlusive events, and blood transfusion in trauma patients with significant haemorrhage (CRASH-2): a randomised, placebo-controlled trial. *Lancet.* 2010;376 (9734):23–32.

35. CRASH-2 collaborators, Roberts I, Shakur H, Afolabi A, et al. The importance of early treatment with tranexamic acid in bleeding trauma patients: an exploratory analysis of the CRASH-2 randomised controlled trial. *Lancet.* 2011;377(9771):1096–101, 1101. e1–2.

36. Morrison JJ, Dubose JJ, Rasmussen TE, Midwinter MJ. Military application of tranexamic acid in trauma emergency resuscitation (MATTERs) study. *Arch Surg.* 2012;147(2):113–19.

37. Lier H, Krep H, Schroeder S, Stuber F. Preconditions of hemostasis in trauma: a

review. The influence of acidosis, hypocalcemia, anemia, and hypothermia on functional hemostasis in trauma. *J Trauma.* 2008;65:951.

38. Howland WS, Schweizer O, Carlon GC, Goldiner PL. The cardiovascular effects of low levels of ionized calcium during massive transfusion. *Surg Gynecol Obstet.* 1977;145:581.

39. Matsushima K, Benjamin E, Demetriades D. Prothrombin complex concentrate in trauma patients. *Am J Surg.* 2015;209 (2):413–17.

40. Harter K, Levine M, Henderson S. Anticoagulation drug therapy: a review. *West J Emerg Med.* 2015;16 (1):11–17.

41. Ranucci M, Isgro G, Soro G, et al. Efficacy and safety of recombinant activated factor vii in major surgical procedures: systematic review and meta-analysis of randomized clinical trials. *Arch Surg.* 2008;143 (3):296–304.

42. Semon G, Cheatham M. Thromboelastography in trauma. Surgical Critical Care Evidence-Based Guidelines Committee. 2014. Available at: www.surgicalcriticalcare.net/Guidelines/TEG%202014.pdf. Accessed December 12, 2017.

43. Cotton B, Faz G, Hatch Q, et al. Rapid thromboelastography delivers real-time results that predict transfusion within 1 hour of admission. *J Trauma.* 2011;71:407–17.

44. Teodoro da Luz L, Nascimento B, Rizoli S. Thromboelastography (TEG): practical considerations on its clinical use in trauma resuscitation. *Scand J Trauma Resusc Emerg Med.* 2013;21:29.

45. Bollinger D, Seeberg M, Tanaka K. Principles and practice of thromboelastography in clinical coagulation management and transfusion practice. *Transfus Med Rev.* 2012:26 (1):1–13.

46. Thakur M, Ahmed A. A review of thromboelastography. *Int J Periop Ultrasound Apply Technol.* 2012;1 (1):25–29.

47. da Luz LT, Nascimento B, Rizoli S. Thrombelastography (TEG®): practical considerations on its clinical use in trauma resuscitation. *Scand J Trauma, Resusc Emerg Med.* 2013;21:29.

48. Hickey M, Gatien M, Taljaard M, et al. Outcomes of urgent warfarin reversal with frozen plasma versus prothrombin complex concentrate in the emergency department. *Circulation.* 2013;128 (4):360–64.

49. Mattu A, Smith S, Lugassy D. Clinical toxicology. *Emerg Med Clin.* 2014;32 (1):1–276.

50. Guyatt G, Akl E, Crowther M, Gutterman D, Schunemann H. Antithrombotic therapy and prevention of thrombosis 9th ed: American College of Chest Physicians evidence-based clinical practice guidelines. *Chest.* 2012;141(2):7S–47S.

51. Awad N, Cocchio C. Activated prothrombin complex concentrates for reversal of anticoagulant-associated coagulopathy. *P T.* 2013;38(11):696–98, 701.

52. Fawole A, Crowther M, Daw H. Practical management of bleeding due to the anticoagulants dabigatran, rivaroxaban, and apixaban. *CCJM.* 2013;80(7):443–51.

53. Pineda AA, Taswell HF. Transfusion reactions associated with anti-IgA antibodies: report of four cases and review of the literature. *Transfusion.* 1975;15 (1):10–15.

54. Finlay HE, Cassorla L, Feiner J, Toy P. Designing and testing a computer-based screening system for transfusion-related acute lung injury. *Am J Clin Pathol.* 2005;124(4):601.

55. Toy P, Gajic O, Bacchetti P, et al. TRALI study group blood. Transfusion-related acute lung injury: incidence and risk factors. *Blood.* 2012;119 (7):1757.

56. Tinmouth A, Fergusson D, Yee IC, Hebert PC: Clinical consequences of red cell storage in the critically ill. *Transfusion.* 2006;46:2014–27.

57. Pidcoke HF, McFaul SJ, Ramasubramanian AK, et al. Primary hemostatic capacity of whole blood: a comprehensive analysis of pathogen reduction and refrigeration effects over time. *Transfusion.* 2013;53 (Suppl 1):137S–149S.

58. Fisher AD, Miles EA, Cap AP, Strandenes G, Kane SF. Tactical damage control resuscitation. *Mil Med.* 2015;180 (8):869–75.

59. Spinella PC, Perkins JG, Grathwohl JG, et al. Warm fresh whole blood is independently associated with improved survival for patients with combat-related traumatic injuries. *J Trauma.* 2009;66: S69–76.

60. Butler FK, Holcomb JB, Schreiber MA, et al. Fluid resuscitation for hemorrhagic shock in tactical combat casualty care: TCCC guidelines change 14-01– 2 June 2014. *J Spec Oper Med.* 2014;14 (3):13–38.

61. Spinella PC, Cap AP. Whole blood: back to the future. *Curr Opin Hematol.* 2016;23 (6):536–42.

62. Strandenes G, Berséus O, Cap AP, et al. Low titer group O whole blood in emergency situations. *Shock.* 2014;41(Suppl 1):70–75.

Trauma in Pregnancy

Michael D. April and R. Erik Connor

Trauma accounts for nearly half of all deaths of pregnant women.[1] Pregnant women have distinct physiologic and anatomic characteristics which complicate their management following major trauma. Furthermore, the presence of a fetus means there are effectively two patients, both of whom require evaluation and potentially treatment. The priority in resuscitation of pregnant trauma patients is maternal stabilization.[2]

Epidemiology

Domestic violence is the most common cause of trauma during pregnancy,[3–6] affecting 11.1% of pregnant women,[7] with a homicide rate of 2.9 per 100,000 live births.[8] Other relatively common mechanisms of injury include motor vehicle crashes and falls (Table 4.1).[8–11]

Anatomical Changes in Pregnancy

- 1st trimester: Uterus is small, thick-walled, confined to bony pelvis.
- 2nd trimester: Uterus rises out of pelvis and fills with amniotic fluid which protects the fetus, but may lead to post-trauma embolism or disseminated intravascular coagulation.[12]
- 3rd trimester: Uterus fully enlarges and is thin-walled. This places it at risk for injury from abdominal trauma; however, it displaces the diaphragm and bowel cephalad, protecting against penetrating visceral injuries (Figure 4.1).[13]
- Throughout pregnancy, the pelvic vasculature dilates, and pelvic injuries may lead to exsanguination.[14] Rapid drops in maternal intravascular volume can lead to fetal hypoxia, with a potentially minimal impact on maternal vital signs.[15]

Table 4.1 Incidence of major traumatic injuries sustained in pregnancy

Mechanism of Injury	Estimated Incidence in Pregnancy/100,000 Births
Domestic violence	8,307
Motor vehicle crashes	207
Falls	48.9
Suicide (completed)	2.0
Burns	0.17

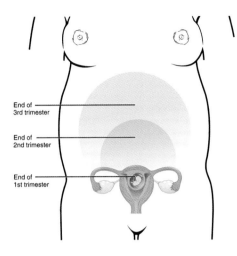

Figure 4.1 Uterine anatomy during pregnancy (image from: https://commons.wikimedia.org/wiki/File:2917_Size_of_Uterus_Throughout_Pregnancy-02.jpg)

End of 3rd trimester

End of 2nd trimester

End of 1st trimester

Physiologic Changes in Pregnancy

There are a myriad of physiologic changes in pregnancy with important implications for trauma management (Table 4.2).[16–21]

Overview of Initial Evaluation and Management

As with all trauma patients, the resuscitation of pregnant trauma patients should start with the primary survey. This includes assessments of the patient's airway, breathing, circulation, disability (neurologic status), and complete exposure of the patient. The unique anatomy and physiology of pregnancy have important implications for each step of the primary survey.[22]

Airway

- As with all trauma patients, maintain cervical spine immobilization in patients who may have sustained spinal cord trauma.
- Anticipate challenging airway characteristics related to pregnancy such as mucosal edema and decreased gastroesophageal sphincter function by developing a difficult airway management plan to include airway adjuncts such as bougie, video laryngoscopy, laryngeal mask airway, and set-up for cricothyrotomy.[23]
- Aggressively pre-oxygenate and consider apneic oxygenation to maintain oxygen saturation >95% to prevent fetal hypoxia.[24,25]
- Place a nasogastric or orogastric tube early in the management of unconscious patients to further minimize the risk of aspiration.[24]
- Though data regarding efficacy are limited,[26] guidelines recommend consideration of cricoid pressure during intubation to minimize risk of aspiration.[24]

Breathing

- Recognize that a "normal" $PaCO_2$ of 35–40 mm Hg may portend impending respiratory failure in pregnant women who often have lower baseline $PaCO_2$ due to hyperventilation.

Table 4.2 Physiologic changes in pregnancy and the potential implications for trauma management

Organ System	Effects of Pregnancy	Implications for Trauma Management
Pulmonary	• Progesterone-mediated hyperventilation with respiratory alkalosis • Increased oxygen demand due to fetus	• Higher susceptibility to acidosis due to fall in plasma bicarbonate • $PaCO_2$ of 30 mm Hg can be normal; $PaCO_2$ of 35–40 mm Hg may portend respiratory failure • Increased risk of hypoxia
Cardiovascular	• Higher cardiac output due to rise in blood volume and heart rate with decreased vascular resistance • Potential compression of inferior vena cava by gravid uterus in the supine position	• Baseline heart rate 10–15 beats per minute faster than pre-pregnancy • Susceptible to hypotension in supine position
Gastrointestinal	• Progesterone-mediated gastroesophageal sphincter relaxation • Progesterone-mediated delayed gastric emptying • Increased intra-abdominal pressure due to gravid uterus	• Increased aspiration risk
Hematologic	• Increase in blood volume with concomitant rise in fraction of plasma volume • Increase in concentrations of fibrinogen and other clotting factors	• Decreased baseline hematocrit (32–42%) • Pregnant patients can lose up to 1,500 mL before showing signs or symptoms of hypovolemia • Pro-coagulant state
Musculoskeletal	• Widening of the symphysis pubis by 4–8 mm in late pregnancy • Widening of the sacroiliac joints	• Altered normal parameters for interpretation of pelvic radiography
Neurologic	• Eclampsia is a known complication of late pregnancy	• Risk of seizures due to non-traumatic etiologies

- Mechanical ventilation settings should target $PaCO_2$ appropriate for the patient's stage of pregnancy: approximately 30 mm Hg in late pregnancy.[27]
- Given the superior displacement of the diaphragm (Figure 4.2), some authors recommend chest tube thoracostomy placement in the third or fourth intercostal space rather than the fifth intercostal space, commonly used in non-pregnant patients.[6,28]

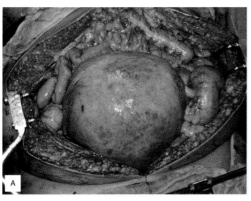
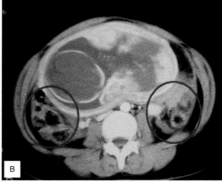

Figure 4.2 Images showing superior displacement of intestine by enlarged uterus intraoperatively (A) and on CT scan (B) (reproduced with permission from *Color Atlas of Emergency Trauma, Second Edition*)

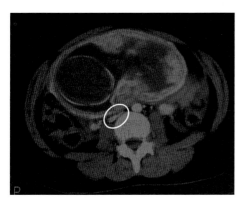

Figure 4.3 Compression of IVC by enlarged uterus on CT scan (highlighted in circle) (reproduced with permission from *Color Atlas of Emergency Trauma, Second Edition*)

Circulation

- Due to the intravascular volume expansion of pregnancy, women may lose up to 1,500 mL of blood before showing signs or symptoms of hypovolemia.[20]
- Guidelines advise against vasopressors given the risk of diminishing uterine blood flow.[24]
- Patients with hypotension should undergo 30–45°+ left lateral tilt to displace the uterus off the inferior vena cava; studies using magnetic resonance imaging and computer modeling suggest that less tilt yields inadequate decompression (Figure 4.3).[29,30]

Cardiopulmonary Resuscitation

- Cardiopulmonary resuscitation via chest compression is thought to be less effective in pregnant patients due to aortocaval compression by the uterus.[31]
- Peri-mortem cesarean section may improve outcomes for the mother and fetus alike by alleviating this compression.[32]
- The mother may hemodynamically benefit from this procedure even if the fetus is non-viable.[31]

Table 4.3 Percentage of peri-mortem cesarean section with neurologic insults compared to the time since maternal arrest

Time Since Maternal Arrest (min)	No. Patients	Neurologic Sequelae (%)
0–5	42	0 (0%)
6–10	8	1 (12.5%)
11–15	7	1 (14.3%)
16–25	4	3 (75.0%)

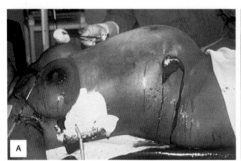
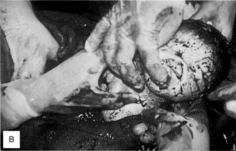
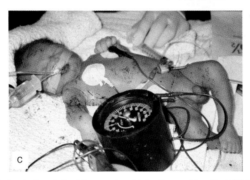

Figure 4.4 Penetrating abdominal and chest trauma in a blatantly gravid patient (A) that resulted in C-section delivery of the term infant (B). This resulted in neonatal resuscitation of the infant (C) but ultimately mother and child survived (reproduced with permission from *Color Atlas of Emergency Trauma, Second Edition*)

- While data are limited, they suggest optimization of maternal and fetal outcomes when performing peri-mortem cesarean section within 4 minutes of cardiac arrest (Table 4.3).[31,32]

Peri-Mortem Cesarean Section Procedure

1. Sterilization by brief application of betadine to the incision site is appropriate, but should not come at the expense of rapid initiation of the procedure (Figure 4.4).
2. Use a No. 10 scalpel to make a midline vertical incision through the abdominal wall spanning from the umbilicus to the symphysis pubis.
3. Expose the uterus, ideally with assistants using retractors to draw the abdominal wound edges laterally and reflect the bladder inferiorly.

4. Make a 5 cm vertical midline incision into the uterus, taking care to avoid fetal injury; stop incision upon achieving amniotic fluid return or visualization of the internal aspect of the uterine cavity.
5. Insert index finger into incision to pull uterine wall away from the fetus and use bandage scissors to extend incision superiorly to the uterine fundus.
6. Deliver the infant ideally by controlling the head; alternatively, if the head is inaccessible, deliver by grasping the infant's feet.
7. Immediately suction the infant's nose and mouth, then clamp and cut the cord.

Secondary Survey

Following the primary survey comes the secondary survey. This comprises a complete history and physical examination from head to toe. Unique considerations in pregnant women include:

- Respiratory distress in absence of traumatic findings may reflect pulmonary edema due to pre-eclampsia[33] or amniotic fluid embolism.[34]
- Assess fundal height as a measure of gestational age and, hence, fetal viability.
- The distance between the symphysis pubis and the uterine fundus in centimeters is a reasonable approximation of the weeks of gestation; approximately 24 cm distance suggests fetal viability.[35]
- Carefully assess the abdomen for trauma and tenderness; by acting as a barrier between the abdominal wall the peritoneum, the gravid uterus may theoretically mask peritonitis.
- Vaginal examination to assess for bleeding, amniotic fluid (confirm by Nitrazine paper color change from yellow to blue), and cervical dilation or effacement.
- A constellation of vaginal bleeding, abdominal pain, contractions, and uterine rigidity are suggestive of placental abruption or uterine rupture and require immediate obstetrics consultation. Ultrasonography is useful if positive, but will be negative for many abruptions.[36]
- Signs of pre-eclampsia, including hypertension, pulmonary edema, neurologic findings, and visual deficits.[33]
- Signs of eclampsia, namely neurologic examination, with recognition that seizures in a pregnant patient with head trauma may represent either intracranial hemorrhage or eclampsia.

Fetal Assessment

Pregnant women must also undergo evaluation of the pregnancy via fetal and uterine monitoring.[24,37] Fetal assessment depends upon whether the fetus has reached viability. The literature generally suggests that fetal viability is ≥24 weeks gestation, though this cut-off is highly situation and setting specific, and may be as low as 22–23 weeks.[38–40] In situations of ambiguity regarding gestational dates, some authors advocate considering as viable any fetus at approximately 20 weeks gestation or greater with the uterine fundus at the level of the umbilicus.[41]

- Prior to viability, fetal assessment should include measurement of fetal heart rate by Doppler or ultrasound; normal is 120–160 beats per minute.
- Past the date of viability, pregnant women sustaining even ostensibly minor abdominal trauma should undergo at least 4 hours of continuous monitoring of fetal heart rate and uterine contractions, ideally under the care of an obstetrician (Figure 4.5).[42]

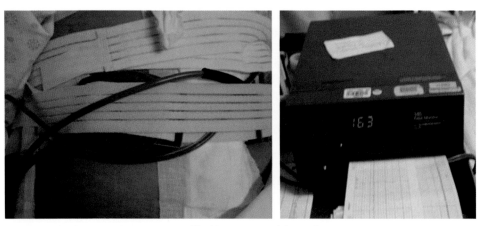

Figure 4.5 Cardiotocographic monitoring of fetal heart rate variability and uterine contractions (reproduced with permission from *Color Atlas of Emergency Trauma, Second Edition*)

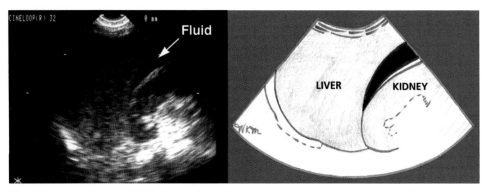

Figure 4.6 View of positive FAST in Morrison's Pouch (reproduced with permission from *Color Atlas of Emergency Trauma, Second Edition*)

- Signs of impending maternal or fetal decompensation include abnormal fetal heart rate, repetitive late or variable decelerations, absence of fetal heart rate variability, and frequent uterine contractions.[43]
- Any signs of ruptured membranes or impending labor in the setting of fetal viability mandates obstetrics consultation for further monitoring and management.

Ultrasound Examination

Ultrasound provides an increasingly available non-radiating imaging modality which may supplement the physical examination of the pregnant woman and her fetus. Potential applications include:

- A focused assessment with sonography for trauma (FAST) examination remains the cornerstone of diagnostic ultrasonography in trauma, but has imperfect sensitivity for intra-peritoneal bleeding (Figure 4.6).[44]
- It is sometimes possible to identify signs of placental abruption such as sub-chorionic hemorrhage, though ultrasound has poor sensitivity for this disease process.[36]

- The literature reports cases of detection of fetal injuries such as intracranial hematomas and skull fractures in utero via ultrasound, though absence of ultrasound findings should again not be considered to definitively rule out injuries.[45,46]
- Evaluation of fetal heart rate when this remains undetectable by other mechanisms. The provider places an M-mode cursor beam over the fetal heart, then determines the heart rate by measuring the distance between heart beats.

Diagnostic Evaluation

As with all trauma patients, providers should order those laboratory and imaging tests which, based upon clinical suspicion, they believe are likely to change management. Considerations specific to pregnant trauma patients include:

- Providers should not refrain from ordering diagnostic imaging modalities involving radiation based upon their clinical suspicion for traumatic disease, as the radiation exposure to the fetus is minimal and fetal survival depends upon maternal well-being.[47]
- All pregnant trauma patients should undergo Rh(D) testing.
- Women who are Rh(D) negative should undergo Kleihauer-Betke testing to quantify fetomaternal hemorrhage and so guide dosing for Rh(D) immune globulin to prevent isoimmunization in the event the fetus is Rh(D) positive.[48]
- Laboratory studies in conjunction with blood pressure measurements to investigate pre-eclampsia including urinalysis, complete blood count, renal function panel, and liver function tests (Table 4.4).[33]

Therapeutic Considerations

- In consultation with obstetrics, consider administration of corticosteroids to pregnant women at increased risk for preterm birth with gestations of viable age but prior to 34/35 weeks to optimize fetal lung development (betamethasone 12 mg intramuscular vs. dexamethasone 6 mg intramuscular).[49]
- Any Rh(D) negative woman experiencing significant trauma should receive 300 μg of Rh(D) immune globulin intravenous[50]; Kleihauer–Betke testing should guide whether higher doses are necessary to prevent isoimmunization.[48]
- There is no contraindication to tetanus toxoid in pregnancy, and pregnant trauma patients meeting standard indications should receive this vaccination.[51]
- Providers should have a high index of suspicion for placental abruption, as it remains the most common complication associated with trauma in pregnancy. Incidence has been reported as high as 5% in minor traumatic injuries and up to 65% with more severe mechanisms (Figure 4.7).[52]

Other Considerations

- Given the high proportion of pregnant trauma patient sustained injuries due to intimate partner violence, be sure to screen these patients for domestic violence in a private setting without partners present.[53]
- Have a low threshold for transfer to tertiary care centers, as there are correlations between even seemingly isolated trauma (e.g., single extremity fractures) and adverse maternal and fetal outcomes.[54,55]

Table 4.4 Diagnostic criteria for pre-eclampsia

Component	Criteria
Blood Pressure	• Systolic blood pressure ≥140 mmHg or diastolic blood pressure ≥90 mm Hg confirmed on two occasions at least 4 hours apart after 20 weeks gestation in woman with previously normal blood pressure, *or* • Systolic blood pressure ≥160 mmHg or diastolic blood pressure ≥110 mm Hg confirmed within minutes
and	
Proteinuria	• ≥300 mg per 24-hour urine collection (or extrapolated from timed collection), *or* • Protein/creatinine ratio ≥0.3, *or* • Urine dipstick reading 1+ protein (used only if quantitative methods unavailable
Or, in the absence of proteinuria, new-onset hypertension with new onset of any of the following:	
Thrombocytopenia	• Platelet count <100,000/μL
Renal insufficiency	• Serum creatinine >1.1 mg/dL or doubling of serum creatinine in the absence of other renal disease
Impaired liver function	• Serum concentrations of liver transaminases twice normal levels
Pulmonary edema	• Clinical diagnosis
Cerebral or visual symptoms	• Clinical diagnosis

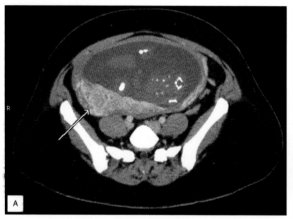
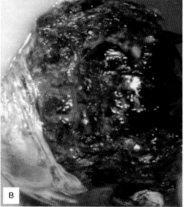

Figure 4.7 CT representation of placental abruption (A). Placental abruption specimen obtained after emergency C-section (reproduced with permission from *Color Atlas of Emergency Trauma, Second Edition*)

Pitfalls in ED Evaluation and Management

• Assuming a $PaCO_2$ of 35–40 mm Hg is normal; these levels may portend impending respiratory failure in pregnant women who generally have a lower baseline $PaCO_2$ due to hyperventilation, particularly in the later stages of pregnancy.

- Relying solely upon maternal vital signs and symptoms to guide volume resuscitation; given the intravascular volume expansion of pregnancy, women may lose up to 1,500 mL of blood before showing signs or symptoms of hypovolemia.
- Applying less than 30° of left lateral tilt in hypotensive pregnant women; tilt less than this amount may not yield clinically significant decompression of the inferior vena cava.
- Delayed initiation of peri-mortem cesarean section; maternal and fetal outcomes are optimized by performing this procedure within 4 minutes of cardiac arrest.
- Failure to consider pre-eclampsia in pregnant women seizing after head trauma.
- Relying upon ultrasonography to rule out placental abruption.
- Refraining from diagnostic imaging modalities entailing ionizing radiation given concerns for fetal radiation exposure at the expense of potentially missing maternal injuries.
- Failure to obtain Kleihauer-Betke testing to guide Rh(D) immune globulin dosing in Rh(D) negative women status post-significant trauma, placing them at high risk for fetomaternal hemorrhage.
- Failing to screen pregnant trauma patients for domestic violence in a private setting without partners present.

Key Points

- Trauma is a common cause of morbidity and mortality in pregnant women.
- Focus resuscitation efforts on the mother, starting with the primary survey.
- Obtain obstetrics consultation early if signs of impending labor in setting of fetal viability (≥24 weeks gestation), but recognize need to simultaneously manage any traumatic injuries.
- Maintain a low threshold for transfer to a tertiary care center given correlations between even isolated and relatively minor traumatic injuries and adverse fetal and maternal outcomes.

References

1. Fildes J, Reed L, Jones N, Martin M, Barrett J. Trauma: the leading cause of maternal death. *J Trauma*. 1992;32:643–45.

2. Esposito TJ. Trauma during pregnancy. *Emerg Med Clin North Am*. 1994;12:167–99.

3. Eisenstat SA, Bancroft L. Domestic violence. *N Engl J Med*. 1999;341:886–92.

4. Kyriacou DN, Anglin D, Taliaferro E, et al. Risk factors for injury to women from domestic violence. *N Engl J Med*. 1999;341:1892–98.

5. Lutgendorf MA, Busch JM, Doherty DA, et al. Prevalence of domestic violence in a pregnant military population. *Obstet Gynecol*. 2009;113:866–72.

6. Mendez-Figueroa H, Dahlke JD, Vrees RA, Rouse DJ. Trauma in pregnancy: an updated systematic review. *Am J Obstet Gynecol*. 2013;209:1–10.

7. Cokkinides VE, Coker AL, Sanderson M, Addy C, Bethea L. Physical violence during pregnancy: maternal complications and birth outcomes. *Obstet Gynecol*. 1999;93:661–66.

8. Palladino CL, Singh V, Campbell J, Flynn H, Gold KJ. Homicide and suicide during the perinatal period: findings from the National Violent Death Reporting System. *Obstet Gynecol*. 2011;118:1056–63.

9. Kvarnstrand L, Milsom I, Lekander T, Druid H, Jacobsson B. Maternal fatalities, fetal and neonatal deaths related to motor vehicle crashes during pregnancy: a national population-based study. *Acta Obstet Gynecol Scand.* 2008;87:946–52.

10. Maghsoudi H, Samnia R, Garadaghi A, Kianvar H. Burns in pregnancy. *Burns.* 2006;32:246–50.

11. Schiff MA. Pregnancy outcomes following hospitalisation for a fall in Washington State from 1987 to 2004. *BJOG.* 2008;115:1648–54.

12. Shah AJ, Kilcline BA. Trauma in pregnancy. *Emerg Med Clin North Am.* 2003;21:615–29.

13. Awwad JT, Azar GB, Seoud MA, Mroueh AM, Karam KS. High-velocity penetrating wounds of the gravid uterus: review of 16 years of civil war. *Obstet Gynecol.* 1994;83:259–64.

14. Stone IK. Trauma in the obstetric patient. *Obstet Gynecol Clin North Am.* 1999;26:459–67, viii.

15. Jensen A, Kunzel W, Kastendieck E. Repetitive reduction of uterine blood flow and its influence on fetal transcutaneous PO2 and cardiovascular variables. *J Dev Physiol.* 1985;7:75–87.

16. Baggish MS, Hooper S. Aspiration as a cause of maternal death. *Obstet Gynecol.* 1974;43:327–36.

17. Berry MJ, McMurray RG, Katz VL. Pulmonary and ventilatory responses to pregnancy, immersion, and exercise. *J Appl Physiol (1985).* 1989;66:857–62.

18. Weissgerber TL, Wolfe LA, Hopkins WG, Davies GA. Serial respiratory adaptations and an alternate hypothesis of respiratory control in human pregnancy. *Respir Physiol Neurobiol.* 2006;153:39–53.

19. Adler G, Duchinski T, Jasinska A, Piotrowska U. Fibrinogen fractions in the third trimester of pregnancy and in puerperium. *Thromb Res.* 2000;97:405–10.

20. American College of Surgeons, Trauma in pregnancy and intimate partner violence. In: C.o. Trauma, ed. *Advanced Trauma Life Support.* Chicago, IL: American College of Surgeons; 2012.

21. Stead LG. Seizures in pregnancy/eclampsia. *Emerg Med Clin North Am.* 2011;29:109–16.

22. Nash P, Driscoll P. ABC of major trauma. Trauma in pregnancy. *BMJ.* 1990;301:974–76.

23. Rocke DA, Murray WB, Rout CC, Gouws E. Relative risk analysis of factors associated with difficult intubation in obstetric anesthesia. *Anesthesiology.* 1992;77:67–73.

24. Jain V, Chari R, Maslovitz S, et al. Guidelines for the management of a pregnant trauma patient. *J Obstet Gynaecol Can.* 2015;37:553–74.

25. Pavlov I, Medrano S, Weingart S. Apneic oxygenation reduces the incidence of hypoxemia during emergency intubation: a systematic review and meta-analysis. *Am J Emerg Med.* 2017;35(8):1184–89.

26. Salem MR, Khorasani A, Zeidan A, Crystal GJ. Cricoid pressure controversies: narrative review. *Anesthesiology.* 2017;126:738–52.

27. Templeton A, Kelman GR. Maternal blood-gases, PAo2–Pao2), hysiological shunt and VD/VT in normal pregnancy. *Br J Anaesth.* 1976;48:1001–4.

28. Brown HL. Trauma in pregnancy. *Obstet Gynecol.* 2009;114:147–60.

29. Higuchi H, Takagi S, Zhang K, Furui I, Ozaki M. Effect of lateral tilt angle on the volume of the abdominal aorta and inferior vena cava in pregnant and nonpregnant women determined by magnetic resonance imaging. *Anesthesiology.* 2015;122:286–93.

30. Summers RL, Harrison JM, Thompson JR, Porter J, Coleman TG. Theoretical analysis of the effect of positioning on hemodynamic stability during pregnancy. *Acad Emerg Med.* 2011;18:1094–98.

31. Katz VL, Dotters DJ, Droegemueller W. Perimortem cesarean delivery. *Obstet Gynecol.* 1986;68:571–76.

32. Katz V, Balderston K, DeFreest M. Perimortem cesarean delivery: were our assumptions correct? *Am J Obstet Gynecol.* 2005;192:1916–20; discussion 1920–21.

33. American College of Obstetricians and Gynecologists, Task Force on Hypertension

in Pregnancy. Hypertension in pregnancy. Report of the American College of Obstetricians and Gynecologists' Task Force on Hypertension in Pregnancy. *Obstet Gynecol.* 2013;122:1122–31.

34. Benson MD. Amniotic fluid embolism mortality rate. *J Obstet Gynaecol Res.* 2017;43(11):1714–18.

35. Deeluea J, Sirichotiyakul S, Weerakiet S, et al. Fundal height growth curve for Thai women. *ISRN Obstet Gynecol.* 2013;2013:463598.

36. Kuhlmann RS, Warsof S. Ultrasound of the placenta. *Clin Obstet Gynecol.* 1996;39:519–34.

37. American College of Obstetricians and Gynecologists. Trauma during pregnancy. ACOG Technical Bulletin Number 161– November 1991. *Int J Gynaecol Obstet.* 1993;40:165–70.

38. Group E, Fellman V, Hellstrom-Westas L, et al. One-year survival of extremely preterm infants after active perinatal care in Sweden. *JAMA.* 2009;301:2225–33.

39. Stoll BJ, Hansen NI, Bell EF, et al. Trends in care practices, morbidity, and mortality of extremely preterm neonates, 1993–2012. *JAMA.* 2015;314:1039–51.

40. Tyson JE, Parikh NA, Langer J, et al. Intensive care for extreme prematurity – moving beyond gestational age. *N Engl J Med.* 2008;358:1672–81.

41. Smith KA, Bryce S. Trauma in the pregnant patient: an evidence-based approach to management. *Emerg Med Pract.* 2013;15:1–18; quiz 18–19.

42. Pearlman MD, Tintinallli JE, Lorenz RP. A prospective controlled study of outcome after trauma during pregnancy. *Am J Obstet Gynecol.* 1990;162:1502–7; discussion 1507–10.

43. Nageotte MP. Fetal heart rate monitoring. *Semin Fetal Neonatal Med.* 2015;20:144–48.

44. Richards JR, Ormsby EL, Romo MV, Gillen MA, McGahan JP. Blunt abdominal injury in the pregnant patient: detection with US. *Radiology.* 2004;233:463–70.

45. Ellestad SC, Shelton S, James AH. Prenatal diagnosis of a trauma-related fetal epidural hematoma. *Obstet Gynecol.* 2004;104:1298–300.

46. Hartl R, Ko K. In utero skull fracture: case report. *J Trauma.* 1996;41:549–52.

47. Mann FA, Nathens A, Langer SG, Goldman SM, Blackmore CC. Communicating with the family: the risks of medical radiation to conceptuses in victims of major blunt-force torso trauma. *J Trauma.* 2000;48:354–57.

48. Kim YA, Makar RS. Detection of fetomaternal hemorrhage. *Am J Hematol.* 2012;87:417–23.

49. Roberts D, Brown J, Medley N, Dalziel SR. Antenatal corticosteroids for accelerating fetal lung maturation for women at risk of preterm birth. *Cochrane Database Syst Rev.* 2017;3:CD004454.

50. Committee on Practice Bulletins-Obstetrics. Practice Bulletin No. 181: prevention of Rh D alloimmunization. *Obstet Gynecol.* 2017;130:e57–e70.

51. Blencowe H, Lawn J, Vandelaer J, Roper M, Cousens S. Tetanus toxoid immunization to reduce mortality from neonatal tetanus. *Int J Epidemiol.* 2010;39(Suppl 1): i102–9.

52. Demetriades D, Newton E. Abdominal trauma in pregnancy. *Color Atlas of Emergency Trauma*, 2nd ed. Cambridge: Cambridge University Press; 2011, pp. 154–59.

53. McFarlane J, Parker B, Soeken K, Bullock L. Assessing for abuse during pregnancy. Severity and frequency of injuries and associated entry into prenatal care. *JAMA.* 1992;267:3176–78.

54. Cannada LK, Pan P, Casey BM, et al. Pregnancy outcomes after orthopedic trauma. *J Trauma.* 2010;69:694–98; discussion 698.

55. El Kady D, Gilbert WM, Xing G, Smith LH. Association of maternal fractures with adverse perinatal outcomes. *Am J Obstet Gynecol.* 2006;195:711–16.

Chapter 5

Pediatric Trauma

Manpreet Singh and Timothy Horeczko

Trauma evaluation and management often focuses on protocols, especially in adults. In children, however, special considerations are made based on *epidemiology, physiology,* and *mechanisms of injury* on the location affected.

Epidemiology

Trauma is the leading cause of death of children >1 year old, with unintentional injury accounting for the majority (Figure 5.1).[1] Injuries predominantly include MVCs, followed by homicide/suicide and drowning.[1] Most pediatric trauma is blunt; penetrating trauma in children accounts for 10–20% of trauma-related deaths. This number is likely to rise in the future.[1]

Anatomy and Physiology

Children demonstrate several anatomic and physiologic differences compared to adults, which must be considered in the evaluation and management of the pediatric trauma patient.

Anatomical Differences

Airway

- *Head*: Children have a relatively large head in proportion to the body. When supine, the prominent occiput causes the neck to flex, which may lead to airway obstruction; always place a rolled towel or sheet under the scapulae to help align airway axes.[2]
- *Tongue*: Usually large and may impede entrainment of air or laryngoscopy.[2]
- *Larynx*: Located anterior and superior in position. The laryngoscopist can look from below up into the airway to aid visualization.[2]
- *Epiglottis*: U-shaped, short, and stiff. As a result, a straight (Miller) blade helps to displace the anterior epiglottis for better visualization.[2] A curved (Macintosh) blade may be used in school-aged children and up.[2]
- *Vocal Cords*: Unlike adult vocal cords, which have a horizontal slant, pediatric vocal cords slant vertically.[2]
- *Trachea*: Tends to be short, leading to an increased likelihood of right mainstem intubation.[2]
- *Airway diameter*: Funnel-shaped with the narrowest portion at the cricoid ring. Cricoid pressure can cause collapse of the delicate trachea, causing obstruction and poor visualization.[2]
- *Lung Capacity*: Small lung capacity, leading to a short time to desaturation.[2]

Developing musculoskeletal system

- Flexible cartilaginous skeleton and open growth plates cause children to suffer more avulsion injuries, rather than fractures (less calcified, less rigid skeleton).[2]
- With less calcification and added flexibility, children have greater incidence of abdominal, chest, and spinal cord injuries without fracture.[2]

Physiological differences

Age-Specific Vitals (Table 5.1)

Traumatic situations make vital sign interpretation difficult. Heart rate may be variably tachycardic in a frightened, screaming child in a traumatic situation, so a proper blood pressure cuff is essential to prevent an artificially low reading.[3]

Table 5.1 Age-specific vital signs

Age Group	HR (beats/min)		R	Leukocyte Count × 10³/mm³	SBP
	↑	↓			
Newborn	>180	<100	>50	>19.5 or <5	<65
Infant	>180	<90	>34	>17.5 or <5	<100
Toddler	>160	NA	>29	>16.5 or <5	<100
Preschool	>140	NA	>22	>15.5 or <6	<94
School age child	>130	NA	>18	>13.5 or <4.5	<105

					Age Groups						
Rank	<1	1-4	5-9	10-14	15-24	25-34	35-44	45-54	55-64	65+	Total
1	Congenital Anomalies 4,825	Unintentional Injury 1,235	Unintentional Injury 755	Unintentional Injury 763	Unintentional Injury 12,514	Unintentional Injury 19,795	Unintentional Injury 17,818	Malignant Neoplasms 43,054	Malignant Neoplasms 116,122	Heart Disease 507,138	Heart Disease 633,842
2	Short Gestation 4,084	Congenital Anomalies 435	Malignant Neoplasms 437	Malignant Neoplasms 428	Suicide 5,491	Suicide 6,947	Malignant Neoplasms 10,909	Heart Disease 34,248	Heart Disease 76,872	Malignant Neoplasms 419,389	Malignant Neoplasms 595,930
3	SIDS 1,568	Homicide 369	Congenital Anomalies 181	Suicide 409	Homicide 4,733	Homicide 4,863	Heart Disease 10,387	Unintentional Injury 21,499	Unintentional Injury 19,488	Chronic Low. Respiratory Disease 131,804	Chronic Low. Respiratory Disease 155,041
4	Maternal Pregnancy Comp. 1,522	Malignant Neoplasms 354	Homicide 140	Homicide 158	Malignant Neoplasms 1,469	Malignant Neoplasms 3,704	Suicide 6,936	Liver Disease 8,874	Chronic Low. Respiratory Disease 17,457	Cerebro-vascular 120,156	Unintentional Injury 146,571
5	Unintentional Injury 1,291	Heart Disease 147	Heart Disease 85	Congenital Anomalies 156	Heart Disease 997	Heart Disease 3,522	Homicide 2,895	Suicide 8,751	Diabetes Mellitus 14,166	Alzheimer's Disease 109,495	Cerebro-vascular 140,323
6	Placenta Cord. Membranes 910	Influenza & Pneumonia 88	Chronic Low. Respiratory Disease 80	Heart Disease 125	Congenital Anomalies 386	Liver Disease 844	Liver Disease 2,861	Diabetes Mellitus 6,212	Liver Disease 13,278	Diabetes Mellitus 56,142	Alzheimer's Disease 110,561
7	Bacterial Sepsis 599	Septicemia 54	Influenza & Pneumonia 44	Chronic Low Respiratory Disease 93	Chronic Low Respiratory Disease 202	Diabetes Mellitus 798	Diabetes Mellitus 1,986	Cerebro-vascular 5,307	Cerebro-vascular 12,116	Unintentional Injury 51,395	Diabetes Mellitus 79,535
8	Respiratory Distress 462	Perinatal Period 50	Cerebro-vascular 42	Cerebro-vascular 42	Diabetes Mellitus 196	Cerebro-vascular 567	Cerebro-vascular 1,788	Chronic Low. Respiratory Disease 4,345	Suicide 7,739	Influenza & Pneumonia 48,774	Influenza & Pneumonia 57,062
9	Circulatory System Disease 428	Cerebro-vascular 42	Benign Neoplasms 39	Influenza & Pneumonia 39	Influenza & Pneumonia 184	HIV 529	HIV 1,055	Septicemia 2,542	Septicemia 5,774	Nephritis 41,258	Nephritis 49,959
10	Neonatal Hemorrhage 406	Chronic Low Respiratory Disease 40	Septicemia 31	Two Tied: Benign Neo./Septicemia 33	Cerebro-vascular 166	Congenital Anomalies 443	Septicemia 829	Nephritis 2,124	Nephritis 5,452	Septicemia 30,817	Suicide 44,193

Figure 5.1 Ten leading causes of death by age group, United States in 2015 (data source: Nation Vital Statistics System, National Center for Health Statistics, CDC. Produced by: National Center for Injury Prevention and Control, CDC using WISQARS™)

- Vasoconstriction is a compensatory mechanism to hypovolemia, specifically hemorrhagic shock in trauma. Children compensate for a loss of cardiac output by increasing their heart rate. Thus, tachycardia is the first sign of shock in children, while hypotension is an ominous, late finding.
- *Shock Index*: Shock index is defined as HR/systolic BP. Though it has been around for some time, it is underutilized. It is most useful as a reference for physicians before the BP drops, especially in the occult shock patient.[4,5]
  . Shock Index, Pediatric Adjusted (SIPA)[4,5]
    - 4–6 years = 1.2
    - 6–12 years = 1
    - >12 years = 0.9

Breathing
Pediatric patients are more prone to hypoxia for a variety of reasons.[6]
- Extrathoracic Airway Differences:
  . Obligate nasal breathers
  . Smaller oral airway
  . Cephalic larynx
  . Epiglottis larger
  . Enlarged adenoid tissue
  . Congenital abnormalities

- Intrathoracic Airway Differences:
  . Fewer, smaller alveoli
  . Poor collateral ventilation
  . Smaller intrathoracic airways collapse
  . Cartilaginous support lacking
  . Residual damage from birth leads to decreased pulmonary compliance
  . Chest wall musculature not fully developed
  . Lower functional residual capacity

- Respiratory Drive Differences:
  . Immature respiratory center
  . Higher metabolic rates

Thermoregulation
- Children readily lose heat through convection (high body surface area), conduction (wet diaper), and radiation (large, well perfused head).[7]
- In addition, a high surface-area-to-mass ratio with thinner skin and less subcutaneous tissue to provide insulation predisposes children to hypothermia, which, in the setting of trauma, may lead to coagulopathy.[7]

Regions

Head

Anatomy

The head is large relative to the body. The occiput is the biggest portion of the head. The open fontanelles (anterior and mastoid) should be evaluated, and clinicians should examine for subgaleal hematomas, which can be a major source of bleeding.

- Caput succedaneum – Extra-periosteal collection. *Crosses suture lines.* Result of birth trauma usually.
- Cephalohematoma – Between skull and periosteum. *Does not cross suture lines.*
- Subgaleal hemorrhage/hematoma – Between skull periosteum and scalp galea aponeurosis. *Crosses suture lines.*

PECARN

The decision to obtain a CT head in a pediatric trauma should be completed with proper risk stratification using validated clinical predictors. The Pediatric Emergency Care Applied Research Network (PECARN) studies provide a set of guidelines to help guide physicians in cases of minor blunt head trauma (Figures 5.2 and 5.3). If a CT head non-contrast is not indicated, observation in the ED or at home is recommended with reassurance, education, and strict return precautions.

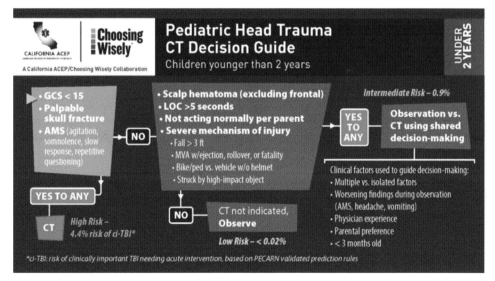

Figure 5.2 Blunt head trauma in children <2 years of age (obtained from Cal ACEP, with permission)

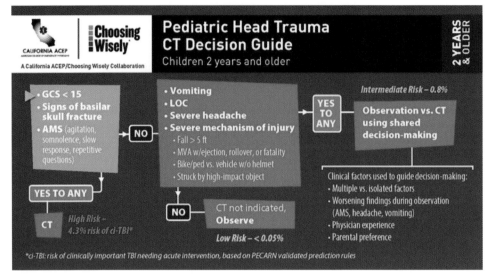

Figure 5.3 Blunt head trauma in children ≥2 years of age (obtained from Cal ACEP, with permission)

Airway Management

If the patient has any subtle changes in mental status, be proactive. Consider intubating early, as the respiratory center is underdeveloped, and hypoxia is associated with mortality in traumatic brain injury.

Neck

Because C2/C3 acts as a fulcrum in children less than 8 years old, they tend to have a higher pattern of cervical spine injury (CSI).[8] For this reason, most pediatric trauma centers include the cervical spine to C3, in an attempt to avoid unnecessary radiation.[8] By age 8, the fulcrum of impact is the C5/C6 level, similar to adults.[8]

C-Spine fractures are usually rare in pediatric patients due to the following differences[9]:

• Ligamentous laxity in facet joints
• Partially cartilaginous endplates (unfused growth plates)
• Intervertebral discs with higher water content and elasticity
• Horizontal facets and shallow facet joints
• Underdeveloped paraspinous muscles

These factors predispose them to more dislocations and ligamentous injuries. Due to this, there may be stretching of cord and nerve roots leading to Spinal Cord Injury Without Radiological Abnormality (SCIWORA) in children >8 years old.[9]

Clearance of the c-spine is typically done via NEXUS or Canadian C-Spine Rule (CCR) if the patient is reliable, awake, and alert. Keep in mind that 9% of NEXUS patients were <18-year-old, where thirty had a c-spine injury (0.98%) of which none were <2 years old and only four were <9 years old; thus it was not powered for children <9 years old.[10] The NEXUS criteria has 100% (87.8%–100%) sensitivity for pediatric patients, but only 19.9% (18.5%–21.3%) specificity.[10] Thus, the low specificity may lead to unnecessary imaging.

CCR on the other hand excluded patients <16 years old.[10] High sensitivity of this rule may also result in false positives, as well as unnecessary imaging.[10]

A recent case-control study of pediatric patients <16 years old shows the following eight factors associated with cervical spine injury[11]:

- AMS
- Focal neurologic findings
- Neck pain
- Torticollis
- Substantial torso injury
- Conditions predisposing to CSI
- Diving
- High risk MVC

Having 1+ factors was 98% sensitive and 26% specific for CSI.

Thorax

Thoracic trauma is the second most common cause of trauma-related death in patients aged <18 years old. Pediatric cases are due to blunt forces with high energy impact causing injury to multiple regions of the body.

The child's chest wall is highly compliant and thin, making it more like an accordion than a cage. Due to this compliance and flexibility of the chest wall, kinetic energy may be transmitted through the chest wall – without much evidence of external trauma – leading to pulmonary contusions or mediastinal injury.[6] As an example, rib fractures in a child require significant focal force and serve as a harbinger of severe injury.

On the other hand, severe thoracic injury in children is very uncommon. In most cases, a screening chest x-ray (CXR) is all that is indicated.[6] The screening "pan scan" seen in adult trauma patients is not recommended for children. Use clinical judgment when deciding to perform a CT chest scan on a child.

CT chest scans are generally overused, with increased cost and radiation, but barely added diagnosis that rarely changes management.[6] Thus, CT should be used judiciously or after screening modalities such as a CXR or ultrasound.

Severe hemo or pneumothoraces are readily picked up by CXR or ultrasound. Rib fractures on CXR predict pulmonary contusions. In general, a widened mediastinum on CXR should be followed by a CT chest to evaluate for greater vessel injuries (e.g. traumatic aortic dissection). Although there is no decision tool, children without predictors listed in Box 5.1 possess a low risk of intrathoracic injuries.[12]

Box 5.1   Predictors of Thoracic Injury (Sensitivity = 98%)

- Low Systolic BP
- Tachypnea
- Abnormal thoracic physical exam
- Abnormal auscultation (including tachypnea)
- Femur fracture
- GCS <15
- Deceleration mechanism

> **Box 5.2 GCS and Abdominal Tenderness Sensitivity**
>
> GCS 15 – abdominal tenderness sensitivity = 79%
> GCS 14 – abdominal tenderness sensitivity = 57%
> GCS 13 – abdominal tenderness sensitivity = 37%

Abdomen

The abdominal wall is thinner, softer, and less muscular in pediatric patients compared to adults, and solid organs are proportionally larger and less protected by the rib cage.[13] These organs are close in proximity, making multiple organ injuries more likely.[13] Unlike being located in the lower pelvis in adults, the bladder is intra-abdominal in younger children.[13]

Evaluation of possible intra-abdominal injuries can be difficult as 50% have no outward sign of trauma. However, the abdominal exam is important. Isolated abdominal pain or tenderness increases the degree of abdominal findings and is associated with risk of injury that warrants evaluation.[13] However, as GCS decreases, the abdominal exam becomes less reliable (Box 5.2).[13]

A seat-belt sign is associated with increased risk for intra-abdominal injuries, especially hollow viscous and mesenteric injuries.[13] Absence of pain or tenderness in its setting connotes a lower risk, but caution should be used.

When evaluating for intra-abdominal injuries, it does not mean all patients require a CT. Risk stratification can be completed by examination of the following:[13]

- Observation with serial abdominal exams
- Bedside ultrasound
- Laboratory studies
  - AST >200 U/L or ALT >125 U/L
  - Hematuria (>5 RBCs/HPF)
  - Initial hematocrit <30%
- In the end, mechanism trumps these laboratory studies.

Focused Assessment with Sonography in Trauma (FAST) is not sensitive enough to rule-out abdominal trauma.[14] One study found a sensitivity of 52% (95% CI = 31–73%).[14] Most splenic or liver lacerations in children are managed non-operatively – for this reason the CT can be an essential tool in assessment. However, with the addition of contrast-enhanced ultrasound, this may change in the near future.[14]

Extremities

Extremity injuries are usually evaluated with physical exam and plain films. Most injuries tend to have ligamentous tears, rather than fractures due to poorly mineralized bone.[15] It is important to consider high-risk anatomically complex areas such as the hand, wrist, tibial plateau, and the midfoot where CT may be useful in finding occult clinically important injuries.[15]

Compartment syndrome is often undiagnosed in children, as "pain out of proportion to the exam" is often difficult to assess in pediatric patients.[15] The key is for frequent re-assessments of compartments, especially in high-impact traumas, and to be suspicious for increasing analgesic requirements or severe patient anxiety.[15]

Pitfalls in ED Evaluation and Management

- Failure to understand differences in anatomy and physiology when dealing with pediatric trauma patients.
- Hypotension is usually a late finding of hemorrhagic shock in children, where vasoconstriction is a compensatory mechanism with tachycardia.
- The CT "panscan" should not be ordered routinely for children, and risk stratification is recommended using decision tools, screening imaging and labs, and observation.
- Over-reliance of FAST to rule-out intra-abdominal traumatic injuries.

Key Points

- Anatomical differences in the pediatric airway should be considered when managing the airway.
- Pediatric patients compensate with tachycardia over perfusion. Hypotension suggests decompensated shock in pediatric patients.
- Selective intentional work-up is important in pediatric trauma patients, where the pan-CT scan is rarely indicated.

References

1. CDC Injury Prevention & Control. Available at: www.cdc.gov/injury/wisqars/LeadingCauses.html. Last updated April 13, 2018. Accessed June 8, 2018.

2. Kissoon N, Dreyer J, Walia M. Pediatric trauma: differences in pathophysiology, injury patterns and treatment compared with adult trauma. *CMAJ*. 1990;142(1):27.

3. De Caen AR, Berg MD, Chameides L, et al. Pediatric advanced life support: 2015 American Heart Association guidelines update for cardiopulmonary resuscitation and emergency cardiovascular care. *Circulation*. 2015;132(18 suppl 2): S526–542.

4. Acker SN, Ross JT, Partrick DA, et al. Pediatric specific shock index accurately identifies severely injured children. *J Pediatr Surg*. 2015;50(2):331–34.

5. Acker SN, Bredbeck B, Partrick DA, et al. Shock index, pediatric age-adjusted (SIPA) is more accurate than age-adjusted hypotension for trauma team activation. *Surgery*. 2017;161(3):803–7.

6. Reynolds SL. Pediatric thoracic trauma: recognition and management. *Emerg Med Clin North Am*. 2018;36(2):473–83.

7. Bernardo LM, Henker R. Thermoregulation in pediatric trauma: an overview. *Int J Trauma Nursing*. 1999;5 (3):101–5.

8. Booth, TN. Cervical spine evaluation in pediatric trauma. *Am J Roentgenol*. 2012;198(5):W417–W425.

9. Kramer DR, Kiehna EN. Spinal cord injury without radiographic abnormality in children – the SCIWORA Syndrome. In: Vaccaro AR, Wilson JR, Fisher CG, eds. *50 Landmark Papers Every Spine Surgeon Should Know*. London: Routledge; 2018, p. 241.

10. Anderson RC, Scaife ER, Fenton SJ, et al. Cervical spine clearance after trauma in children. *J Neurosurg*. 2006;105 (5):361–64.

11. Leonard JC, Kuppermann N, Olsen C, et al. Factors associated with cervical spine injury in children after blunt trauma. *Ann Emerg Med.* 2011;58 (2):145–55.

12. McNamara C, Mironova I, Lehman E, et al. Predictors of intrathoracic injury after blunt torso trauma in children presenting to an emergency department as trauma activations. *J Emerg Med.* 2017;52 (6):793–800.

13. Lynch T, Kilgar, J, Al Shibli A. Pediatric abdominal trauma. *Curr Pediat Rev.* 2018;14(1):59–63.

14. Armstrong LB, Mooney DP, Paltiel H, et al. Contrast enhanced ultrasound for the evaluation of blunt pediatric abdominal trauma. *J Pediat Surg.* 2018;53(3):548–52.

15. Rickert KD, Hosseinzadeh P, Edmonds EW. What's new in pediatric orthopaedic trauma: the lower extremity. *J Pediat Orthopaed.* 2018;38(8):e434–e439.

Geriatric Trauma

Matthew R. Levine

Importance

According to 2010 US Census data, adults >65 years old account for 14% of the population, and one in five US residents will be elderly by 2050.[1,2] Approximately one million Americans of 65 years and older are affected by trauma each year.[3]

Trauma in elders accounts for $12 billion in medical costs and $25 billion in total costs yearly.[4]

While elderly patients comprise a small percentage of total major trauma patients (8–12%), they represent a disproportionate percentage of trauma mortalities and costs (15–30%, Figures 6.1 and 6.2).

Older age is an independent risk factor for morbidity and mortality, despite lesser severity of injuries.[1,2] The Major Trauma Outcome Study (1989), which included 3,833 patients aged >65 and 42,944 patients aged <65, showed that mortality rose sharply between 45–55 years and doubled by 75 years of age. This pattern occurred at all Injury Severity Scores (ISS), mechanisms, and body regions.[5] Other literature reports various inflection points between the ages of 45 and 70 years, where trauma mortality increases.[6,7]

While age has value in mortality projections for geriatric trauma patients, there is no specific age cutoff for prediction of in-hospital mortality. Furthermore, literature suggests favorable functional outcomes for those who survive to hospital discharge (Box 6.1).[8] **Age alone is not a sole criterion for denying or limiting care in elderly.**[9]

Triage of Elderly Trauma Patients

Prehospital

Under-triage is defined as a trauma patient not being transported to a state-designated trauma center. Under-triage keeps patients away from trauma centers who would benefit from trauma center care.

Per the CDC: "Under triage of the older adult population is a substantial problem."[10] Older patients were 34% less likely to die if they presented to centers treating a high vs. low proportion of elderly trauma.[11]

Standard adult EMS triage guidelines provide poor sensitivity for detecting older adults needing trauma center care.[12] The under-triage rate is approximately 50% in patients older than 65, vs. 17.8% for those under 65.[13,14]

Several sources have concluded that there should be an age threshold that mandates triage to a trauma center, with various age ranges (55–70 years) recommended.[6,9,15–17]

Total Traumas

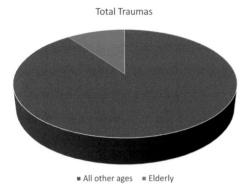

■ All other ages   ■ Elderly

Figure 6.1 Proportion of all trauma patients that are elderly

Trauma Mortalities and Costs

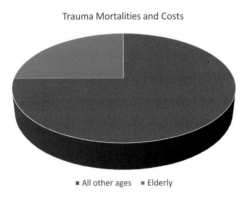

■ All other ages   ■ Elderly

Figure 6.2 Proportion of all trauma mortalities and costs that are elderly

Box 6.1   Limitations of Research in Geriatric Trauma
- Few prospective randomized controlled trials
- No uniform age cutoff criteria for elderly (45–80 years)[6]
- Lack of uniform definition of an elderly trauma patient
- Much of the literature is old

Potential explanations for under-triage of elderly trauma patients are significant injury from low energy mechanisms and altered physiologic response to injury with aging.

The CDC recommends direct transport to a trauma center for any trauma patient age $\geq$65 with SBP $\leq$110.[10] Substituting SBP <110 instead of SBP <90 for patients older than 65 reduced under-triage by 4.4% while only increasing over-triage by 4.3%.[18]

Although patients at level 1 trauma centers may have longer lengths of stay and higher total charges, a higher percentage of patients are discharged home.[19] Elderly patients with femur fractures and those with multiple injuries benefit from trauma center care.

After Arrival at the Trauma Center

Once an elderly patient arrives at a trauma center, trauma team activation occurs significantly less often for elderly patients (14% vs. 29%), despite a similar percentage of severe injuries (defined as ISS >15).[1]

Table 6.1 Triage implications for elderly trauma patients

Location	Recommendation
Prehospital	Low threshold for recommending EMS transport of elderly trauma patients to a designated trauma center, especially for patients with SBP <110
After hospital arrival	Low threshold for activating the trauma team after arrival at a trauma center for elderly trauma patients

Table 6.2 Comorbidities that contribute to poor outcome in geriatric trauma

Comorbidity	Effects
Diabetes Mellitus	Poor wound healing
End Stage Renal Disease	Unclear fluid resuscitation goals Platelet dysfunction
Osteoporosis	Higher fracture risk
Congestive Heart Failure	Medications obscure interpretation of vitals Poor cardiac output augmentation
Dementia	Poor participation in physical and occupational therapy

The Eastern Association for the Surgery of Trauma (EAST) recommends a lower threshold for trauma team activation for patients 65 and older evaluated at trauma centers (level 3 evidence).[20]

Some trauma centers use age as mandatory criteria for trauma team activation. This is supported by data that 63% of elderly trauma patients with ISS >15 had no standard physiologic activation criteria (Table 6.1).

Pathophysiology Concerns in the Elderly

The elderly are more susceptible to serious injury from low-energy mechanisms (particularly falls) and are less able to compensate from the stress of injury. They also are more likely to suffer complications during treatment and recovery. Key reasons for this include:

- Less physiologic reserve
- Occult shock/misleading picture of stability
- Comorbid illnesses, not just age, contribute to poor prognoses in geriatric trauma (Table 6.2).

An important point of emphasis in elderly patients is that *profound shock may be present even in the setting of "normal" vital signs*. The window to intervene may be narrow, and delayed recognition of shock will delay needed resuscitation and interventions.

- While common medications in the elderly, such as beta blockers and calcium channel blockers, may prevent typical tachycardic responses in shock, these medications do not need to be on board for an elderly patient to have "normal" vital signs in the setting of perfusion deficits.
- The elderly myocardium has decreased sensitivity to endogenous catecholamines.

- Blood pressures that would be considered normal in young patients may be relatively hypotensive compared to the baseline BP of an elderly patient. In fact, HR >90 and SBP <110 have been correlated with increased mortality in elderly trauma patients.[18,21]

Supporting Evidence

A landmark article by Scalea et al.[22] in 1990 that involved early invasive (PA catheter) monitoring in elderly trauma patients with "stable" vitals demonstrated that many of these patients have profound perfusion deficits despite "normal" vital signs.

Multiple subsequent studies have demonstrated that elevated lactate levels (>2) or abnormal base deficit (<−6) are associated with major injury and mortality both in elderly and non-elderly patients.[23–25]

In one study, venous lactate >2.5 helped diagnose occult hypoperfusion in 20% of 1987 geriatric trauma patients.[26] Lactate levels and/or base deficit should be used as an adjunct to vital signs for early identification of perfusion deficits in elderly trauma patients.

These factors have several clinical implications:

- Avoid being falsely reassured by normal vitals
- Consider systolic blood pressure ≤110 mm Hg to be hypotension
- Use lactate levels or base deficit as adjuncts to detect occult shock and guide resuscitation in unclear cases
- Use ECG to detect silent ischemia as a response to the physiologic stress of trauma
- Have a lower threshold for admitting elderly trauma patients to an ICU

Mechanisms and Injuries That are More Concerning in the Elderly

While the elderly are at increased risk for injury from all forces compared to younger adults exposed to the same force, mechanisms that have a disproportionate burden on elderly patients are:

- Falls from a ground level (Figure 6.3)
- Head trauma
- Chest wall injuries
- Cervical spine injuries
- Pedestrian struck by vehicle

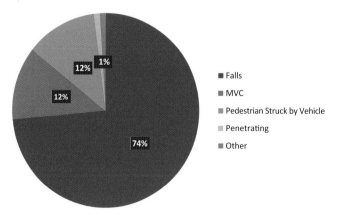

Figure 6.3 Mechanisms of injury in elderly trauma patients (data from Labib et al.[27])

- Falls
- MVC
- Pedestrian Struck by Vehicle
- Penetrating
- Other

Box 6.2 Elements That Must Be Assessed After an Elderly Patient Falls
- Sudden disturbance in cardiovascular/neurologic function
- New/progression of underlying conditions or emerging infection
- Intoxicants/medication effects
- Environmental safety, especially at home
- Impact of injury on functional status/ability to care for self
- *Complete history and physical exam*

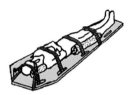

Figure 6.4 A rigid cervical collar and spine board immobilization can greatly impair respiratory status in elderly patients, especially in the setting of a chest wall injury (image by Christophe Dang Ngoc Chan, reproduced under CC BY-SA 3.0 license https://creativecommons.org/licenses/by-sa/3.0/)

Falls
- The most frequent cause of injury in age >65 years.[27]
- The most common fatal accident in age >80 years.
- More than one third of older adult ED fall patients had an ED revisit or died within one year![28]
- Same level falls must not be minimized, as they are 10× more likely to cause death than in a non-elderly patient (25% vs. 2.5%).[29]
- Even falls that seem purely mechanical can be a sign of occult illness and require advanced assessment (Box 6.2).

Head Injury
- Age related atrophy of the brain leads to more potential space and shearing forces of the intracranial bridging veins when exposed to trauma.
- The risk of intracranial bleeding is markedly increased with medications common in the elderly like anticoagulants and anti-platelet agents.[30,31]
- Elderly patients are typically excluded from studies that tell us who does *not* need brain imaging in trauma.

Chest Wall Injuries
- Even "minor" chest injuries impair the elderly. These are poorly tolerated due to a stiffer chest wall, loss of alveolar surface area, impaired lung defenses, and bacterial colonization.
- A rigid cervical collar and backboard can further impair chest wall expansion (Figure 6.4).
- The morbidity and mortality from rib fractures is much higher in geriatric populations. Studies have shown that each additional rib fracture in the elderly increases mortality by 19%![32] Elderly patients with rib fractures are at increased risk for pneumonia

> **Box 6.3** Clinical Implications of Mechanisms and Injuries That Disproportionately Affect the Elderly
>
> - Heightened suspicion for significant injury, even from ground level falls
> - Assess for medical impairments that could have led to the fall
> - Liberal use of CT scanning for elderly head and neck trauma
> - Inquire about the use of anticoagulant and anti-platelet medication
> - Ensure adequate analgesia and oxygenation for chest wall injuries
> - Remove the cervical collar and backboard as early as safely possible
> - Lower threshold for admitting elderly patients with rib fractures (even one)

(31% vs. 17%, with a 16% increase per rib fractured), pulmonary contusion, and delayed hemothorax.[32]

Cervical Spine Injuries

- The elderly spine is more vulnerable to fracture from minor mechanisms such as falls from standing.[33] This is due to common conditions such as cervical stenosis, osteoporosis, and arthritis (degenerative, rheumatoid, and osteoarthritis).
- High cervical fractures (type 2 odontoid being the most common) and central cord syndromes are more frequent in the elderly.[34]

Pedestrian Struck by Vehicle

- Perhaps the most devastating common mechanism of injury to disproportionately affect this population.
- Age >65 years accounts for 22% of pedestrian struck deaths.
- 46% occur in crosswalks.
- Factors that may make elderly susceptible are decreased ability to raise or turn the head from cervical arthropathy and less speed and agility (crosswalk timers often allow for a pedestrian speed of 4 ft/sec).

Box 6.3 discusses key trauma considerations in geriatric patients.

Trauma Survey Principles in the Elderly

The principles of diagnosis and management in trauma are the same regardless of age. However, certain aspects of the trauma assessment require special attention and emphasis (Table 6.3).

Elder Abuse

Elder abuse can be very difficult to detect for several reasons:

- Patient reluctance to get a loved one in trouble.
- Frail status makes the patient feel helpless to seek help.
- Cognitive impairment limits the history or the ability to self-report abuse.
- Patient dependence on the abuser.
- Abuse in the form of neglect can mimic cachexia from comorbidities.

Table 6.3 Special trauma survey applications to elderly patients

Airway	Early airway control Edentulous patients may be difficult to bag Remove dentures for intubation
Breathing	Avoid respiratory decompensation by use of O_2, analgesia for chest injuries, suction/pulmonary toilet, clearing the cervical spine, and removing the back board as early as possible to prevent respiratory impairment
Circulation	Early transfusion to minimize fluid overload from crystalloids Recognizing that "normal" BP may be relative hypotension for an elderly patient Recognizing that occult hypoperfusion can be present with normal vital signs Seek anticoagulant use and consider reversal early
Disability	Liberal use of head and cervical spine CT GCS less reliable to rule in or rule out brain injury
Exposure	Seek clues of comorbidities that may not have been reported (i.e. surgical scars, pacemakers, medication bottles or lists in patient belongings, medical alert tags, bruising from anticoagulants)

Steps the clinician can take to detect elder abuse:

- When the scenario has stabilized, assess the patient's social situation.
- Be wary of wounds or injuries that are suspicious for abuse or do not seem to match the reported mechanism of injury.
- Ask the patient, preferably in private.

Anticoagulants

- Anticoagulant use is far more prevalent in the elderly population.
- Make sure to ask the patient right away if he/she is on a blood thinner, aspirin, clopidogrel, or other anti-platelet agents. An irregular heartbeat may be a clue to chronic atrial fibrillation and suggests use of these medications.
- Sustained reversal of warfarin is best achieved with vitamin K. More immediate reversal is achieved with prothrombin complex concentrates or fresh frozen plasma.
- Greater numbers of elderly patients are on direct oral anticoagulants (DOACS) which are not as readily reversible as warfarin and have no universally accepted protocol for reversal.
- Know your institution's reversal protocol for DOACs. If your institution does not have one, then know which prothrombin complex concentrates (PCCs) are available to you. PCCs seem to be the preferred agents for DOAC reversal until definitive antidotes are readily available.
- There are two types of DOACs: direct factor II inhibitors (dabigatran) and direct factor Xa inhibitors (rivaroxaban, apixaban, edoxaban).
- Dabigatran can be removed by dialysis. In 2015, a monoclonal antibody to dabigatran, idarucizumab, was introduced for dabigatran reversal.
- A recombinant modified decoy molecule, andexanet-alpha, is currently approved by the FDA for reversal of factor Xa inhibitors. Further clinical studies are underway evaluating efficacy.

Pitfalls

- Withholding initial aggressive care based solely on advanced age
- Delayed recognition of hypoperfusion because of normal vital signs
- Giving too much crystalloid before starting blood
- Underestimating the impact of a ground level fall
- Not fully investigating a seemingly mechanical fall for decompensation of a comorbid condition
- Respiratory embarrassment from prolonged spine board and cervical collar immobilization
- Underappreciation of the impact of a rib fracture on an elderly patient
- Under-triage of an injured elderly patient away from a trauma center
- Not fully investigating for comorbidities and anticoagulant use
- Missing elder abuse as a cause of injury

Key Points

- Resuscitation of the elderly trauma patient must be thoughtful but aggressive
- Heighten awareness that with age, signs and symptoms may be minimal, and that the outcome is often initially unclear and commonly *but not necessarily* poor
- Up to 85% of survivors return to baseline or independent function[9]
- This justifies an *initial aggressive approach* which can be reassessed later when patient and family wishes and prognosis become more clear[9]
- Less physiologic reserve leaves little room for delays in diagnosis and under- or over-resuscitation
- Blood is the fluid of choice
- The principles of diagnosis and management in trauma are the same, regardless of age

---

References

1. Hashmi A, Ibrahim-Zada I, Rhee P, et al. Predictors of mortality in geriatric trauma patients: a systematic review and meta-analysis. *J Trauma Acute Care Surg.* 2014;76:894–901.

2. Vincent GK, Velkoff VA, U.S. Census Bureau. The next four decades the older population in the United States: 2010 to 2050. Population estimates and projections P25–1138. Washington, DC: U.S. Dept. of Commerce, Economics and Statistics Administration, U.S. Census Bureau; 2010. Available from http://purl.access.gpo.gov/GPO/LPS126596. Accessed April 8, 2018.

3. CDC. CDC National Center for Health Statistics (NCHS), National Vital Statistics System. www.cdc.gov/nchs/nvss.htm. Accessed April 8, 2018.

4. CDC. CDC Data and Statistics (WISQARS™): Cost of Injury Reports Data Source: NCHS Vital Statistics System for Numbers of Deaths. http://wisqars.cdc.gov/8080/costT/. Accessed April 8, 2018.

5. Champion HR, Copes WS, Buyer D, et al. Major trauma in geriatric patients. *Am J Public Health.* 1989;79:1278–82.

6. Bonne S, Schuerer D. Trauma in the older adult – epidemiology and evolving geriatric trauma principles. *Clin Geriatr Med.* 2013;29:137–50.

7. Goodmanson NW, Rosengart MR, Barnato AE, et al. Defining geriatric trauma: when does age make a difference? *Surgery.* 2012;152:668–75.

8. Grossman MD, Ofurum U, Stehly CD, et al. Long-term survival after major

trauma in geriatric trauma patients: the glass is half full. *J Trauma.* 2012;72:1181–85.

9. Jacobs DG, Plaisier BR, Barie PS, et al. Practice management guidelines for geriatric trauma. The EAST practice management guidelines work group. *J Trauma.* 2003;54:391–416.

10. Sasser SM, Hunt RC, Faul M, et al. Guidelines for field triage of injured patients: recommendations of the National Expert Panel on Field Triage, 2011. *MMWR Recomm Rep.* 2012;61(RR-1):1–20.

11. Zafar SN, Obirieze A, Schneider EB, et al. Outcomes of trauma care at centers treating a higher proportion of older patients: the case for geriatric trauma centers. *Acute Care Surg.* 2015;78:852–59.

12. Ichwan B, Subrahmanyam D, Shah MN, et al. Geriatric-specific triage criteria are more sensitive than standard adult criteria in identifying need for trauma center care in injured older adults. *Ann Emerg Med.* 2015;65:92–100.

13. Chang DC, Bass RR, Cornwell EE, et al. Undertriage of elderly trauma patients to state-designated trauma centers. *Arch Surg.* 2008;143:776–81.

14. Kodadek LM, Selvarajah S, Velopulos CG, et al. Undertriage of older trauma patients: is this a national phenomenon? *J Surg Res.* 2015;199:220–29.

15. Caterino JM, Valasek T, Werman HA. Identification of an age cutoff for increased mortality in patients with elderly trauma. *Am J Emerg Med.* 2010;28:151–58.

16. Lehmann R. The impact of advanced age on trauma triage decisions and outcomes: a statewide analysis. *Am J Surg.* 2009;197 (5):571–74.

17. ATLS Subcommittee; American College of Surgeons Committee on Trauma; International ATLS working group. Advanced trauma life support (ATLS®): the ninth edition. *J Trauma Acute Care Surg.* 2013;74(5):1363–66.

18. Brown JB, Gestring ML, Forsythe RM, et al. Systolic blood pressure criteria in the National Trauma Triage Protocol for geriatric trauma: 110 is the new 90. *J Trauma Acute Care Surg.* 2015;78:352–59.

19. Maxwell CA, Miller RS, Dietrich MS, et al. The aging of America: a comprehensive look at over 25,000 geriatric trauma admissions to United States hospitals. *Am Surg.* 2015;81(6):630–36.

20. Calland JF, Ingraham AM, Martin N, et al. Evaluation and management of geriatric trauma: an Eastern Association for the Surgery of Trauma practice management guideline. *J Trauma Acute Care Surg.* 2012;73:S345–350.

21. Heffernan DS, Thakkar RK, Monaghan SF, et al. Normal presenting vital signs are unreliable in geriatric blunt trauma victims. *J Trauma.* 2010;69(4):813–20.

22. Scalea TM, Simon HM, Duncan AO, et al. Geriatric blunt multiple trauma: improved survival with early invasive monitoring. *J Trauma.* 1990;30:129–36.

23. Zehtabchi S, Baron BJ. Utility of base deficit for identifying major injury in elder trauma patients. *Acad Emerg Med.* 2007;14:829–31.

24. Callaway DW, Shapiro NI, Donnino MW, et al. Serum lactate and base deficit as predictors of mortality in normotensive elderly blunt trauma patients. *J Trauma.* 2009;66:1040–44.

25. Paladino L, Sinert R, Wallace D, et al. The utility of base deficit and arterial lactate in differentiating major from minor injury in trauma patients with normal signs. *Resuscitation.* 2008;77:363–68.

26. Salottolo KM, Mains CW, Offner PJ, et al. A retrospective analysis of geriatric trauma patients: venous lactate is a better predictor of mortality than traditional vital signs. *Scand J Trauma Resusc Emerg Med.* 2013;21:1–7.

27. Labib N, Nouh T, Winocour S, et al. Severely injured geriatric population: Morbidity, mortality, and risk factors. *J Trauma.* 2011;71(6):1908–14.

28. Liu SW, Obermeyer Z, Chang Y, et al. Frequency of ED revisits and death among older adults after a fall. *Am J Emerg Med.* 2015;33:1012–18.

29. Sterling DA, O'Connor JA, Bonadies J. Geriatric falls: injury severity is high and disproportionate to mechanism. *J Trauma.* 2001;50(1):116–19.

30. Rathlev NK, Medzon R, Lowery D, et al. Intracranial pathology in elders with blunt head trauma. *Acad Emerg Med.* 2006;13 (3):302–7.

31. Li J, Brown J, Levine M. Mild head injury, anticoagulants, and risk of intracranial injury. *Lancet.* 2001;357 (9258):771–72.

32. Bulger EM. Rib fractures in the elderly. *J Trauma.* 2000;48(6):1040.

33. Bonne S, Schuerer DJ. Trauma in the older adult: epidemiology and evolving geriatric trauma principles. *Clin Geriatr Med.* 2013;29(1):137–50.

34. Reinhold M, Bellabarba C, Bransford R, et al. Radiographic analysis of type II odontoid fractures in a geriatric patient population: description and pathomechanism of the "Geier"-deformity. *Eur Spine J.* 2011;20(11):1928–39.

Head Trauma

Brit Long

Head trauma is a significant cause of death around the world, especially in patients 1–45 years old.[1–5] Close to 80% of patients are managed in the emergency department (ED).[1,2] Head injury not only causes initial primary injury, but it is associated with several secondary injuries.[1–5]

Neurologic Injuries

The goal of resuscitation and management of the patient with head trauma is to target normal ICP, while preserving cerebral blood flow and perfusion.[2,6–10]

$$\text{Cerebral Perfusion Pressure (CPP)} = \text{Mean Arterial Pressure (MAP)} - \text{Intracranial Pressure (ICP)}$$

- ICP is a function of the brain parenchyma, blood, and cerebrospinal fluid (CSF).[2,7–13] An increase of one component requires a decrease in another.[2,7–13]
- Once compensatory methods are exhausted, further volume leads to increases in ICP.
- Increases in ICP and decreases in cerebral perfusion are difficult to measure directly in the ED, and physicians should assess for clinical findings.
- An increase in ICP may result in herniation and decreased blood flow (Table 7.1, Figures 7.1 and 7.2).[2,7,14,15]
- Head injury is classified most commonly based on the Glasgow Coma Scale (GCS). Mild (GCS 14–15) is most common, followed by moderate TBI (GCS 9–13) and severe (GCS ≤8), which has mortality approaching 40% (Table 7.2).[2,7,14,15]
- Blunt impact to the head causes acceleration and deceleration of the brain, resulting in compression, distortion, and shearing of the tissues.[2,7,10,14–17]
- Penetrating injury is less common, though it has a more severe mortality, with 9% survival.[2,7,14,15,18,19] Most penetrating TBI is due to firearm projectiles, which not only penetrate brain matter but are associated with a wavelike pattern of tissue injury (Figures 7.9 and 7.10).[2,15,18,19]
- Blast injury is rare in civilians, with the majority occurring in war. Any explosion can cause energy transmission through the cranium and central vasculature.[18,19] Cerebral edema may occur, which occurs within one hour of injury. Vasospasm occurs in 50% of patients.[2,14,15,18,19]

Physiologic Goals

A goal systolic blood pressure of at least 100 mm Hg (ages 50–69) and 110 mm Hg for 15–49 years and >70 years is recommended per the Brain Trauma Foundation.[2,7,8,14]

Table 7.1 Herniation syndromes

Herniation	Pathophysiology	Presentation
Uncal	• Parasympathetic fibers of cranial nerve III compression • Pyramidal tract compression	• Ipsilateral fixed and dilated pupil • Contralateral motor paralysis
Subtype: Kernohan's notch	• Compression of cerebral peduncle in uncal herniation • Secondary condition caused by primary injury on opposite hemisphere	• Ipsilateral hemiplegia/hemiparesis, called Kernohan's sign • False localizing sign
Central transtentorial	• Midline lesion with compression of midbrain	• Bilateral nonresponsive midpoint pupils, bilateral Babinski, increased muscular tone
Cerebellotonsillar	• Cerebellar tonsil herniation through foramen magnum	• Pinpoint pupils, flaccid paralysis, sudden death
Upward posterior fossa/ transtentorial	• Cerebellar and midbrain movement upwards through tentorial opening	• Pinpoint pupils, downward conjugate gaze, irregular respirations • Death

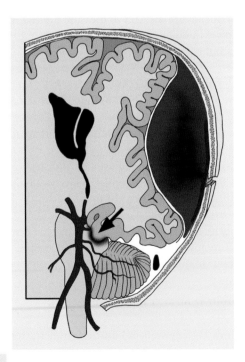

Figure 7.1 Brainstem herniation. Illustration of an epidural hematoma with acute mass effect and compression of the ipsilateral cerebral peduncle resulting in uncal herniation and compression of the brain stem (arrow) (illustration by Robert Amaral, reproduced with permission from *Color Atlas of Emergency Trauma, Second Edition*)

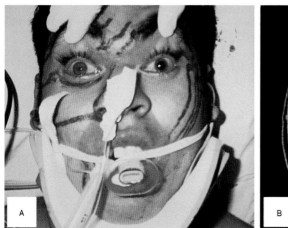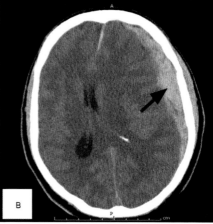

Figure 7.2 Brainstem herniation. (A) Patient with transtentorial herniation from blunt head trauma. The right pupil is constricted normally; the left pupil is fixed and dilated. (B) CT scan shows a large left subdural hematoma (arrow) with midline shift. This compression resulted in brainstem herniation (reproduced with permission from *Color Atlas of Emergency Trauma, Second Edition*)

Otherwise, a MAP of 70–80 mm Hg is advised (Box 7.1).[14,15] Normal oxygen saturation is vital, as hypoxemia results in a significant increase in mortality.

Secondary Injuries

Secondary injuries must be prevented to avoid worsened patient outcome.[2,7,15,20–23]

- Hypotension: Occurs in 1/3 of patients, resulting in worse outcome (OR = 2.67).
- Hypoxia: Occurs in 50% of patients, resulting in worse outcome (OR = 2.14).
- Hyperoxia: PaO_2 levels above 300–470 mm Hg are associated with worse outcome.
- Fever: Elevated body temperature furthers central brain injury.
- Coagulopathy: May cause worsening of the neurologic injury and death.
- Glucose: Hyper- and hypoglycemia are predictors of poor neurologic status.

ED Evaluation and Management

Focus on airway, breathing, circulation, disability, and exposure in the primary survey, with spinal precautions.[2,14,24,25] Avoid secondary complications (Box 7.2).[2,14]

- Markers of worse outcome include poor GCS motor score, pupillary dysfunction, and increased ICP. Abnormal pupillary response and altered motor function are markers of severity.[2,7,14,15]
- Decorticate posturing (arm flexion and leg extension) is due to injury above the midbrain, and decerebrate posturing (arm extension and internal rotation, wrist and finger flexion, leg internal rotation and extension) is a sign of midbrain injury.[2,14]
- Abnormal pupils, decreased mental status, abnormal GCS, penetrating injury, abnormal motor status, and severe injury require neuroimaging after initial stabilization.
- Severe head trauma requires consultation with neurosurgery.[2,7,10,14]
- Constant reassessment is required due to the risk of intracranial pathology worsening, especially with intracerebral hemorrhage. If worsening, emergent neuroimaging is required.[14,26–28]

Table 7.2 Head injuries

Injury	Pathophysiology	Common locations	Characteristics
Contusion (Figure 7.3)	• Coup and contrecoup injury from trauma	• Orbitofrontal region • Anterior temporal region	• Up to one third may expand
Epidural hematoma (Figure 7.4)	• Middle meningeal artery and vein injury	• Close to site of skull fracture	• Convex shape • Does not cross suture lines • Commonly not associated with brain injury
Subdural hematoma (Figure 7.5)	• Bridging vein injury	• Cerebral convexities • Tentorium and falx	• Concave shape • Crosses suture lines • Associated with brain injury • More common in those with brain atrophy
Subarachnoid hemorrhage (Figure 7.6)	• Pial vessel injury or laceration	• Cerebral convexities • Interpeduncular cisterns • Ventricles	• May be present in a few sulci or fissures, more diffuse if severe • Most common CT finding in moderate TBI
Diffuse axonal injury (Figure 7.7)	• Shearing mechanism results in white matter damage • Diffuse axonal swelling	• Gray-white matter junction in hemispheres • Severe injuries may affect corpus callosum and midbrain	• May present in profound coma without elevated ICP • Poor outcome common
Depressed skull fracture (Figure 7.8)	• Fracture through cranial vault	• Any site of cranial trauma	• Often associated with underlying damage to central vasculature or parenchyma

Tiers of ICP management are suggested per the Brain Trauma Foundation (Table 7.3).[2,7,14,15] Tier 0 therapies should be initiated immediately, with head of bed elevation and pain and agitation treatment. Hyperventilation should only be used in patients with concern for active herniation.[2,7,14]

Airway Management

- Airway protection and blood pressure support for severe head trauma with first pass success are priorities.

Box 7.1 Goal Physiologic Parameters

- Pulse oximetry 94–98% (avoid hypoxemia and hyperoxemia)
- $PaCO_2$ 35–45 mm Hg
- SBP $\geq$100 mm Hg (50–69 years), and $\geq$110 mm Hg (15–49, >70 years)
- pH 7.35–7.45
- ICP $\leq$20 mm Hg
- Glucose 80–180 mg/dL
- CPP $\geq$60 mm Hg
- Serum Na 135–145, (Hypertonic saline goal is 145–160)
- INR $\leq$1.4
- Platelets $\geq$75 × 10^3/mm^3
- Hgb >8 mg/dL

Box 7.2 ED Management Goals

- Maintain spinal precautions
- Conduct primary and secondary surveys; address life-threatening injuries
- Advanced airway management may be needed for airway protection, hypoxia, and control of ventilation
- Obtain rapid IV access
- Optimize oxygenation, blood pressure, and ventilation
- Target oxygen saturation >94%, with systolic blood pressure >100–110 mm Hg
- Focused neurologic exam: GCS, motor function, and pupillary function
- Obtain head CT noncontrast
- Any sign of worsening neurologic status warrants hyperosmolar therapy

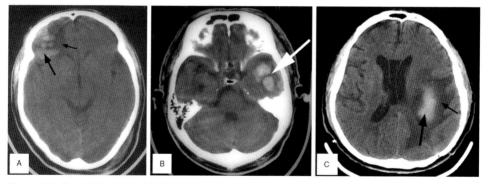

Figure 7.3 Cerebral Contusion. (A) CT right frontal lobe contusion (large arrow) with surrounding edema (small arrow). (B) Axial CT scan showing a left temporal lobe contusion (arrow) with surrounding edema. (C) Axial CT scan with large left hemispheric contusion (large arrow) and surrounding edema (small arrow) (reproduced with permission from *Color Atlas of Emergency Trauma, Second Edition*)_

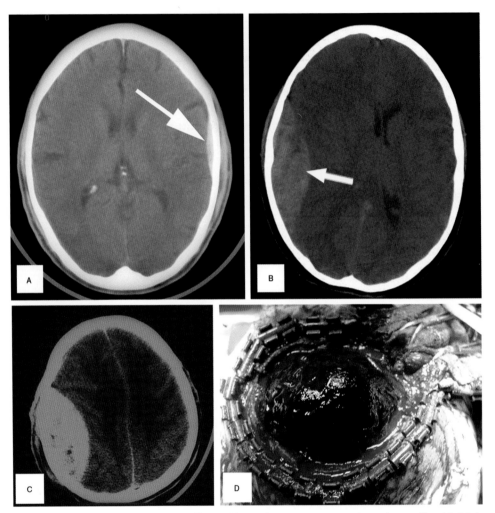

Figure 7.4 Epidural hematoma. CT scans of epidural hemorrhages progressing in size and mass effect. (A) Subtle left parietal EDH without mass effect; arrow reveals lenticular space occupying hyperdense lesion. (B) EDH in the right parietal area (arrow) with narrowing of right ventricle and midline shift. (C) Massive acute right parietal EDH with a mass effect and increased intracranial pressure. (D) Intraoperative appearance of a large EDH. The hematoma is on top of the dura mater (reproduced with permission from *Color Atlas of Emergency Trauma, Second Edition*)

- Rapid sequence intubation with in-line stabilization of the cervical spine may be necessary (Box 7.3).[2,11,18–20]
- Preoxygenation is important to avoid desaturation.[21,22]

Pretreatment

Eighty percent of patients experience hypertension to laryngoscopy or suctioning. Lidocaine does not reduce ICP or improve neurologic outcome.[25,31,32] Fentanyl (2–5 µg/kg IV prior to intubation) can reduce the hyperdynamic response to intubation, as can esmolol at 1.5 mg/kg IV. Esmolol should be avoided in patients with hypotension, hemorrhagic shock, or signs of multiple trauma.[25,31,32]

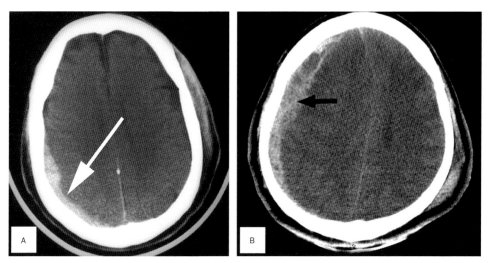

Figure 7.5 Subdural hematoma. Axial CT scans of subdural hemorrhages. (A) Small right parieto-occipital acute SDH without mass effect (arrow). (B) Right SDH (arrow) with left cephalohematoma demonstrating coup–contrecoup injury. Note the significant midline shift (reproduced with permission from *Color Atlas of Emergency Trauma, Second Edition*)

Induction

Ketamine, propofol, or etomidate can be used. The key for an induction agent is utilizing lower doses in patients with hypotension, as any agent at full dose will worsen hypotension.[33–37]

- Ketamine can be used for induction, as it improves cerebral blood flow, and evidence suggests it does not raise ICP.[33,34]
- Etomidate may result in less hypotension and cardiac dysfunction. It can reduce ICP and maintain CPP, but it also may lower the seizure threshold and increase the risk of vomiting and myoclonic movements.[33,35]
- Propofol has high lipid solubility and rapid onset of action that can reduce ICP and oxidative stress, though it may cause hypotension.[33,36,37]

Paralysis

Improves first pass success, including succinylcholine or rocuronium. Succinylcholine allows faster time to recovery and neurologic status assessment. Both are safe and efficacious.[14,33,38–40] Defasciculating doses of paralytics do not reduce ICP and are not recommended.[33,40]

Post Intubation

Inadequate analgesia and sedation may increase ICP due to sympathomimetic response.[2,14,33] Post intubation medications should be ordered at the same time as paralytic and induction agents.[41,42]

- Analgesics including fentanyl (1 mcg/kg IV) and remifentanil are fast and predictable. Hydromorphone and morphine have a longer duration of effect but may accumulate with longer infusions.

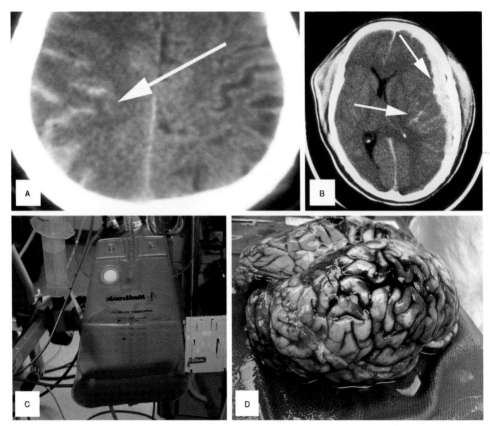

Figure 7.6 Subarachnoid hemorrhage. (A) CT scan of SAH appears like fingerlike projections of hyperdense blood as it tracks along the sulci of the posterior parietal lobe (arrow). (B) CT scan showing left parietal SAH (lower arrow), acute left SDH (upper arrow). Note the effacement of the posterior horn of the left lateral ventricle and midline shift. (C) Bloody CSF drainage from a ventriculostomy catheter in a patient with SAH. (D) Autopsy specimen of a brain with SAH seen here tracking along the sulci of the brain beneath the arachnoid membrane (reproduced with permission from *Color Atlas of Emergency Trauma, Second Edition*)

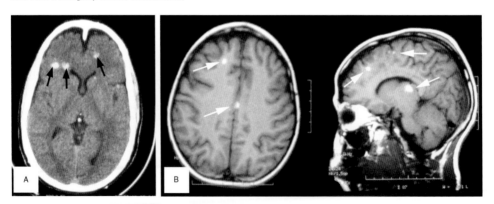

Figure 7.7 Diffuse axonal injury. (A) CT showing focal petechial hemorrhages in the frontal lobes at the gray–white matter junction (arrows) in a patient with diffuse axonal injury. (B) MRI showing multiple high-intensity focal hemorrhages (arrows) including those at the gray–white matter interface in a patient with diffuse axonal injury (reproduced with permission from *Color Atlas of Emergency Trauma, Second Edition*)

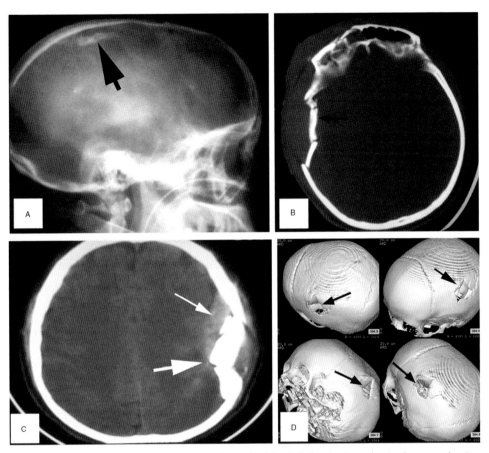

Figure 7.8 Depressed skull fracture. (A) Lateral radiograph of the skull showing hyperdensity due to overlapping bone fragments (arrow) at the apical–parietal skull. (B) CT scan bone windows showing right temporoparietal comminuted depressed fracture (arrow) and associated soft tissue swelling. This patient suffered a concomitant epidural hematoma. (C) CT scan showing depressed fracture of the left parietal bone (large arrow) with underlying epidural hematoma (small arrow). (D) CT scan showing 3-D reconstruction of a skull with left parietal depressed comminuted skull fracture (arrow) (reproduced with permission from *Color Atlas of Emergency Trauma, Second Edition*)

- Sedative medications include propofol, which possesses fast onset and offset. Side effects include hypotension. Infusion rather than bolus will decrease the risk of hypotension. Benzodiazepines are less reliable and will decrease BP and respiratory status.[41,42] Tolerance may develop and accumulation may occur. Dexmedetomidine is a selective alpha-2 receptor agonist with anxiolytic and sedative effects.[42]

Target oxygen saturations 94–98% with $PaCO_2$ levels of 35–40 mm Hg, or end tidal CO_2 30–40 mm Hg.[2,14,33,43]

Blood Pressure Control

Maintaining adequate MAP is vital to patient outcome.

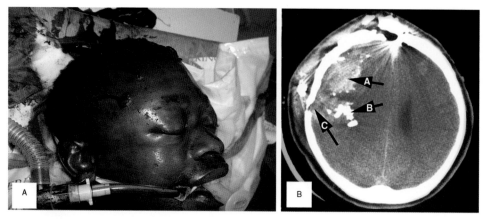

Figure 7.9 Gunshot wound to the head. Gunshot wounds to the brain. (A) Patient with multiple gunshot wounds to the head. Note the cephalohematoma and periorbital ecchymosis. (B) CT scan of a gunshot wound showing a SDH, intraparenchymal hemorrhage (arrow A) and intraparenchymal bullet fragments (arrow B), and an open frontotemporal skull fracture (arrow C) (reproduced with permission from *Color Atlas of Emergency Trauma, Second Edition*)

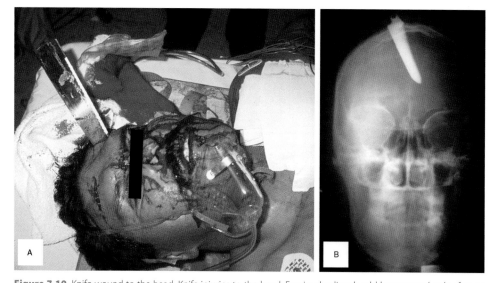

Figure 7.10 Knife wound to the head. Knife injuries to the head. Foreign bodies should be removed only after an angiogram or in the operating room. (A) Stab wound to the head with an embedded knife in the frontal area. The patient was awake and alert. (B) Anteroposterior radiograph revealing the knife blade within the cranium. The knife was pulled out in the operating room without any complication (reproduced with permission from *Color Atlas of Emergency Trauma, Second Edition*)

Hypotension

Defined by SBP less than 90 mm Hg, hypotension increases mortality two-fold.[2,14,43–46] Hypotension does not occur until herniation is imminent. Permissive hypotension is not recommended. ATLS recommends MAP >80 mm Hg. Minimum SBP should be 100 mm Hg.[5]

Table 7.3 Management tiers

Tier	Options
0	• Head of bed elevation • Control fever, pain, and agitation • Optimize physiologic parameters such as blood pressure and oxygen • Target $PaCO_2$ to 35–38 mm Hg
1	• Osmotic therapy includes mannitol, hypertonic saline, or sodium bicarbonate • External ventricular drainage system should be placed if acute obstruction is present
2	• Propofol drip titration • Optimize other parameters
3	• Barbiturate coma • Surgical decompression if ICP refractory to treatment • Therapeutic hypothermia • Moderate hyperventilation (only if active herniation)

Box 7.3 Keys in Airway Management

- Preparation: Proper positioning, preoxygenate, and use apneic oxygenation with nasal cannula, facemask, or noninvasive positive pressure ventilation
- Elevate head of bed to improve CPP and decrease aspiration
- Premedication regimens are controversial. Fentanyl at 2–5 µg/kg IV or esmolol 1.5 mg/kg IV may decrease catecholamine surge and control the hemodynamic response to intubation
- Induction agents may include ketamine or etomidate – these agents have less hemodynamic effects
- Propofol has neuroprotective effects, but hypotension may occur
- Post-intubation analgesia and sedation are essential – have your drips ready to go at the time of intubation[29,30]

For treatment, IV fluids should be started with NS. Albumin and hypo-osmotic fluid should be avoided. Start first with fluids, specifically normal saline or blood.[2,14,43–46] Avoid hypo-osmotic fluids, which can increase cerebral edema and ICP.[14,43]

Neurogenic Shock
Neurogenic shock occurs with injury above T6 spinal level, caused by a loss of sympathetic tone.[47–49] This presents with hypotension and bradycardia, though hypovolemic shock should be assumed in the trauma patient. Management includes IV fluids and vasopressors as needed in neurogenic shock, with goal MAP above 80 mm Hg.[47–49]

Vasopressors
SBP of at least 100–110 mm Hg is recommended by the Brain Trauma Foundation.[14] Patients with neurogenic shock require a higher MAP target for spinal cord perfusion.[47–49]

Norepinephrine will increase afterload and inotropy, while phenylephrine will improve vascular tone and can be used in patients who are not bradycardic.

Hypertension

Hypertension is common as the body attempts to autoregulate. A rapid decrease in blood pressure is not advised. Levels less than 180/100 mm Hg are recommended (target 140–180/70–100 mm Hg), and lower target levels do not improve outcomes. Options for blood pressure management include nicardipine (bolus and infusion) and labetalol.[2,14,43]

Hyperosmolar Therapy

This reduces ICP and improve cerebral blood flow.[2,7,14,50–58] These agents should be used with signs of increased ICP, pupillary change, a decrease in GCS ≥ 2 points, or posturing.[2,7,14,43,50] For ICP reduction, a 2015 meta-analysis finds no difference in neurologic outcome or mortality between mannitol and HTS.[50]

Mannitol

Administered as a 20% solution, 0.25–1 g/kg IV over 5 minutes. Mannitol deforms RBCs and decreases blood viscosity. The blood–brain barrier should be intact if using mannitol. If not intact, mannitol will worsen outcomes. Following mannitol, rebound increases in ICP may occur. However, mannitol can result in significant diuresis and hypotension. Fluids should be provided and a Foley catheter placed to monitor mannitol's diuretic effect.[2,14,43,50–58]

HTS

Concentrations range from 2% to 23.4%, which also improves cerebral blood flow and reduces brain water content. The most common solution is 3% HTS 250 mL over 10 minutes (23.4% 30 mL can be used through central line). In patients with hypotension, HTS can improve blood pressure as a volume expander. Risk of rebound ICP is less with HTS. Hyperchloremic metabolic acidosis is the most common side effect.[2,14,43,50–58]

ICP Monitoring

Placement of an ICP monitor allows continuous assessment of ICP and may assist in management. This should be completed in consultation with a neurosurgeon.[2,7,14,59,60] Invasive placement of a ventricular catheter or intraparenchymal monitor is most reliable (Box 7.4). Ventriculostomy or external ventricular drain (EVD) allows drainage of CSF, which can be therapeutic.[2,14,59,60]

Box 7.4   Indications For ICP Monitor Placement

- GCS 3–8 with abnormal CT scan
- GCS 3–8 with normal CT and two of the following: Age >40 years, motor posturing, SBP <90 mm Hg
- GCS 9–15 with CT showing mass lesion (>1 cm contusion, ICH >3 cm), effaced cisterns, or midline shift >5 mm
- Following craniectomy for ICP monitoring
- Inability to follow neurologic examination (such as with sedation)

Table 7.4 Surgical interventions for specific injuries

Lesion	Surgical Indication
Epidural hematoma	• GCS <9 with anisocoria • EDH >30 cm^3
Subdural hematoma	• SDH thickness >10 mm or midline shift >5 mm regardless of GCS • GCS decline by >2 • Fixed and dilated or asymmetric pupils • ICP >20 mm Hg
Parenchymal lesion	• Lesion ≥50 cm^3 • GCS 6–8 with midline shift ≥5 mm, cistern compression, or frontal/temporal contusion ≥20 cm^3 • Continued neurologic decline, refractory intracranial hypertension, or mass effect on CT due to lesion
Posterior fossa lesion	• Mass effect on CT • Neurologic decline due to lesion
Depressed skull fracture	• Open fracture greater than cranium thickness • Open fracture with dural penetration, significant associated intracranial hematoma, depression >1 cm, frontal sinus involvement, gross deformity, wound infection, pneumocephalus, gross wound contamination

Utility of US in ICP Evaluation

Optic nerve sheath diameter (ONSD) correlates with ICP, evaluated by US. Normal ONSD is up to 5 mm in diameter, and values greater than 5 mm suggest increased ICP (sensitivity and specificity >90%). This should be measured 3 mm posterior to the globe.[61–63]

Surgical Indications

Decompressive craniectomy may be needed for refractory intracranial hypertension, though it does not improve functional outcome (DECRA, RESCUE-ICP trials) (Table 7.4).[64–68]

Coagulopathy Reversal in Traumatic Intracerebral Hemorrhage

Close to one third of patients will have a coagulopathy.[2,7,14] Coagulation panel and TEG or ROTEM are recommended. Vitamin K, PCC/FFP, and novel antidotes may be required.[69–72] Platelet transfusion for ICH in patients on antiplatelet medication with ICH may be harmful and should be discussed with neurosurgery.[73]

Seizure Management

Seizures occur in close to 30% of patients. Early posttraumatic seizures occur within 7 days of injury, with late seizures beyond 7 days.[2,7,14,74,75]

- Benzodiazepines should be provided as first line therapy for active seizure.
- Prophylaxis is recommended for GCS < 10, cortical contusion, any intracranial hematoma, depressed skull fracture, penetrating head injury, or seizure within 24 hours of injury.[14]
- Levetiracetam is recommended as first line for prophylaxis.[74,75]

Tranexamic Acid in Head Trauma

CRASH-2 and MATTERs studies show survival benefit within three hours of trauma for TXA.[76,77] The CRASH-2 Intracranial Bleeding Study suggests a trend towards reduction in ICH size and lower mortality, with another study finding reduced bleeding.[78] CRASH-3 evaluating TXA in head trauma is ongoing.[79]

Hypothermia and pharmacologically-induced coma (barbiturates) may be used for extreme refractory ICP elevations, but no improvement in outcomes has been suggested in the literature.[80–82]

Pitfalls in ED Evaluation and Management

- Several medications have not demonstrated improvement in outcomes in head trauma, including corticosteroids, progesterone, magnesium, hyperbaric oxygen, and cyclosporine.[2,7,14]
- Hyperventilation can reduce ICP for short periods, but hyperventilation may result in secondary ischemia, increasing the risk of cerebral edema. A $PaCO_2$ less than 30 mm Hg for six hours up to five days is associated with worse outcome.[2,7,14,43]

Key Points

- Head trauma is common. Primary and secondary injuries result in severe morbidity and mortality.
- Injuries include head contusion, epidural hematoma, subdural hematoma, subarachnoid hemorrhage, diffuse axonal injury, skull fracture, and traumatic spinal cord injury.
- Cerebral perfusion pressure requires adequate cerebral blood flow.
- Evaluation and management in the emergency department entails initial stabilization and resuscitation while assessing neurologic status.
- Targeting MAP, oxygen levels, and neurologic status are key components. ICP management should follow a tiered approach.
- Intubation of the patient with head trauma should be completed with several considerations.
- Hyperosmolar treatments include HTS and mannitol.

References

1. Faul M, Xu L, Wald MM, et al. *Traumatic Brain Injury in the United States: Emergency Department Visits, Hospitalizations and Deaths 2002–2006.* Atlanta, GA: Centers for Disease Control and Prevention, National Center for Injury Prevention and Control; 2010.

2. Wan-Tsu WC, Badjatia N. Neurotrauma. *Emerg Med Clin N Am.* 2014;32:889–905.

3. Rutland-Brown W, Langlois JA, Thomas KE, Xi YL. Incidence of traumatic brain injury in the United States, 2003. *J Head Trauma Rehabil.* 2006;21:544.

4. Tagliaferri F, Compagnone C, Korsic M, et al. A systematic review of brain injury epidemiology in Europe. *Acta Neurochir (Wien).* 2006;148:255.

5. Thurman DJ, Alverson C, Dunn KA, et al. Traumatic brain injury in the United States: a public health perspective. *J Head Trauma Rehabil.* 1999;14:602.

6. Oddo M, Le Roux PD. What is the etiology, pathogenesis and pathophysiology of

elevated intracranial pressure? In: Neligan P, Deutschman CS, eds. *The Evidenced Based Practice of Critical Care.* Philadelphia: Elsevier Science; 2009.

7. Swadron SP, LeRoux P, Smith WS, Weingart SD. Emergency neurological life support: traumatic brain injury. *Neurocrit Care.* 2012;17:S112–121.

8. Brainline. TBI Statistics. https://www.brainline.org/identifying-and-treating-concussionmtbi-service-members-and-veterans/about-concussionmtbi/tbi. Accessed June 16, 2016.

9. Barr RM, Gean AD, Le TH. Craniofacial trauma. In: Brant WE, Helms CA, eds. *Fundamentals of Diagnostic Radiology.* Philadelphia: Lippincott, Williams & Wilkins; 2007, p. 69.

10. Gruen P. Surgical management of head trauma. *Neuroimag Clin N Am.* 2002;12 (2):339–43.

11. Smith J, Tiandra JJ, Clupie GJA, Kaye AH. *Textbook of Surgery.* Hoboken, NJ: Wiley-Blackwell; 2006, p. 446.

12. Bouma GJ, Muizelaar JP. Cerebral blood flow, cerebral blood volume, and cerebrovascular reactivity after severe head injury. *J Neurotrauma.* 1992;9(Suppl 1): S333.

13. Bouma GJ, Muizelaar JP, Bandoh K, Marmarou A. Blood pressure and intracranial pressure-volume dynamics in severe head injury: relationship with cerebral blood flow. *J Neurosurg.* 1992;77:15.

14. Carney N, Totten AM, O'Reilly C, et al. Guidelines for the management of severe traumatic brain injury, *fourth edition.* Neurosurgery. 2017;80(1):6–15.

15. Stevens RD, Huff JS, Duckworth J, et al. Emergency neurological life support: intracranial hypertension and herniation. *Neurocrit Care.* 2012;17(Suppl 1):S60–65.

16. Robertson CS, Valadka AB, Hannay HJ, et al. Prevention of secondary ischemic insults after severe head injury. *Crit Care Med.* 1999;27:2086.

17. Howells T, Elf K, Jones PA, et al. Pressure reactivity as a guide in the treatment of

cerebral perfusion pressure in patients with brain trauma. *J Neurosurg.* 2005;102:311.

18. Aarabi B, Tofighi B, Kufera JA, et al. Predictors of outcome in civilian gunshot wounds to the head. *J Neurosurg.* 2014;120 (5):1138–46.

19. Magnuson J, Leonessa F, Ling GS. Neuropathology of explosive blast traumatic brain injury. *Curr Neurol Neurosci Rep.* 2012;12(5):570–79.

20. Chestnut RM, Marshall LF, Klauber MR, et al. The role of secondary brain injury in determining outcome from severe head injury. *J Trauma.* 1993;34(2):216–22.

21. Marmarou A, Anderson RL, Ward JD, et al. Impact of ICP instability and hypotension on outcome in patients with severe head trauma. *J Neurosurg.* 1991;75(Suppl): S59–66.

22. McHugh GS, Engel DC, Butcher I, et al. Prognostic value of secondary insults in traumatic brain injury: results from the IMPACT study. *J Neurotrauma.* 2007;24:287.

23. Harhangi BS, Kompanje EJ, Leebeek FW, Maas AI. Coagulation disorders after traumatic brain injury. *Acta Neurochir (Wien).* 2008;150:165.

24. Perkins ZB, Wittenberg MD, Nevin D, et al. The relationship between head injury severity and hemodynamic response to tracheal intubation. *J Trauma Acute Care Surg.* 2013;74:1074.

25. Bucher J, Koyfman A. Intubation of the neurologically injured patient. *JEM.* 2015;49(6):920–27.

26. Chang EF, Meeker M, Holland MC. Acute traumatic intraparenchymal hemorrhage: risk factors for progression in the early post-injury period. *Neurosurgery.* 2006;58:647.

27. Oertel M, Kelly DF, McArthur D, et al. Progressive hemorrhage after head trauma: predictors and consequences of the evolving injury. *J Neurosurg.* 2002;96:109.

28. Narayan RK, Maas AI, Servadei F, et al. Progression of traumatic intracerebral hemorrhage: a prospective observational study. *J Neurotrauma.* 2008;25:629.

29. Weingart SD, Levitan RM. Preoxygenation and prevention of desaturation during emergency airway management. *Ann Emerg Med.* 2012;59:165–175.e1.

30. Dixon BJ, Dixon JB, Carden JR, et al. Preoxygenation is more effective in the 25 degrees head-up position than in the supine position in severely obese patients: a randomized controlled study. *Anesthesiology.* 2005;102:1110–15, discussion 1115A.

31. Robinson N, Clancy M. In patients with head injury undergoing rapid sequence intubation, does pretreatment with intravenous lignocaine/lidocaine lead to an improved neurological outcome? A review of the literature. *Emerg Med J.* 2001;18 (6):453–57.

32. Ugur B, Ogurlu M, Gezer E, et al. Effects of esmolol, lidocaine and fentanyl on haemodynamic responses to endotracheal intubation: a comparative study. *Clin Drug Invest.* 2007;27: 269–77.

33. Seder DB, Riker RR, Jagoda A, Smith WS, Weingart SD. Emergency neurological life support: airway, ventilation, and sedation. *Neurocrit Care.* 2010;17:S4–20.

34. Cohen L, Athaide V, Wickham ME, et al. The effect of ketamine on intracranial and cerebral perfusion pressure and health outcomes: a systematic review. *Ann Emerg Med.* 2015;65:43–51.

35. Moss E, Powell D, Gibson RM, McDowall DG. Effect of etomidate on intracranial pressure and cerebral perfusion pressure. *Br J Anaesth.* 1979;51:347–52.

36. Rossaint J, Rossaint R, Weis J, et al. Propofol: neuroprotection in an in vitro model of traumatic brain injury. *Crit Care.* 2009;13:R61.

37. Hug CC Jr, McLeskey CH, Nahrwold ML, et al. Hemodynamic effects of propofol: data from over 25,000 patients. *Anesth Analg.* 1993;77:S21–29.

38. Kovarik WD, Mayberg TS, Lam AM, et al. Succinylcholine does not change intracranial pressure, cerebral blood flow velocity, or the electroencephalogram in patients with neurologic injury. *Anesth Analg.* 1994;78:469–73.

39. Brown MM, Parr MJ, Manara AR. The effect of suxamethonium on intracranial pressure and cerebral perfusion pressure in patients with severe head injuries following blunt trauma. *Eur J Anaesthesiol.* 1996;13:474–77.

40. Koenig KL. Rapid-sequence intubation of head trauma patients: prevention of fasciculations with pancuronium versus minidose succinylcholine. *Ann Emerg Med.* 1992;21:929–32.

41. Otterspoor LC, Kalkman CJ, Cremer OL. Update on the propofol infusion syndrome in ICU management of patients with head injury. *Curr Opin Anaesthesiol.* 2008;21:544.

42. Jakob SM, Ruokonen E, Grounds RM, et al. Dexmedetomidine vs. midazolam or propofol for sedation during prolonged mechanical ventilation: two randomized controlled trials. *JAMA.* 2012;307:1151–60.

43. Weingart S. EMCrit: Podcast 78 – Increased intra-cranial pressure (ICP) and herniation, aka brain code. Available at: http://emcrit.org/podcasts/high-icp-herniation/. Accessed November 16, 2016.

44. Berry C, Ley EJ, Bukur M, et al. Redefining hypotension in traumatic brain injury. *Injury.* 2012;43(11):1833–37.

45. Brenner M, Stein DM, Hu PF, et al. Traditional systolic blood pressure targets underestimate hypotension-induced secondary brain injury. *J Trauma Acute Care Surg.* 2012;72(5):1135–39.

46. Butcher I, Murray GD, McHugh GS, et al. Multivariable prognostic analysis in traumatic brain injury: results from the IMPACT study. *J Neurotrauma.* 2007;24 (2):329–37.

47. ATLS Subcommittee; American College of Surgeons' Committee on Trauma; International ATLS working group. Advanced trauma life support (ATLS®): the ninth edition. *J Trauma Acute Care Surg.* 2013;74(5):1363–66.

48. Hadley MN, Walters BC, Grabb PA, et al. Blood pressure management after acute spinal cord injury. *Neurosurgery.* 2002;50: S58–62.

49. Guidelines for the management of acute cervical spine and spinal cord injuries: Available at: www.aans.org/en/Education%20and%20Meetings/*/media/Files/Education%20and%20Meetingf/Clinical%20Guidelines/TraumaGuidelines.ashx. 2007. Accessed May, 2016.

50. Boone MD, Oren-Grinberg A, Robinson TM, et al. Mannitol or hypertonic saline in the setting of traumatic brain injury: what have we learned? *Surg Neurol Int.* 2015;6:177.

51. Freshman S, Battistella F, Matteucci M, et al. Hypertonic saline (7.5%) versus mannitol: a comparison for treatment of acute head injuries. *J Trauma.* 1993;35(3):344–48.

52. Thenuwara K, Todd MM, Brian JE. Effect of mannitol and furosemide on plasma osmolality and brain water. *Anesthesiology.* 2002;96(2):416–21.

53. Wang LC, Papangelou A, Lin C, et al. Comparison of equivolume, equiosmolar solutions of mannitol and hypertonic saline with or without furosemide on brain water content in normal rats. *Anesthesiology.* 2013;118(4):903–13.

54. Scalfani M, Dhar R, Zazulia A, et al. Effect of osmotic agents on regional blood flow in traumatic brain injury. *J Crit Care.* 2012;27(5):526.e7–1.

55. Battison C, Andrews PJ, Graham C, Petty T. Randomized, controlled trial on the effect of a 20% mannitol solution and a 7.5% saline/6% dextran solution on increased intracranial pressure after brain injury. *Crit Care Med.* 2005;33:196.

56. Vialet R, Albanèse J, Thomachot L, et al. Isovolume hypertonic solutes (sodium chloride or mannitol) in the treatment of refractory posttraumatic intracranial hypertension: 2 mL/kg 7.5% saline is more effective than 2 mL/kg 20% mannitol. *Crit Care Med.* 2003;31:1683.

57. Muizelaar JP, Wei EP, Kontos HA, et al. Mannitol causes compensatory cerebral vasoconstriction and vasodilation in response to blood viscosity changes. *J Neurosurg.* 1983;59(5):822–28.

58. Palma L, Bruni G, Fiaschi A, et al. Passage of mannitol into the brain around gliomas: a potential cause of rebound phenomenon. A study on 21 patients. *J Neurosurg Sci.* 2006;50(3):63–66.

59. Brain Trauma Foundation, American Association of Neurological Surgeons, Congress of Neurological Surgeons, et al. Guidelines for the management of severe traumatic brain injury. VI. Indications for intracranial pressure monitoring. *J Neurotrauma.* 2007;24(Suppl 1);S37.

60. Narayan RK, Kishore PR, Becker DP, et al. Intracranial pressure: to monitor or not to monitor? *J Neurosurg.* 1982;56(56):650–59.

61. Potgieter DW, Kippin A, Ngu F, McKean C. Can accurate ultrasonographic measurement of the optic nerve sheath diameter (a non-invasive measure of intracranial pressure) be taught to novice operators in a single training session? *Anaesth Intensive Care.* 2011;39(1):95–100.

62. Sekhon MS, McBeth P, Zou J, et al. Association between optic nerve sheath diameter and mortality in patients with severe traumatic brain injury. *Neurocrit Care.* 2014;21(2):245–52.

63. Hassen GW, Bruck I, Donahue J, et al. Accuracy of optic nerve sheath diameter measurement by emergency physicians using bedside ultrasound. *J Emerg Med.* 2015;48(4):450–57.

64. Cooper DJ, Rosenfeld JV, Murray L, et al. Decompressive craniectomy in diffuse traumatic brain injury. *N Engl J Med.* 2011;364(16):1493–502.

65. Honeybul S, Ho KM, Lind CR. What can be learned from the DECRA study. *World Neurosurg.* 2013;79(1):159–61.

66. Fehlings MG, Vaccaro A, Wilson JR, et al. Early versus delayed decompression for traumatic cervical spinal cord injury: results of the surgical timing in acute spinal cord injury study (STASCIS). *PLoS One.* 2012;7(2):e32037.

67. Hutchinson PJ, Kolias AG, Timofeev IS, et al. Trial of decompressive craniectomy for traumatic intracranial hypertension. *N Engl J Med.* 2016;375(12):1119–30.

68. Bullock MR, Chestnut R, Ghajar J, et al. Guidelines for the surgical management of

traumatic brain injury. *Neurosurgery.* 2006;58(Suppl):S2-1-3.

69. Morgenstern LB, Hemphill JC 3rd, Anderson C, et al. Guidelines for the management of spontaneous intracerebral hemorrhage: a guideline for healthcare professionals from the American Heart Association/American Stroke Association. *Stroke.* 2010;41:2108.

70. Manno EM, Atkinson JL, Fulgham JR, et al. Emerging medical and surgical management strategies in the evaluation and treatment of intracerebral hemorrhage. *Mayo Clin Proc.* 2005;80:420.

71. Eller T, Busse J, Dittrich M, et al. Dabigatran, rivaroxaban, apixaban, argatroban and fondaparinux and their effects on coagulation POC and platelet function tests. *Clin Chem Lab Med.* 2014;52:835.

72. Dickneite G, Hoffman M. Reversing the new oral anticoagulants with prothrombin complex concentrates (PCCs): what is the evidence? *Thromb Haemost.* 2014;111:189.

73. Baharoglu MI, Cordonnier C, Al-Shahi Salman R, et al. Platelet transfusion versus standard care after acute stroke due to spontaneous cerebral haemorrhage associated with antiplatelet therapy (PATCH): a randomised, open-label, phase 3 trial. *Lancet.* 2016;387(10038):2605-13.

74. Inaba K, Menaker J, Branco BC, et al. A prospective multicenter comparison of levetiracetam versus phenytoin for early posttraumatic seizure prophylaxis. *J Trauma Acute Care Surg.* 2013;74 (3):766-71, discussion: 771-73.

75. Torbic H, Forni A, Anger KE, et al. Use of antiepileptics for seizure prophylaxis after

traumatic brain injury. *Am J Heal Pharm.* 2013;70(9):759-66.

76. Morrison JJ, Dubose JJ, Rasmussen TE, Midwinter MJ. *Military Application of Tranexamic Acid in Trauma Emergency Resuscitation (MATTERs) study. Arch Surg.* 2012;147(2):113-19.

77. Perel P, Al-Shahi Salman R, Kawahara T, et al. CRASH-2 (Clinical Randomisation of an Antifibrinolytic in Significant Haemorrhage) intracranial bleeding study: the effect of tranexamic acid in traumatic brain injury – a nested randomised, placebo-controlled trial. *Health Technol Assess.* 2012;16(13):iii–xii, 1–54.

78. Roberts I, Shakur H, Coats T, et al. The CRASH-2 trial: a randomised controlled trial and economic evaluation of the effects of tranexamic acid on death, vascular occlusive events and transfusion requirement in bleeding trauma patients. *Health Technol Assess.* 2013;17(10):1–79.

79. Dewan Y, Komolafe EO, Mejía-Mantilla JH, et al. CRASH-3 - tranexamic acid for the treatment of significant traumatic brain injury: study protocol for an international randomized, double-blind, placebo-controlled trial. *Trials.* 2012;13:87.

80. Sydenham E, Roberts I, Alderson P. Hypothermia for traumatic head injury. *Cochrane Database Syst Rev,* 2009;(2): CD00104.

81. Peterson K, Carson S, Carney N. Hypothermia treatment for traumatic brain injury: a systematic review and meta-analysis. *J Neurotrauma.* 2008;25(1):62–71.

82. Roberts I, Sydenham E. Barbiturates for acute traumatic brain injury. *Cochrane Database Syst Rev.* 2012;(12):CD000033.

Facial Trauma

Norah Kairys and Zachary Repanshek

Introduction

Facial trauma is a common presentation in the Emergency Department. As the face is vital to both physical appearance and the ability to eat, speak, and perform other important functions, proper management of patients presenting with facial trauma is critical. Initial treatment must focus on life-threatening injuries, but careful attention to long-term function and cosmesis must also be considered. Any patient presenting with facial trauma must also be evaluated for other traumatic injuries, as more than 50% of these patients will have injuries in multiple systems.[1] As with any trauma patient, ATLS guidelines should be followed, and the initial evaluation of injuries should begin with management of the airway, breathing, and circulation.

Facial injuries commonly occur secondary to sport injuries, assault, and motor vehicle collisions. Interestingly, in developing countries severe facial trauma most commonly results from motor vehicle collisions, while in the developed world assault is the most common cause (Figure 8.1).[2] As with all patients presenting with traumatic injuries, careful documentation for forensic purposes plays an important part of patient care, especially when injuries occur secondary to assault.[3]

The ABCs

- Facial trauma can complicate the early management of a trauma patient due to its close proximity to the brain, cervical spine, and airway.[4]
- Even minor maxillofacial injuries can pose a significant threat to the airway, as broken teeth, avulsed tissues, mandibular fractures, glottis edema, and foreign bodies all have the potential to compromise the airway.[4]
- Facial fractures can make bag-mask-valve techniques more challenging by impeding jaw-thrust maneuvers.[4]
- The fundamental strategy of look, listen, and feel can help to determine causes of airway obstruction and anticipate potential complications.[4]
- All maxillofacial trauma patients should receive adequate oxygenation and uninterrupted saturation monitoring.[4]
- Spinal collars should be applied with caution to prevent any posterior displacement of the mandible which could further compromise the airway.[4]
- If intubation is necessary, nasotracheal intubation may be contraindicated in patients with comminuted mid-face fractures due to fear of iatrogenic penetration of the skull base.[5] A study by Crewdson and Jerry[5] demonstrated a 12% unsuccessful intubation rate in trauma patients with noisy or clogged airways.[5-7]

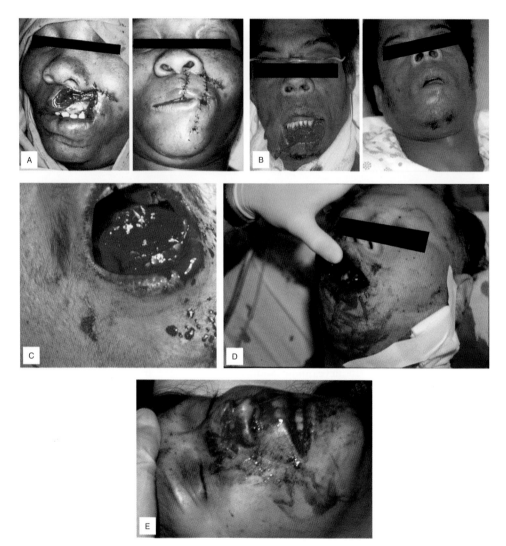

Figure 8.1 Image of patient with facial trauma. (A) Photographs of a patient with a complex facial laceration involving loss of tissue from the upper lip with avulsion of almost half the upper lip (left). After careful alignment of the vermilion border and restoration of the "cupid's bow," an acceptable cosmetic result is obtained (right). (B) Photographs before (left) and after (right) repair of a complex laceration of the lower lip caused by a human bite. An acceptable cosmetic result is obtained. (C) Amputation of the distal tongue caused by a human bite from the patient's girlfriend. (D) Patient with gunshot wound to the mouth and missing teeth. This patient should undergo radiological evaluation of the neck, chest, and abdomen to locate the missing teeth. (E) Photograph of a laceration through the nasal cartilage (reproduced with permission from *Color Atlas of Emergency Trauma, Second Edition*)

- A "difficult intubation" tray should always be present so that a surgical airway can quickly be obtained if oral intubation is unsuccessful.[4]

After stabilization of the airway and addressing breathing problems, attention must switch to circulation. Maxillofacial trauma predisposes a patient to significant hemorrhage. Studies have shown life threatening hemorrhage rates in these patients range anywhere from 1.4% to 11% (Box 8.1).[8–11]

Table 8.1 Facial anatomy

Zone of the Face	Structures Included	Bones Often Fractured
Upper face	Hairline to the glabella	Frontal bone and frontal sinus
Mid-face	Glabella to the base of the columella	Maxilla, nasal bones, nasoethmoidal complex, zygomaticomaxillary complex, and the orbital floor
Lower face	Columella to the soft tissue menton	Dentoalveolar segments and the mandible

---

Box 8.1   Affected Vessels in Facial Trauma

Common origins of hemorrhage after maxillofacial trauma:
- Ethmoid artery
- Ophthalmic artery
- Vidian branch of the internal carotid artery
- Maxillary artery*

   * cause of most severe epistaxis.[4,10]

- Hemostasis is necessary to reduce blood loss and, in supine patients, to protect the airway.[4]
- Patients with oral bleeding who require c-spine precautions may require head elevation in order to reduce the risk of aspiration.[4]
- Control of bleeding can be achieved by urgent suturing of lacerations, pressure packing, manual reduction of fractures, administration of tranexamic acid, balloon tamponade, or angiography with trans-arterial embolization or ligation.[12–14] Ligation of these commonly implicated vessels carries a relatively low risk of tissue ischemia due to extensive facial artery collateral flow.[12–14]
- Balloon tamponade must be performed with caution in patients with comminuted mid-face fractures that are at risk for displacement of fractured fragments into the orbit or brain.[4]
- Facial injuries can be associated with traumatic occlusion or dissection of the internal carotid artery or vertebral arteries.[4] Clinical suspicion should be increased if examination demonstrates a bruit/thrill, expanding hematoma, pulse deficit, or any focal or lateralizing neurological deficits.[4]

Anatomy

The posterior portion of the face forms the anterior wall of the calvaria. The face is divided anatomically into three parts (Table 8.1).
- Nasal fractures are the most common facial injuries.
- Nasoethmoidal fractures rarely occur as isolated injuries. Associated injuries often include central nervous system injury, cribriform plate fractures, cerebrospinal fluid

Table 8.2 Cranial nerves involved in facial trauma[16]

Cranial Nerve	Function	Travels Through
Trigeminal nerve (V)	Sensation to the face and motor to muscles of mastication	Several foramina in the middle cranial fossa
Facial nerve (VII)	Motor function to the anterior muscles of the face and muscles of mastication	Narrow canal in temporal bone and courses through the parotid gland
Glossopharyngeal nerve (VIIII)	Motor function to muscles of mastication	Jugular foramen
Vagus nerve (X)	Motor function to muscles of mastication	Jugular foramen

rhinorrhea, lacrimal system injury, and fractures of the frontal bone, orbital floor, and mid-face.[15]
- Up to one third of patients with frontal sinus fractures may have concomitant intracranial injures.[1]
- Alveolar fractures can occur in isolation from a direct blow or as an extension of a fracture through the alveolar portion of the maxilla or mandible.[1]
- The supraorbital rim, maxilla, mandible, and frontal bones require high-impact forces in order to be damaged, but bones such as the zygoma and nasal bone are susceptible to injury with even low-impact forces.[1]
- Facial fractures may be associated with cranial nerve injuries (Table 8.2).

Approach
Clues from the history and physical exam can help to elucidate concern for facial injuries, even when there are minimal external signs of trauma.

History
- As with all trauma patients, it is critical to ask the patient information about the mechanism of injury, and whether or not there is any substance use that could be altering the patient's memory or perception of what has happened to them.
- Additional history should be obtained from EMS, associates, or bystanders whenever possible.
- It is important to note if there was a loss of consciousness associated with the event, if there is difficulty with swallowing or shortness of breath, and to assess for as complete a review of systems as possible.

Examination
- Initial examination must include palpation of the bony prominences for focal tenderness, step-off, crepitus, or abnormal motion.
- It can be helpful to ask the patient to breathe out of each nare separately, and to assess for double vision, hearing changes, difficulty speaking, facial numbness, alignment of the teeth, and to determine if there are any painful or loose teeth.

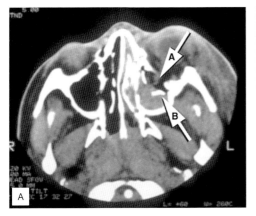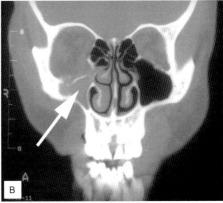

Figure 8.2 CT max/face with fractures. (A) CT scan of the orbits showing fracture of the posterior/inferior orbital wall (arrow A) with herniation of orbital contents into the maxillary sinus on the left (arrow B). (B) CT scan showing fracture of the inferior orbital wall with opacification of the right maxillary sinus (arrow) (reproduced with permission from *Color Atlas of Emergency Trauma, Second Edition*)

- Basilar skull fractures are at high risk for epidural hematomas. These fractures often cause a dural tear, and, therefore, up to 45% of these fractures can cause a CSF leak. Otorrhea or rhinorrhea after facial trauma is considered pathognomonic for a basilar skull fracture. Other clinical signs may include retroauricular ecchymosis (Battle sign), periorbital ecchymosis (raccoon eyes), and/or hemotympanum.[17–19]
- An increased intercanthal distance suggests a naso-orbital-ethmoid fracture which may also indicate the presence of an additional basal skull fracture. Typically, the normal intercanthal distance (telecanthus) in adults ranges from 28 to 34 mm, which is about the horizontal length of one eye.[15,20]
- Assessment for immediate facial paralysis raises concern for transection of the facial nerve, whereas delayed facial paralysis is more often related to nerve edema or facial swelling.[21]

Imaging
- Plain x-rays may be used for screening purposes, but the ideal imaging for facial fractures is computed tomography (CT). Typically, a CT max-face will visualize most of the territory required to screen for facial fractures (Figure 8.2), but occasionally a CT orbit and/or CT head will be needed as well.
- Studies have shown that there is no indication for nasal bone x-ray if both nares are patent, there is no septal deviation or hematoma on inspection, and if the tenderness and swelling is isolated to only the bony bridge.[22]
- A panorex may help to identify any isolated mandibular fractures, dental fractures, or alveolar ridge fractures (Figure 8.3).[22]
- CT angiography should be considered if there is a hematoma or any clinical concern for injury or dissection of the carotid/vertebral artery (Figure 8.4).[22]

Management
- Any patient with trauma to the brow, forehead, or nasal bridge should expect additional periorbital swelling and ecchymosis to occur within 12–36 hours.[23]

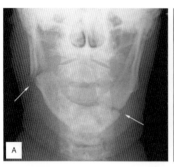
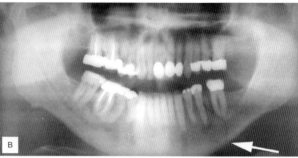

Figure 8.3 Image of panorex with alveolar ridge fracture. (A) Anteroposterior radiograph of the mandible showing bilateral displaced fractures of the angles of the mandible (arrows). (B) Panorex view of the mandible showing an undisplaced fracture of the left mandibular ramus (arrow) (reproduced with permission from *Color Atlas of Emergency Trauma, Second Edition*)

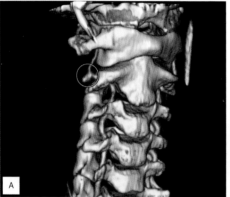
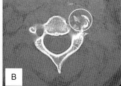
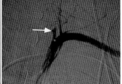
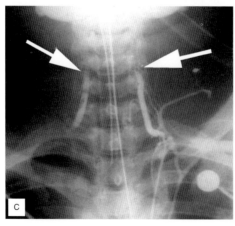

Figure 8.4 CTA neck with dissection of carotid artery. Penetrating injuries to the vertebral artery. (A) Patient with gunshot wound in zone III of the neck. CT angiogram with 3-D reconstruction shows a pseudoaneurysm of the distal vertebral artery (circle). (B) Patient with a gunshot wound to the neck. The CT scan shows a fracture of the vertebral foramen (left, circle). In such cases there is concern of injury to the vertebral artery that travels through the foramen. Angiography confirms injury and thrombosis of the vertebral artery (right, arrow). (C) Patient with a transcervical gunshot wound to the neck and fracture of the cervical spine. Angiography showing thrombosis of both vertebral arteries (arrows). The patient had no neurological deficits from this injury (reproduced with permission from *Color Atlas of Emergency Trauma, Second Edition*)

- Definitive repair of non-displaced facial fractures is typically not required emergently, as adults will typically not develop firm fibrous union until 10 days after the injury. Therefore, most injuries requiring surgical internal fixation are usually performed at 4–10 days post-injury once the swelling has dissipated.[4,9]
- All external wounds should be debrided and repaired for both cosmesis and hemostasis.[24]
- Typically, antibiotics are provided if injuries were secondary to a human or animal bite, and when there is evidence of devascularization, penetration of the buccal mucosa, through-and-through injuries of the lip, exposed cartilage of the nose or ear, gross contamination, or open fractures.[24,25]
- Although controversial, antibiotics do not need to be routinely prescribed for nasal packing that is placed for management of epistaxis.[25]
- Tetanus vaccination should be administered if the patient is not up-to-date, and rabies vaccination is implicated with certain animal bites.[25]

Specific Injuries

Orbit

- Orbital blow out fractures typically occur when direct pressure has been applied to the eye, causing a fracture of the inferior bony structures of the orbit. These fractures can lead to entrapment of the inferior rectus muscle, causing the eye to fixate in a downward position.[26]
- Non-displaced orbital fractures can typically be managed as an outpatient, but any injuries causing entrapment of the orbital muscles or retrobulbar hematoma require urgent ophthalmology consultation.[11,26]
- Orbital injuries can lead to enophthalmos, diplopia, impaired eye movement, or infraorbital hypoesthesia.[26] Furthermore, any anesthesia in the infraorbital nerve distribution is concerning for an orbital floor fracture.[4,26]
- A complete orbital exam includes visual acuity; range of extraocular motion; and inspection for an afferent pupillary defect, hyphema, corneal abrasion, or orbital step-off.[26]

Ear

- Hematoma formation from blunt trauma to the ear can accumulate in the subperichondrial potential space which can lead to formation of a cauliflower ear (wrestler's ear) (Figure 8.5), and therefore any hematoma in this area should be drained (Box 8.2).[27]
- Tympanic membrane perforation can occur with trauma. Although this can lead to conductive hearing loss and an increased risk of infection, most heal spontaneously on their own within 4 weeks.[29]
- Typically, TM perforations are managed by ENT as an outpatient and ultimately require myringoplasty if they do not resolve on their own.[29]
- Patients with TM perforation and severe hearing loss, vertigo, nystagmus, or ataxia should be evaluated urgently by ENT.
- Additionally, post-auricular ecchymosis (battle sign) can indicate a basilar skull fracture (although bruising in this area does not usually develop until 1–2 days after trauma).[30]

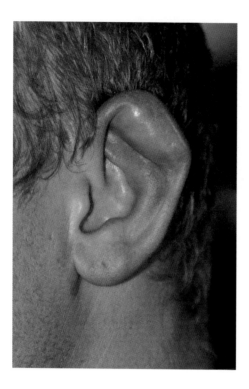

Figure 8.5 Image of cauliflower ear (photograph courtesy of MartialArtsNomad.com, reproduced under CC BY 2.0; https://creativecommons.org/licenses/by/2.0/)

Box 8.2   Steps of Draining a Subperichondrial Hematoma[28]

1. Cleanse the area with an antiseptic solution
2. Provide local anesthesia (epinephrine should be avoided due to the limited blood supply to the external ear) either around the hematoma itself or via a greater auricular nerve block
3. Aspirate from the most fluctuant area of the hematoma with an 18 gauge needle or make a small incision with an #11 blade scalpel
4. Milk the hematoma to ensure complete drainage
5. Apply direct pressure for 5–10 minutes and then place a pressure dressing over the area to prevent reaccumulation

Larger hematomas may require an incision with an 11 blade (best preformed parallel to the helical curve for cosmesis) followed by mattress suturing

---

- Otoscopic evaluation should be performed to evaluate for hemotympanum and otorrhea (Figure 8.6).[30]
- If otorrhea is found, a drop of the fluid can be placed onto filter paper. A rapidly advancing halo, or ring of clear fluid surrounding a circle of dark red fluid, is considered a positive test and may indicate a CSF leak (Figure 8.7).[31–33]
- It is important to note that a false positive can occur if the fluid obtained is actually saline or saliva.[31–33]

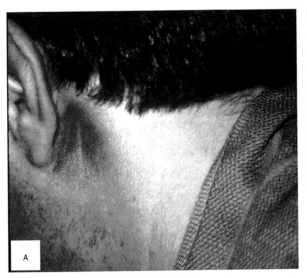
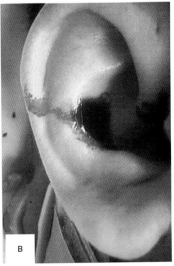

Figure 8.6 Image of battle sign or hemotympanum. Physical exam findings indicative of basilar skull fracture of the middle cranial fossa. (A) Battle's sign – ecchymosis over the mastoid process, indicating basilar fracture and tracking of blood through the mastoid air cells. (B) Bloody otorrhea following basilar skull fracture of the middle cranial fossa with rupture of tympanic membrane (reproduced with permission from *Color Atlas of Emergency Trauma, Second Edition*)

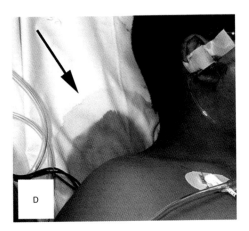

Figure 8.7 Image of halo sign. Bloody otorrhea, arrow reveals the "halo effect" or "double ring sign" of CSF separating from blood when applied to the sheet. This sign can also be seen when the bloody drainage is applied to a paper towel or filter paper (reproduced with permission from *Color Atlas of Emergency Trauma, Second Edition*)

- Although not commonly done, a more specific test to evaluate for a CSF leak is to test the fluid obtained for beta2-transferrin, as this protein is only found in CSF, aqueous humor, and perilymph.[31–33]

Nasal Injury

- Inspection for nasal bone injuries often includes palpitation for tenderness, crepitus, abnormal movement, and a nasal speculum exam to evaluate for a septal hematoma.[34]
- If a septal hematoma is found it will need to be urgently drained as they can quickly progress to necrosis of the septum itself.[34]

- To drain a septal hematoma the patient is positioned supine with the head of the bed elevated. The area should be anesthetized with lidocaine and then the mucosa over the area of greatest fluctuance should be incised with an 11-blade scalpel.
- After incision and drainage is performed, anterior nasal packing is placed for 2–3 days and the patient is scheduled to follow up with ENT as an outpatient.[34]
- As mentioned, routine imaging is not necessary for uncomplicated nasal bone fractures.[35]
- The management of nasal bone fractures includes ice and elevation of the head. Ideally, these fractures should be reduced by ENT within 6 hours if markedly displaced.[23]
- Urgent evaluation for nasoethmoid fractures must be obtained in patients with suspected anterior skull base fractures to monitor for potential cerebrospinal fluid (CSF) leak, as this raises a high concern for complications such as meningitis.[36]
- The presenting complaint for cribriform plate fractures is often anosmia.[35]

Zygomatic Bone Fractures

- Due to the prominence of the zygomatic bone, fractures in this complex occur quite frequently.[37]
- Dislocation of the zygoma initially occurs in the direction of the impact, but this is then further pulled by traction from the masseter muscle.[37]
- Patients with injury to this area must be instructed not to blow their nose, as this may lead to laceration of the mucosa of the maxillary sinus, which can cause increased pressure in the paranasal sinuses. Emphysema in theses tissues can extend into the mediastinum via the neck.[37]
- Fractures of the zygomatic complex can also lead to infraorbital nerve impairment.[37]

Tripod Fracture

- Tripod fractures are a specific type of injury that involves the zygoma, lateral orbit, and maxilla (Figure 8.8).[38] This fracture pattern poses a significant threat of airway compromise.
- Isolated tripod fractures typically occur secondary to a direct blow injury and, since these fractures are frequently displaced, they often require surgical correction.[38]
- This constellation of injuries is often associated with ocular findings, such as abnormal extra-ocular movements. Therefore, ophthalmic consultation is typically obtained for patients with these injuries.[38]

Maxillary Fractures

- Maxilla fractures may be present in patients with dysphonia or edema of oropharynx, suggesting a hematoma or fracture.[4,9,39]
- A fracture of the anterior wall of the maxillary sinus may present with denervation of the maxillary teeth.[4,40]

Maxillary fractures are classified as a LeFort I, II, or III injuries (Table 8.3) (Figure 8.9).

- LeFort II and III fractures are considered to be unstable fractures and have a high risk for concurrent cerebrovascular injury.[4,40]

Table 8.3 LeFort fractures[4,9,40]

Type	Caused By	Fracture Extends Through	Indicates
LeFort I	Horizontal maxillary fracture across the inferior aspect of the maxilla separating the alveolar process from the rest of the maxilla	The lower third of the septum and includes the medial and lateral maxillary sinus walls, extending into the palatine bones and pterygoid plates	Palate-facial separation
LeFort II	Pyramidal fracture originating at the nasal bone	The ethmoid and lacrimal bones into the zygomaticomaxillary suture, through the maxilla, and into the pterygoid plates	Pyramidal disjunction
LeFort III	Full separation of the facial bones from the cranial base	The zygoma, maxilla, and nasal bones	Craniofacial disjunction

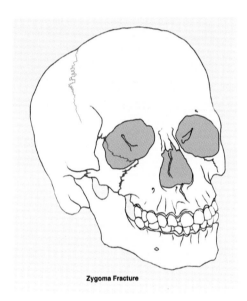

Zygoma Fracture

Figure 8.8 Image of a tripod fracture. Illustration outlining a tripod fracture of the zygoma (reproduced with permission from *Color Atlas of Emergency Trauma, Second Edition*)

- Inspection, palpation, and manipulation (by gasping the superior anterior teeth/alveolar ridge while moving the maxilla anteriorly and posteriorly) may be used to evaluate for unstable LeFort fractures.[4,40]

TMJ

- The temporomandibular joint allows the condyle of the mandible to rotate and translate anteriorly to open the jaw. A meniscus overlies the condyle that enables this motion.[41]
- Disruption of the TMJ from condylar or zygomatic arch fractures can prevent jaw opening, even when the patient is paralyzed.[41]
- Anterior dislocation of the TMJ presents with fixation of the jaw in an open position, and these patients will require reduction of the joint after fractures are ruled out with imaging (Box 8.3).[41]

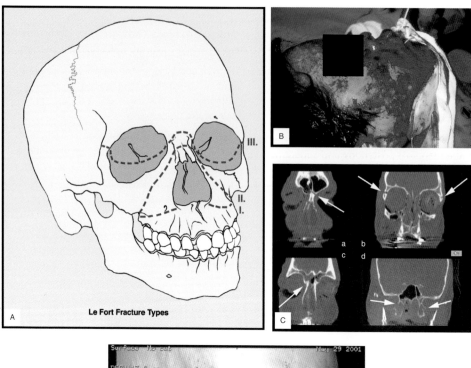

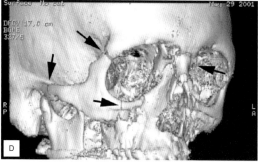

Figure 8.9 Image of LeFort Fractures. (A) Schematic showing three types of Le Fort fracture. (B) Photograph of a patient who had a garage door crush his face. The abnormal concavity of the face ("dish face") is characteristic of a Le Fort III fracture. (C) CT scan of the face showing Le Fort III fracture: (a) anterior ethmoid fracture (arrow); (b) mid ethmoid and lateral orbit fractures (arrows); (c) frontal sinus fracture (arrow); (d) pterygoid fractures (arrows). (D) CT scan 3-D reconstruction of a Le Fort III fracture showing multiple fractures, including a tripod fracture of the zygoma (arrows) (reproduced with permission from *Color Atlas of Emergency Trauma, Second Edition*)

- All TMJ injuries can lead to malpositioning of the jaw, therefore these patients must follow up with oral surgery within two weeks post-injury.[41]

Mandible Fractures

- Malocclusion of the jaw may indicate a mandibular fracture.[44]
- To evaluate for injury, have the patient bite down on a tongue depressor placed between upper and lower molars while the physician twists the blade. A fracture is unlikely if the

Box 8.3 Methods Used to Reduce a Dislocated TMJ[42,43]

Syringe method: A 5–10 mL syringe is placed between the posterior upper and lower molars on one side and the patient is instructed to bite down on the syringe while rolling it back and forth between their teeth until the dislocation on that side is reduced. Repeat on the opposite side if it does not reduce spontaneously.

Intraoral technique: Manual reduction by having the clinician grasp the ridge of the mandible adjacent to the molars and wrap their fingers around the outside of the jaw. The physician can use shortened tongue blades on the upper and lower surfaces of their thumbs for protection. Then the clinician applies downward pressure to the mandible to free the condyles and guide the mandible posteriorly and superiorly into the temporal fossa.

Extraoral technique: On one side the clinician grasps the mandibular angle with his/her fingers and places his/her thumb over the malar eminence of the maxilla. On the other side, the clinician places his/her thumb above the displaced coronoid process and puts his/her fingers behind the mastoid process. At the same time the clinician pulls the mandibular angle forward on one side and pushes the coronoid process backward on the other side.

patient has enough bite strength to crack the blade when it is twisted. Studies have found that this is 95% sensitive and 65% specific for mandibular injuries. This simple test can have a negative predictive value of greater than 92% if the patient is able to crack a tongue depressor on both sides of their jaw.[44–46]

- The mandible is most vulnerable to injury at the ramus. Injuries to the body of the mandible typically occur at the level of the first and second molars. Bilateral mandibular fractures pose an increased risk for airway obstruction secondary to posterior displacement of the tongue.[44]
- Open fractures require antibiotics and immediate oral surgery consultation.

Parotid Duct
- The parotid gland lies anterior to the auricle and posterior to the ramus of the mandible.[47]
- Stenson's duct travels anteriorly in the horizontal plane and opens in the inner wall of the cheek by the second upper molar.[47]
- If blood is expressed from Stenson's duct with manual compression over the parotid gland, a specialized repair over a stent is required to prevent a cutaneous fistula from forming.[47]

Dental Injuries
Dental fractures are often classified using the Ellis scale (Table 8.4).
- Any partially avulsed teeth should be removed, particularly if the patient is altered, to prevent aspiration.[48–51]
- Removed teeth can be stored in culture media or milk.[48–51]
- Fractures through the alveolar ridge may require stabilization with a wire, arch bar, or acrylic splinting after fracture reduction by oral surgery. These fractures often require outpatient antibiotics.[48–51]

Table 8.4 Ellis fracture[48]

Type	Structures Involved	Pain	Management
Ellis I	Enamel of a tooth	No	Outpatient dental follow up, file with emery board
Ellis II	Exposes the dentin of the tooth	Yes	Outpatient follow up (24–48 hours) after the fracture is covered with calcium hydroxide for protection
Ellis III	Exposes the dental pulp (often visualized as a red dot or line in the middle of the fractured tooth)	Yes	Dental or endodontic management within 24 hours, cover with calcium hydroxide

Pitfalls in Facial Trauma

- Although facial trauma can be distracting to both the patient and the physician, maxillofacial injuries are often complicated by a compromised airway, which needs to be the priority in initial management.[4,52]
- Even minor injuries to the face can result in significant airway complications.[4]
- Maxillofacial injuries can be prone to massive and life-threatening hemorrhage (one in ten complicated facial fractures leads to significant bleeding).[13,41]
- In all complex maxillofacial trauma patients, cervical spine fractures should be considered until proven otherwise. The incidence of cervical spine injury in these patients ranges from 1% to 10%.[53]

Key Points

- Facial trauma is a complicated presenting complaint that often requires multidisciplinary management due to the complexity of associated injuries.[4,52]
- Unstable facial fractures, such as tripod fractures and LeFort II and III fractures, require immediate surgical correction. Otherwise, most non-displaced facial fractures are repaired 4–10 days after injury after the swelling has gone down.[40]
- Septal hematomas require immediate incision and drainage to prevent necrosis of the nasal septum. Likewise, auricular hematomas should be drained emergently to prevent cauliflower ear.[23,27,34]

References

1. Tintinalli JE, Kelen GD, Stapczynski JS, et al. *Emergency Medicine: A Comprehensive Study Guide*. 6th ed. New York, NY: McGraw-Hill; 2004.

2. Erdmann D, Follmar KE, Debruijn M, et al. A retrospective analysis of facial fracture etiologies. *Ann Plast Surg.* 2008;60 (4):398–403.

3. Shetty V, Dent DM, Glynn S, Brown KE. Psychosocial sequelae and correlates of orofacial injury. *Dent Clin North Am.* 2003;47(1):141–57, xi.

4. Jose A, Nagori SA, Agarwal B, Bhutia O, Roychoudhury A. Management of

maxillofacial trauma in emergency: an update of challenges and controversies. *J Emerg Trauma Shock*. 2016;9(2): 73–80.

5. Crewdson K, Jerry PN. Management of the trauma airway. *Trauma*. 2011;13 (3):221–32.

6. Rosen CL, Wolfe RE, Chew SE, Branney SW, Roe EJ. Blind nasotracheal intubation in the presence of facial trauma. *J Emerg Med*. 1997;15(2):141–45.

7. Roppolo LP, Vilke GM, Chan TC, et al. Nasotracheal intubation in the emergency department, revisited. *J Emerg Med*. 1999;17(5):791–99.

8. Ardekian L, Samet N, Shoshani Y, Taicher S. Life-threatening bleeding following maxillofacial trauma. *J Craniomaxillofac Surg*. 1993;21(8):336–38.

9. Thaller SR, Beal SL. Maxillofacial trauma: a potentially fatal injury. *Ann Plast Surg*. 1991;27(3):281–83.

10. Buchanan RT, Holtmann B. Severe epistaxis in facial fractures. *Plast Reconstr Surg*. 1983;71(6):768–71.

11. Gwyn PP, Carraway JH, Horton CE, Adamson JE, Mladick RA. Facial fractures – associated injuries and complications. *Plast Reconstr Surg*. 1971;47 (3):225–30.

12. Dakir A, Ramalingam B, Ebenezer V, Dhanavelu P. Efficacy of tranexamic acid in reducing blood loss during maxillofacial trauma surgery – a pilot study. *J Clin Diagn Res*. 2014;8(5):ZC06–8.

13. Bynoe RP, Kerwin AJ, Parker HH, 3rd, et al. Maxillofacial injuries and life-threatening hemorrhage: treatment with transcatheter arterial embolization. *J Trauma*. 2003;55(1):74–79.

14. Shimoyama T, Kaneko T, Horie N. Initial management of massive oral bleeding after midfacial fracture. *J Trauma*. 2003;54 (2):332–36; discussion 336.

15. Sargent LA, Rogers GF. Nasoethmoid orbital fractures: diagnosis and management. *J Craniomaxillofac Trauma*. 1999;5(1):19–27.

16. Crean SJ. Cranial nerves: functional anatomy. *Ann R Coll Surg Engl*. 2007;89 (2):194.

17. Dahiya R, Keller JD, Litofsky NS, et al. Temporal bone fractures: otic capsule sparing versus otic capsule violating clinical and radiographic considerations. *J Trauma*. 1999;47(6):1079–83.

18. Yilmazlar S, Arslan E, Kocaeli H, et al. Cerebrospinal fluid leakage complicating skull base fractures: analysis of 81 cases. *Neurosurg Rev*. 2006;29 (1):64–71.

19. Nosan DK, Benecke JE, Jr, Murr AH. Current perspective on temporal bone trauma. *Otolaryngol Head Neck Surg*. 1997;117(1):67–71.

20. Freihofer HP. Inner intercanthal and interorbital distances. *J Maxillofac Surg*. 1980;8(4):324–26.

21. Chang CY, Cass SP. Management of facial nerve injury due to temporal bone trauma. *Am J Otol*. 1999;20(1): 96–114.

22. Sun JK, LeMay DR. Imaging of facial trauma. *Neuroimaging Clin N Am*. 2002;12 (2):295–309.

23. Mondin V, Rinaldo A, Ferlito A. Management of nasal bone fractures. *Am J Otolaryngol*. 2005;26(3):181–85.

24. Singer AJ, Mach C, Thode HC, Jr, et al. Patient priorities with traumatic lacerations. *Am J Emerg Med*. 2000;18 (6):683–86.

25. Moran GJ, Talan DA, Abrahamian FM. Antimicrobial prophylaxis for wounds and procedures in the emergency department. *Infect Dis Clin North Am*. 2008;22 (1):117–43, vii.

26. McClenaghan FC, Ezra DG, Holmes SB. Mechanisms and management of vision loss following orbital and facial trauma. *Curr Opin Ophthalmol*. 2011;22 (5):426–31.

27. Stuteville OH, Janda C, Pandya NJ. Treating the injured ear to prevent a "cauliflower ear." *Plast Reconstr Surg*. 1969;44(3):310–12.

28. Greywoode JD, Pribitkin EA, Krein H. Management of auricular hematoma and the cauliflower ear. *Facial Plast Surg.* 2010;26(6):451–55.

29. Gao T, Li X, Hu J, et al. Management of traumatic tympanic membrane perforation: a comparative study. *Ther Clin Risk Manag.* 2017;13:927–31.

30. Hough, JVD. Fractures of the temporal bone and associated middle and inner ear trauma. *Proc R Soc Med.* 1970;63;245–56.

31. Dula DJ, Fales W. The 'ring sign': Is it a reliable indicator for cerebral spinal fluid? *Ann Emerg Med.* 1993;22(4):718–20.

32. Friedman JA, Ebersold MJ, Quast LM. Post-traumatic cerebrospinal fluid leakage. *World J Surg.* 2001;25(8):1062–66.

33. McCudden CR, Senior BA, Hainsworth S, et al. Evaluation of high resolution gel beta (2)-transferrin for detection of cerebrospinal fluid leak. *Clin Chem Lab Med.* 2013;51(2):311–15.

34. Olsen KD, Carpenter RJ 3rd, Kern EB. Nasal septal injury in children. Diagnosis and management. *Arch Otolaryngol.* 1980;106(6):317–20.

35. Rohrich RJ, Adams WP Jr. Nasal fracture management: minimizing secondary nasal deformities. *Plast Reconstr Surg.* 2000;106 (2):266–73.

36. Bell RB, Dierks EJ, Homer L, Potter BE. Management of cerebrospinal fluid leak associated with craniomaxillofacial trauma. *J Oral Maxillofac Surg.* 2004;62(6):676–84.

37. Kuhnel TS, Reichert TE. Trauma of the midface. *GMS Curr Top Otorhinolaryngol Head Neck Surg.* 2015;14:10.

38. Jacoby CG, Dolan KD. Fragment analysis in maxillofacial injuries: the tripod fracture. *J Trauma.* 1980;20(4):292–96.

39. Motamedi MH, Dadgar E, Ebrahimi A, et al. Pattern of maxillofacial fractures: a 5-year analysis of 8,818 patients. *J Trauma Acute Care Surg.* 2014;77(4):630–34.

40. Fraioli RE, Branstetter BF 4th, Deleyiannis FW. Facial fractures: beyond Le Fort.

41. Yanagisawa E. Symposium on maxillofacial trauma. 3. Pitfalls in the management of zygomatic fractures. *Laryngoscope.* 1973;83(4):527–46.

42. Gorchynski J, Karabidian E, Sanchez M. The "syringe" technique: a hands-free approach for the reduction of acute nontraumatic temporomandibular dislocations in the emergency department. *J Emerg Med.* 2014;47(6):676–81.

43. Shorey CW, Campbell JH. Dislocation of the temporomandibular joint. *Oral Surg Oral Med Oral Pathol Oral Radiol Endod.* 2000;89(6):662–68.

44. Schwab RA, Genners K, Robinson WA. Clinical predictors of mandibular fractures. *Am J Emerg Med.* 1998;16(3):304–5.

45. Caputo ND, Raja A, Shields C, Menke N. Re-evaluating the diagnostic accuracy of the tongue blade test: still useful as a screening tool for mandibular fractures? *J Emerg Med.* 2013;45(1):8–12.

46. Alonso LL, Purcell TB. Accuracy of the tongue blade test in patients with suspected mandibular fracture. *J Emerg Med.* 1995;13 (3):297–304.

47. Lazaridou M, Iliopoulos C, Antoniades K, et al. Salivary gland trauma: a review of diagnosis and treatment. *Craniomaxillofac Trauma Reconstr.* 2012;5(4):189–96.

48. Belmonte FM, Macedo CR, Day PF, Saconato H, Fernandes Moca Trevisani V. Interventions for treating traumatised permanent front teeth: luxated (dislodged) teeth. *Cochrane Database Syst Rev.* 2013; (4):CD006203.

49. Day P, Duggal M. Interventions for treating traumatised permanent front teeth: avulsed (knocked out) and replanted. *Cochrane Database Syst Rev.* 2010;(1):CD006542.

50. Petrovic B, Markovic D, Peric T, Blagojevic D. Factors related to treatment and outcomes of avulsed teeth. *Dent Traumatol.* 2010;26(1):52–59.

Otolaryngol Clin North Am. 2008;41 (1):51–76, vi.

51. Schatz JP, Hausherr C, Joho JP.
A retrospective clinical and radiologic
study of teeth re-implanted following
traumatic avulsion. *Endod Dent Traumatol.*
1995;11(5):235–39.

52. Perry M. Advanced trauma life support
(ATLS) and facial trauma: can one size fit
all? Part 1: dilemmas in the management of

the multiply injured patient with coexisting
facial injuries. *Int J Oral Maxillofac Surg.*
2008;37(3):209–14.

53. Merritt RM, Williams MF. Cervical spine
injury complicating facial trauma:
incidence and management. *Am
J Otolaryngol.* 1997;18(4):235–38.

Chapter

Eye Trauma

Brandon Morshedi, John D. Pemberton, R. Grant Morshedi, and Brit Long

Introduction and Epidemiology

According to the United States Eye Injury Registry, eye injury is the leading cause of monocular blindness, and there are approximately 2.4 million eye injuries occurring annually in the US, resulting in 500,000 years of lost eyesight annually.[1] These injuries occur more often in males (>70%), and 95% of occupational injuries occur in males.[2,3] This chapter will describe the approach to the patient with eye trauma in the emergency department (ED), including how to perform a detailed history and physical examination related to eye injuries, as well as covering the traumatic presentations in Table 9.1.

There are multiple possible mechanisms for ocular trauma, outlined in Table 9.2.

Table 9.1 Eye trauma

Vision-Threatening Conditions	Other Traumatic Eye Presentations
• Ocular chemical burns	• Eyelid lacerations
• Orbital compartment syndrome	• Corneal abrasions and corneal foreign bodies
• Carotid-cavernous fistula	• Conjunctival injuries
• Open globe injury	• Orbital fractures
• Traumatic hyphema	
• Vitreous hemorrhage	
• Retinal trauma	
• Optic nerve injury	

Table 9.2 Mechanisms of ocular trauma

Blunt	Penetrating	Other
• Assault (i.e. punched)	• Bullets, BBs	• Fireworks
• Airbag deployment	• Scissors or knives	• Blast injuries
• Falls	• Projectiles related to cutting, hammering, or nailing	• Acid and alkali burns
• Bungee cord recoil	• Tree branches	• Welding
• Paintball or pellet gun		• Fingernails
• Sports-related		• Curling irons

Approach to the Patient With Eye Trauma

Treat Life-Threatening Conditions First

Ocular trauma may be isolated or in combination with multisystem trauma. Given that there is a high association of ocular trauma with other facial trauma, the initial approach should focus on adequate airway management, if necessary, followed by respiratory and circulatory support. Once acute life threats are excluded, then history, examination, and intervention focus on the injured eye.

Involve the Ophthalmologist Early

It is important to involve the ophthalmologist early, as there is a higher chance for improved visual acuity with early involvement. In one study of serious injuries in 11,320 eyes, 27% of patients had initial visual acuity <20/200. However, with treatment, 61% of patients had improvements in their visual acuity.[4] The authors noted specific positive and negative risk factors for improvement in visual acuity, detailed in Table 9.3.

Focused History

The clinician should take a focused history, concentrating on the mechanism of injury to determine the likelihood of open vs. closed globe injuries. The timing of the injury should be elicited, as injuries that present early may have an improved chance of recovery and lower risk of infection or other complications compared to those that present later. Any associated symptoms should be noted, as they provide clues to the underlying injury. Diplopia, painful ocular motion, and facial numbness may indicate orbital wall fracture, while excessive tearing and photophobia may indicate traumatic iritis. Obtain any relevant information related to past ocular history, especially any previous surgical procedures, contact lens wear, and baseline visual status. For occupational injuries, document whether protective eyewear was being utilized at the time of injury – this may become an important medicolegal and/or worker's compensation consideration. Finally, obtain relevant past medical history, active medications, allergies, and status of last tetanus immunization.

Immediately Identify Acute Visual Threats

In some cases, the history may lead the clinician to discover immediate threats to vision that require intervention prior to beginning a detailed examination of the eye. Examples include chemical injury requiring immediate irrigation, orbital compartment syndrome requiring lateral canthotomy/cantholysis, a protruding intraocular foreign body requiring stabilization and immediate referral without any further manipulation, and an open globe that may limit further aspects of the physical examination.

Table 9.3 Factors associated with positive or negative visual acuity outcomes in traumatic eye injury

Positive Risk Factors	Negative Risk Factors
• <60 years of age	• >60 years of age
• Eye contusions	• Injured by assault, street/highway, fall, or gunshot
• Intraocular foreign bodies	• Left eye injury
	• Involvement of posterior segment

Examination of the Injured Eye

Visual Acuity

Visual acuity is often considered the primary "vital sign" of the eye. It should be performed on every ocular injury. Visual acuity is often obtained by use of a bedside "near card" or a Snellen Chart (Figure 9.1). Visual acuity should be tested with the patient's corrective lenses in place, if possible. The clinician should test each eye individually. If the visual acuity is decreased to 20/40, worse than the patient's baseline, or one line lower on the Snellen Chart compared to the patient's baseline, then further evaluation and urgent Ophthalmology consultation are recommended.[5]

Periocular Examination

It is critical to examine all structures surrounding the eye to identify any associated injuries that could lead to increased morbidity or dysfunction, such as orbital blowout fractures, nerve injuries, lacrimal system disruption, and many others. Evaluation should focus on the orbit, orbital rim, lids, lid function, and eyelid and periocular sensation.

Orbit and Orbital Rim

Palpate circumferentially around the orbit and along the orbital rim. Feel for step-off, crepitus, deformity, or elicitation of tenderness. Visually inspect for protrusion of any

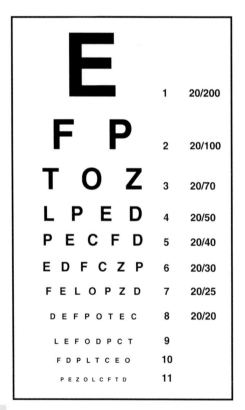

Figure 9.1 Snellen Chart as a visual acuity tool (from: https://upload.wikimedia.org/wikipedia/commons/7/77/1606_Snellen_Chart-02.jpg)

orbital fat through a wound, as this indicates damage to underlying levator muscle, orbital septum, or both.[5]

Lids and Lid Function

Visually inspect the superior and inferior lid and lid margin for any laceration, and give special attention to the area within 6–8 mm of the medial canthus – the expected location of the lacrimal canaliculi. In the case of suspected foreign body, the eyelid should be everted to examine the pretarsal sulcus of the upper lid, where foreign bodies tend to be retained. During evaluation of the lids, if the patient is unable to open the eyelids due to periorbital edema, then care should be taken to gently pull the lids apart or lift the upper lid and avoid exerting pressure on the globe. Additionally, evaluate whether the patient can effectively approximate the lids when closing them. Full-thickness eyelid lacerations are associated with ocular injury in two thirds of cases, and the clinician should have increased suspicion in those instances. The clinician can specifically evaluate for levator palpebrae transection by assessing for eyelid excursion. When the patient demonstrates upgaze, the upper lid will not elevate.[5]

Eyelid and Periocular Sensation

Evaluate sensation along the upper eyelid and forehead, as well as the lower eyelid and upper cheek. Any deficit in the superior aspect indicates a possible injury to the supraorbital nerve along the superior orbital rim. Any deficit in the inferior aspect indicates a possible injury to the infraorbital nerve, suggesting a possible inferior orbital wall fracture.

Ocular Examination

The ocular examination includes the pupils, extraocular motility, the anterior segment (conjunctiva, cornea, anterior chamber, iris, and lens), and the posterior segment (vitreous humor, retina, and optic nerve), as well as intraocular pressure measurement and fluorescein staining. Refer to Figure 9.2 for a review of relevant ocular anatomy.

Pupils

Pupil examination is best conducted using a penlight to evaluate size, shape, and reactivity. The clinician should also evaluate for a relative afferent pupillary defect (rAPD). An rAPD is present when rapidly swinging the penlight to the affected eye causes the pupil to dilate, whereas shining the penlight into the unaffected eye will cause the pupil to constrict. This occurs due to either an optic nerve injury (e.g. traumatic optic neuropathy or avulsion), or possibly to a diffuse retinal injury such as a detachment. If a red reflex is symmetric, the rAPD is likely due to optic nerve injury. If a red reflex is asymmetric, the rAPD is likely due to posterior chamber pathology. A patient may have a pre-existing rAPD in cases of other severe ocular disease such as glaucoma or previous retinal detachment.

Extraocular Motility

The clinician should evaluate extraocular motion in the six cardinal directions of gaze, as well as symmetric gaze when looking straight ahead, up, and down. Figure 9.3 demonstrates the relevant movements with their associated ocular muscles. Asymmetries may be related to ocular muscle damage or entrapment, neuropathies, or retrobulbar hematoma.[5]

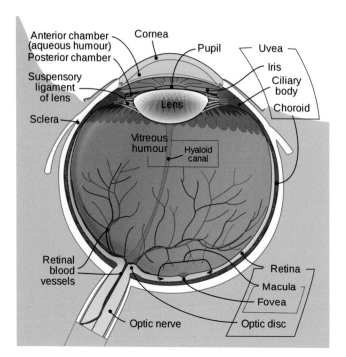

Figure 9.2 Cross-sectional ocular anatomy (image courtesy of Rhcastilhos and Jmarchn. Reproduced under CC BY-SA 3.0 https://creativecommons.org/licenses/by-sa/3.0/)

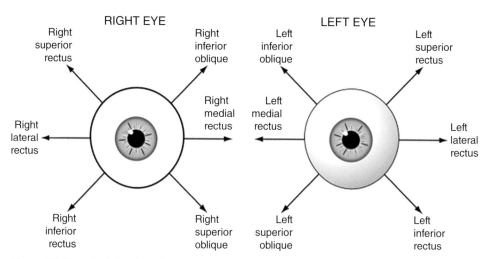

Figure 9.3 Six cardinal directions of gaze (courtesy: http://clinicalexamskills.blogspot.com/2010/10/cranial-nerves-ii-iv-and-vi.html)

Anterior Segment

While the slit lamp is the preferred method of evaluation of the anterior segment, it may not always be feasible. Significant associated trauma and patient condition may limit the evaluation of the anterior segment to that which can only be seen by penlight or Wood's

Lamp. Evaluation of the anterior segment should focus on the conjunctiva, cornea, anterior chamber, and iris.

- *Conjunctiva.* The clinician should inspect the bulbar and the tarsal conjunctiva, evaluating for the presence or absence of subconjunctival hemorrhage, foreign bodies, chemosis, or laceration. Subconjunctival hemorrhage can be classified as flat or bullous, with the latter more suspicious for underlying scleral laceration. Foreign bodies are usually associated with tearing and photophobia. Chemosis appears as serous fluid within the substance of the conjunctiva. Conjunctival lacerations may also be associated with subconjunctival hemorrhages and chemosis and should raise suspicion for possible open globe or penetrating eye injury.
- *Cornea.* The clinician should inspect the cornea for similar findings as the conjunctiva, including the presence of abrasions, foreign bodies, edema, and lacerations. Corneal abrasions are usually diagnosed through slit lamp examination but can be performed with fluorescein staining and Wood's Lamp evaluation as an alternative.
- *Anterior chamber.* The anterior chamber is best visualized with a slit lamp but can also be viewed with a penlight. The anterior chamber is the location of a hyphema, or a collection of red blood cells, in the setting of relevant trauma. A hyphema typically settles to the lower portion of the anterior chamber if the patient is upright for an extended period of time and can then be measured directly. With slit lamp, "cell and flare" may also be discovered, which suggests traumatic uveitis in the setting of trauma. Severe uveitis may result in hypopyon. The depth of the anterior chamber can be assessed by shining a penlight along the temporal portion of the chamber and visualizing the light shining across the flat iris in a normal anterior chamber, or only across a small portion of the temporal iris with a shadow across the nasal iris in a shallow anterior chamber. An asymmetric anterior chamber depth, when compared with the uninjured eye, can be a subtle sign of occult open globe injury.

Retina and Optic Nerve

The retina and optic nerve are best visualized through direct or panoramic ophthalmoscopy, but this can be technically difficult in the traumatized, undilated eye. In the absence of ophthalmoscopy, the red reflex can be used to grossly assess for retinal pathology. In the absence of a relative afferent pupillary defect, a uniform reflex that is symmetric between the two eyes can effectively exclude significant vitreous hemorrhage or large retinal detachments.[5] Color vision testing with standard color plates is a sensitive indicator of optic nerve damage but is not typically performed in the ED. Red desaturation testing may also be helpful when traumatic optic neuropathy is suspected. Red desaturation is assessed by asking the patient to subjectively judge the relative intensity of a red colored object in one eye vs. the other.[5,6]

Intraocular Pressure Measurement

Prior to performing intraocular pressure (IOP) measurement, the clinician must exclude open globe injury, as placing pressure on the globe could further extrude intraocular contents. If open globe is ruled out, the clinician can measure IOP through applanation tonometry (i.e. TonoPen). Pressure should be obtained in both eyes for comparison. Normal IOP is between 10–21 mmHg. Increased IOP could be associated with orbital compartment syndrome, retrobulbar hematoma, hyphema, traumatic iritis, and with some chemical burns.

Table 9.4 Advantages and disadvantages of ocular imaging modalities

	Computed Tomography	Ultrasound	Magnetic Resonance Imaging
Advantages	• Preferred imaging • Rapid • Can identify orbital wall trauma, soft tissue entrapment, fluid collection, and foreign bodies	• Rapid • Can identify organic foreign bodies • Can identify posterior vitreous hemorrhage and retinal detachment	• Better soft tissue definition • Better identification of fluid
Disadvantages	• Radiation exposure	• Contraindicated in suspected or confirmed open globe injury	• Slow to obtain • Contraindicated in metallic foreign bodies

Fluorescein Staining

Fluorescein staining is performed in trauma to evaluate for corneal abrasions, lacerations, and Seidel sign. Fluorescein stain is placed through a drop or moistened strip on the conjunctiva and allowed to distribute across the surface of the eye through blinking. It is taken up by the basement membrane wherever an epithelial defect is present and illuminates under cobalt blue light. Seidel sign can be seen in penetrating trauma and is defined as a streaming of leaking aqueous humor through the fluorescein coating the ocular surface.[5]

Diagnostic Imaging

Computed tomography (CT) is the preferred imaging of choice in ocular trauma. It will effectively identify orbital wall trauma, soft tissue entrapment, fluid collection, and specific foreign bodies. Ultrasound can identify organic foreign bodies that may not appear on CT, but caution is recommended when utilizing ultrasound for intraocular assessment. Placing excessive pressure on the eye from the ultrasound probe may cause further extrusion of intraocular contents in an open globe injury. MRI is not the diagnostic imaging modality of choice in trauma due to the time to obtain the imaging, in addition to the contraindications in the presence of possible metallic foreign bodies. Refer to Table 9.4 for a summary of the imaging modalities with listed advantages and disadvantages.

Vision-Threatening Conditions

Ocular Chemical Burns

Ocular chemical burns are one of the few ocular traumas that require intervention prior to evaluation. Once an ocular chemical burn is identified, the area should immediately be flushed with 1–2 L of normal saline through manual application or a commercial irrigation system (i.e. Morgan Lenses) prior to evaluation. Irrigation should continue until the pH is

Table 9.5 Common acids and alkalis that cause ocular chemical burns

Acids (pH <7)	Alkalis (pH >7)
• Sulfuric acid (i.e. car battery) • Sulfurous acid • Hydrochloric acid (i.e. toilet bowl cleaner) • Nitric acid • Acetic acid (i.e. nail polish remover) • Chromic acid • Hydrofluoric acid (i.e. glass polish)	• Ammonia hydroxide (i.e. cleaning products) • Sodium hydroxide (i.e. oven cleaner) • Lye (i.e. drain cleaners) • Potassium hydroxide (i.e. fertilizers) • Magnesium hydroxide (i.e. fertilizers) • Lime (i.e. plaster and cement)

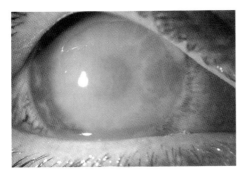

Figure 9.4 Chemical injury to the eye. There is diffuse uptake of fluorescein dye, indicating a large corneal epithelial defect (courtesy: Crimson House Publishing LLC)

neutral for at least 30 minutes after irrigation. Alkaline chemicals with pH >12 and acidic chemicals with pH <2 cause the most damage. However, alkaline chemicals cause more damage than acidic chemicals, due to the fact that alkaline chemicals cause liquefaction necrosis and deeper injury. In contrast, acidic chemicals cause coagulation necrosis, and the coagulum layer protects from further penetration. Table 9.5 lists some of the more common acids and bases implicated in ocular chemical burns.

Following irrigation, perform a detailed examination as described above, with particular attention to visual acuity, intraocular pressure, corneal scarring or clouding, anterior chamber "cell and flare," and conjunctival injection and chemosis. Use of fluorescein staining can determine the presence of any epithelial defects (Figure 9.4).

Obtain ophthalmology consultation for all but minor burns. Any patient with corneal clouding or an epithelial defect after irrigation should receive prompt ophthalmology referral.[7]

Treatment of chemosis without corneal or anterior chamber findings is with erythromycin ointment four times daily and referral for ophthalmologic examination in 24 to 48 hours. Ensure that tetanus vaccination is updated, and provide adequate analgesics if epithelial defect is present.

Orbital Compartment Syndrome

Blunt ocular trauma can lead an orbital (intraconal or extraconal) hemorrhage, which may rapidly elevate orbital pressure, transmitting pressure to the globe and optic nerve, and leading to ischemia and eventual blindness if not corrected in a timely fashion. It is

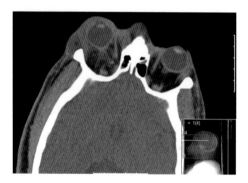

Figure 9.5 CT scan showing right retrobulbar hemorrhage in the intraconal space, causing right proptosis and a visible "tenting" of the globe where the optic nerve is connected (courtesy: Crimson House Publishing LLC)

important to distinguish preseptal from postseptal hemorrhage, given the clinical significance of the latter. Key history and physical exam findings are outlined in Box 9.1.

The most important tool for the emergency physician is high index of suspicion and a low threshold to take action and enlist help of an ophthalmologist. The diagnosis is made through use of tonometry, measuring intraocular pressures greater than 40 mmHg. Additionally, CT of the orbit can reveal retrobulbar or intraorbital hemorrhage as the source of the elevated pressures (Figure 9.5).

If orbital compartment syndrome is suspected, emergency ophthalmology consult should be requested. Management of orbital compartment syndrome is through emergent lateral canthotomy and inferior cantholysis, which reduce globe and intraocular pressure and reestablish retinal artery blood flow.[7] Outside of delay for ABC's of trauma resuscitation, there should be no other delays, including for imaging. The steps for lateral cantholysis are presented in Box 9.2.

After lateral canthotomy and inferior cantholysis, further management of orbital compartment syndrome includes elevation of the head of bed to 45°, pain control, correction of coagulopathy, management of elevated blood pressure after analgesia, prevention of sudden increases in intraocular pressure through use of antiemetics and cough suppression, and hospitalization for definitive management.

Carotid-Cavernous Fistula

An additional vision-threatening diagnosis as a result of blunt trauma is a carotid cavernous fistula (CCF). Seen in up to 4% of basilar skull fractures and other blunt facial trauma, a

Box 9.2 Steps For Lateral Canthotomy and Inferior Cantholysis[8]

1. Cleanse the area with povidone-iodine solution, hibiclense, or alcohol.
2. Using a 25 g needle, perform field block with infiltration of 1% or 2% lidocaine with epinephrine above and below the lateral canthus 1–2 cm.
3. Clamp a straight hemostat horizontally at the lateral canthal crus (between the upper and lower eyelid) for approximately 1 minute. This helps with hemostasis.
4. Remove the clamp, and with blunt-tipped scissors, cut between the upper and lower eyelid at the lateral canthus approximately 1 cm (called a lateral canthotomy).
5. Grasp the lower lid at the lid margin with forceps (i.e. Adsons) and provide upward traction toward the ceiling.
6. Identify the lateral canthal tendon with a strumming motion using closed scissors.
7. Once identified, cut the tendon until the eyelid is fully mobile (called an inferior cantholysis). The procedure is successful if the lateral lower eyelid can be mobilized to the superolateral orbital rim and to the temporal limbus.
8. Reassess visual acuity and intraocular pressure immediately after the procedure.
9. If intraocular pressure remains elevated, a superior cantholysis is needed. Identify and cut the superior crus of the canthal tendon.
10. Continue to provide hemostasis through direct compression of the wound at the orbital rim without further compression of the globe itself. Bipolar cautery may need to be used if bleeding at the canthotomy incision cannot be controlled.

Box 9.3 Signs and Symptoms of Carotid-Cavernous Fistula With Associated Percent of Patients With Findings

- Subjective bruit (80%), bruits may also be auscultated over the globe
- Blurred vision (25–29%)
- Headache (53–75%)
- Diplopia (50–85%)
- Ocular and/or orbital pain (35%)
- Proptosis (72–87%)
- Chemosis and conjunctival injection (55–89%)
- Cranial nerve VI palsy (50–85%)
- Cranial nerve III palsy (67%)
- Cranial nerve IV palsy (49%)
- Fundoscopic exam findings including dilated retinal veins and intraretinal hemorrhages

direct, high-flow CCF results from a direct connection between the carotid artery and the surrounding cavernous sinus.[9,10] Symptoms may manifest immediately or be delayed by days to weeks.[9] Symptoms are usually sudden in onset when they do occur and are the result of arterialization of orbital and ocular venous systems. Signs and symptoms are included in Box 9.3.[9,11–13]

The arterialization of conjunctival and episcleral vessels results from blood forced into the venous drainage of the orbit, leading to elevated episcleral venous pressure (Figures 9.6a and 9.6b), secondary glaucoma, and, rarely, catastrophic central retinal artery occlusion.[9,14]

If identified in the ED, CCF closure is the definitive treatment and should proceed without delay in consultation with neurosurgery or interventional radiology. However,

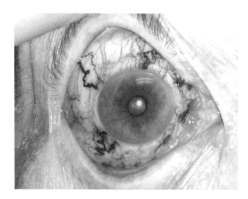

Figure 9.6a Photo showing typical appearance of enlarged "corkscrew" episcleral vessels (courtesy: Crimson House Publishing LLC)

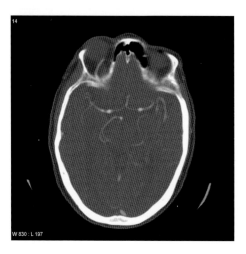

Figure 9.6b In the same patient as Figure 9.6a, the axial contrasted CT shows enlargement of the superior ophthalmic vein in the right orbit (courtesy: Crimson House Publishing LLC)

medical management of ocular sequelae is recommended. Since elevated intraocular pressures are seen in up to two-thirds of patients with CCF, treatment should proceed similar to that of open-angle glaucoma, through the use of acetazolamide, intravenous corticosteroids, and topical beta-blockers as adjuncts to reduce intraocular pressure.[9]

Open Globe Injury

An open globe injury can be one of the more dramatic ocular trauma emergencies, but it can also be more occult in nature. Open globe injuries can occur as a result of blunt or penetrating trauma. In the case of blunt trauma, the sudden increase in intraocular pressure will cause the globe to rupture at its thinnest points, such as the limbus or behind the insertion of extraocular muscles. In the case of penetrating trauma, any projectile has the potential to penetrate the eye.[7] The smaller the diameter of the projectile, the higher the likelihood of an occult globe rupture. Corneal abrasions associated with high-speed projectiles or mechanisms (i.e. machinery, hammering, weed-eaters, etc.) should raise suspicion for globe penetration as well. A classic historical feature is hammering "metal on metal."

At any step during examination of the eye, if open globe is suspected, then examination should be stopped, a protective shield should be placed over the eye, and an emergency

Box 9.4 Key Physical Exam Findings of an Open Globe Injury[7,8]

- Obvious corneal or scleral laceration
- Volume loss to eye
- Uveal (iris or ciliary body) prolapse
- Iris abnormalities (peaked or eccentric pupil)
- Extrusion of vitreous
- Seidel sign
- Hyphema
- Lens dislocation

- 360-degree, bullous subconjunctival hemorrhage
- Intraocular or protruding foreign body
- Decreased visual acuity
- Relevant afferent pupillary defect
- Increased (posterior rupture) or decreased (anterior rupture) anterior chamber depth
- Tenting of cornea or sclera at site of puncture

ophthalmology consult should be placed. Key physical exam findings of an open globe are included in Box 9.4. It should be noted that the examination might be normal or have minimal findings (i.e. small subconjunctival hemorrhage) in the setting of a tiny, high-speed projectile.

Diagnostic evaluation of an open globe injury should be via non-contrast CT scan with 1–2 mm axial and coronal images. CT cannot exclude open globe injury. Ultrasound, use of tonometry, and forced eyelid retraction should be avoided, as these result in increased pressure to the orbit and could lead to further extrusion of vitreous contents. There should be no medications placed into the eye, and protruding foreign bodies should not be removed. MRI is contraindicated if a metallic foreign body is suspected.

Management of an open globe injury includes emergent ophthalmology consultation, updated tetanus vaccination, and broad-spectrum antibiotics. If intubation is indicated due to additional associated injuries, the clinician should avoid high-dose ketamine (>4 mg/kg IV) or depolarizing neuromuscular blocking agents, as these may increase intraocular pressure. Ketamine with induction doses of 1–2 mg/kg IV is safe and does not raise intraocular pressure.

Traumatic Hyphema

A hyphema is a layering of red blood cells in the anterior chamber and is usually caused by blunt trauma to the eye, but it can also be spontaneous, such as in the case of sickle cell disease. Hyphemas are usually visible to the naked eye of the clinician but can be viewed easier and measured by slit lamp (Figure 9.7). The presence of a hyphema or microhyphema (seen only on slit lamp, but not visible to the naked eye) in the setting of a foreign body suggests open globe injury. In a supine patient, the hyphema may not be evident, due to the posterior layering of red blood cells. The anterior chamber may appear as red and hazy in this case. If the patient is placed in the upright position, the hyphema will layer out inferiorly and will be more evident on exam.

Hyphema should be evaluated in the ED by ophthalmology, particularly for those with associated open globe injuries, those with sickle cell disease, or those taking anticoagulants, as these patients tend to have more complications. Complications of hyphema include increased intraocular pressure, rebleeding, peripheral anterior synechiae, corneal blood

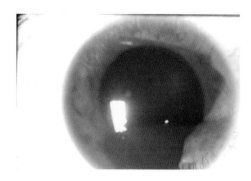

Figure 9.7 Grossly visible hyphema in the anterior chamber following blunt ocular injury. The hyphema is visible as a layering of red blood cells in the anterior chamber (courtesy: Crimson House Publishing LLC)

staining, optic atrophy, and accommodative impairment. Acute management includes elevating the head of the bed to 45° to promote inferior layering of red blood cells and avoid occlusion of trabecular meshwork.[7] In collaboration with an ophthalmologist, consider pupil dilation to avoid "pupillary play," the phenomenon of constriction and dilation movements of the iris in response to changing lighting conditions which stretch the involved iris vessel and causing rebleeding. Because the risk of rebleeding after initial injury is high, ophthalmologists may choose to admit and observe these patients or have close outpatient follow up. In general, patients with hyphema occupying one-third or less of the anterior chamber can be followed closely as outpatients.[7] Patients discharged from the ED should have eye shielding, instructions for limited activity, and cycloplegics, if appropriate. They should be instructed to maintain a head-elevated position at all times and to avoid anticoagulants. Glucocorticoids have been shown to decrease the risk of rebleeding but should only be prescribed in consultation with an ophthalmologist.[15]

Vitreous Hemorrhage

The vitreous is avascular and attached anteriorly at the ora serrata, posteriorly at the optic nerve head, and along the major retinal vessels.[7] Separation can cause bleeding of the retinal vessels, and the blood accumulates in the posterior vitreous. Patients describe "flashes," "floaters," and "cobwebs" in their visual fields. In cases of large vitreous hemorrhages, the red reflex may be obscured or asymmetric when compared to the uninvolved eye. Most cases of vitreous hemorrhage are spontaneous, caused by proliferative diabetic retinopathy or posterior vitreous detachments in the elderly. However, vitreous hemorrhages are seen often in infants as a result of non-accidental trauma. In the pediatric and adult population, vitreous hemorrhages seen in the setting of trauma could indicate worsening underlying intracranial trauma, such as subarachnoid or subdural bleeding, and further workup may be indicated. Vitreous hemorrhages can be viewed with direct or indirect ophthalmoscopy or through the use of ultrasound.

Retinal Trauma

Traumatic injuries to the retina result in loss of vision that can be partial or complete. They are often difficult to diagnose, as they are rarely isolated, and indirect ophthalmoscopy is challenging in the setting of an injured anterior chamber with a hyphema or otherwise hazy cornea. In this instance, ultrasound may be a better modality to view a retinal tear or detachment. Retinal injuries can be classified as retinal breaks, retinal detachments, retinal

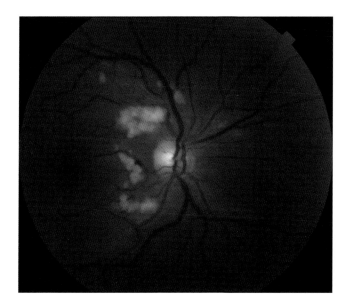

Figure 9.8 A fundus photograph of the right fundus of a patient following a severe thoracic crush injury, showing typical findings of Purtscher retinopathy: cotton-wool spots and flame-shaped intraretinal hemorrhages in a pattern radiating outward from the optic nerve (courtesy: Crimson House Publishing LLC)

edema, and Purtscher retinopathy, which is bilateral superficial retinal injuries around the optic nerve from compressive injuries of the head, chest, or lower extremities (Figure 9.8).

Optic Nerve Injury

The optic nerve can be injured directly or indirectly. Direct injury can occur from nerve laceration, contusion, or avulsion, or from direct puncture wounds. Indirect optic nerve injuries are much more common and occur from contusions within the optic canal from direct blows to the temple or brow.[8] Further evaluation of optic nerve injury is through complete ophthalmologic examination and CT imaging of the orbit. Management of optic nerve injury is guided by the underlying etiology and in conjunction with ophthalmology or neurology.

Other Traumatic Eye Presentations

Traumatic Uveitis

Anterior uveitis typically affects patients aged 20–50 years, with the traumatic form associated with blunt trauma. Patients most commonly present with unilateral pain, photophobia, and blurred vision.[16] Examination often reveals circumcorneal or limbic redness, with little conjunctival redness. The pupil is often poorly reactive or constricted. Slit lamp will demonstrate cell and flare, which represents inflammatory debris. If severe, a hypopyon may be present. Consensual photophobia is common. Treatment includes cycloplegics and oral anti-inflammatory agents. Steroids should only be used with ophthalmologist consultation. Complications include cataracts, glaucoma, macular edema, and band keratopathy. If IOP is elevated, the patient should be treated similarly to those with acute angle closure glaucoma. Most cases will resolve in 6 weeks.[16]

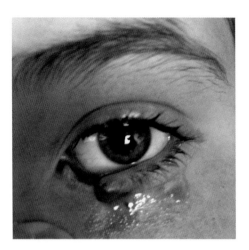

Figure 9.9 Full-thickness laceration of the left lower eyelid, crossing the lid margin medial to the punctum and involving the lower canaliculus (courtesy: Crimson House Publishing LLC)

Box 9.5 Types of Lacerations That Warrant Repair by Specialist[5,7,8]

- Involvement of lid margin
- Within 6–8 mm of medial canthus
- Involvement of the lacrimal duct or sac
- Involvement of inner surface of lid
- Associated with ptosis
- Involvement of tarsal plate or levator palpebrae
- Full-thickness of the eyelid
- Associated with orbital fat prolapse
- Associated with poor alignment and/or avulsion
- Associated with open globe injury or foreign body

Eyelid Lacerations

Eyelid lacerations are a common finding in ocular trauma. While not vision-threatening, they are often associated with other conditions that can be considered vision-threatening, such as open globe, traumatic hyphema, or corneal abrasions in up to two-thirds of cases.[8] In general, the emergency physician can carefully repair wounds that are superficial or those that are parallel to the lid margin. Repair of all other eyelid lacerations should be performed only by an ophthalmologist or others with special expertise in repair of the eyelid such as an ophthalmic plastic surgeon. The emergency physician should carefully evaluate for involvement of the medial canthus or canalicular structures, demonstrated in Figure 9.9. In many cases the lid laceration is inconspicuous, and the canalicular/lacrimal involvement may be overlooked. All eyelid lacerations medial to the puncta should be evaluated by an ophthalmologist or ophthalmic plastic surgeon within 24 hours. Other specific types of lacerations that should be repaired by a specialist are included in Box 9.5.

Corneal Abrasions and Corneal Foreign Bodies

Corneal abrasions and foreign bodies are common eye injuries. A recent review of 1400 ED ocular emergencies identified that 27% were related to trauma, of which 73% involved

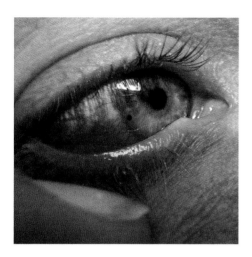

Figure 9.10 Corneal foreign body located at 9:00 position of right eye. Note the associated conjunctival injection (photo courtesy of E van Herk, reproduced under CC BY-SA 3.0 license https://creativecommons.org/licenses/by-sa/3.0/)

corneal abrasions, and 5% involved corneal foreign bodies.[6,17] A patient with corneal abrasion or foreign body will likely have severe photophobia, pain, diffuse injection, tearing, and a foreign body, or "scratchy" sensation (Figure 9.10). Visual acuity is usually retained except for the case of corneal abrasion or foreign body in the central visual axis or if the patient has associated iritis. Use of a topical anesthetic can facilitate an accurate physical examination with slit lamp or Wood's lamp and assessment of visual acuity. Use fluorescein staining to assess for corneal abrasions with cobalt blue filter on slit lamp, or with Wood's lamp. Caution should be exercised in use of Wood's lamp as the single examination tool due to increased chances of missing microscopic or punctate abrasions. Fluorescein staining can also be used to determine Seidel sign in the setting of full-thickness corneal lacerations, although it can be negative if a diagonally avulsed corneal flap closes the laceration, or if the full-thickness laceration is small and has closed spontaneously. Discovery of multiple corneal abrasions in parallel vertical lines at the upper edge of the cornea is suspicious for retained upper palpebral conjunctival foreign body as the source.

Foreign bodies may or may not be obvious to the patient initially, as they may not recall a specific incident for which the foreign body may have entered the eye. In the case of potential for high velocity foreign body introduction to the eye (i.e. metal grinding, compressed air tools, lawn equipment, etc.), the emergency physician should have high index of suspicion for penetrating eye injury or intraocular foreign body. In most instances, corneal foreign bodies are easy to identify on slit lamp exam. Special care should be taken to evaluate for retained foreign bodies on the palpebral conjunctiva through inversion and sweeping of the upper and lower lids. Corneal foreign bodies may be removed in the ED, with the exception of full-thickness corneal foreign bodies, which should be removed by an ophthalmologist. Attempts to remove superficial corneal foreign bodies may be attempted through use of saline irrigation, moistened cotton applicator, a 25-gauge needle with the beveled edge up, or a sterile foreign body spud on an Alger brush. This should be performed in conjunction with the slit lamp for magnification. After removal of a metallic foreign body, a rust ring may be present which will require removal. It may be removed via ophthalmic burr or spud, but often reaccumulates within 24 hours. Therefore, it is not necessary to remove a rust ring in the ED if a patient can be seen by ophthalmology the

Table 9.6 Suggested ophthalmic antibiotics for corneal abrasions[6]

Situation	Antibiotic
Not related to contact lens wearer	Erythromycin ophthalmic ointment 3–4 times daily
Related to contact lens wearer	Ciprofloxacin, ofloxacin, or tobramycin 3–4 times daily
Organic source	Erythromycin ointment 3–4 times daily

following day.[7] No ED drill burring should take place if the rust ring is located in the visual axis (pupil) owing to the risk of visually significant scarring.[7]

After successful removal of a corneal foreign body, the patient may be discharged with topical antibiotics, cycloplegics, and oral analgesics, with consideration of coverage for *Pseudomonas aeruginosa* infections in contact lens wearers. The same treatment applies for corneal abrasions. Suggested antibiotics are listed in Table 9.6. Patients should be instructed to discontinue contact lens wear in the affected eye until they are cleared to resume by their ophthalmologist.

The decision to prescribe a limited supply of topical anesthetic (i.e. less than 72 hours) to aid in analgesia for patients following a simple corneal abrasion is a topic of debate. While it has been shown to improve patient comfort and decrease oral analgesic requirements,[18,19] abuse of topical anesthetics has been associated with severe and potentially sight-threatening corneal complications. The potential risks must be carefully weighed with the benefit for each individual patient.

Conjunctival Injury

Conjunctival injuries include subconjunctival hemorrhage and conjunctival laceration, foreign bodies, and abrasions. The patient will likely be complaining of photophobia, pain, diffuse injection, tearing, and a foreign body or "scratchy" sensation. Consider use of topical anesthetic to facilitate thorough evaluation, except for cases where there is strong suspicion for open globe injury. The slit lamp is the preferred tool for evaluation in conjunctival injuries.

Subconjunctival Hemorrhages

These are usually benign and not associated with underlying intraocular injury. They usually heal spontaneously and may be evaluated by ophthalmology on a non-urgent outpatient basis. However, in the setting of bullous, elevated subconjunctival hemorrhage, there may be a hidden underlying laceration.[8]

Conjunctival Lacerations

Conjunctival lacerations (Figure 9.11), if identified, should raise suspicion for open globe injury or traumatic hyphema. CT of the orbit can better evaluate for this condition. Consider urgent ophthalmology consultation to evaluate for additional retinal trauma and to definitively rule out open globe injury.[20] All patients with conjunctival lacerations should be discussed with an ophthalmologist if available, and those greater than 1 cm in length require urgent ophthalmology consultation for repair.[20] If a conjunctival laceration is determined to be superficial, not associated with any other serious intraorbital or ocular injury, and is small (<1 cm), the patient may receive treatment with an antibiotic ointment (Table 9.6) and be referred for ophthalmologic evaluation in 1–3 days.[20,21]

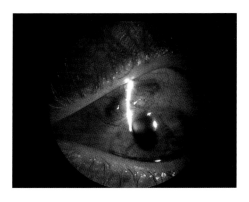

Figure 9.11 Occult scleral laceration following blunt ocular trauma. The pupil is peaked superiorly, and the dark uveal tissue is seen bulging through a scleral rupture into the subconjunctival space. Since the uveal tissue "plugged" the scleral rupture, the patient's visual acuity and intraocular pressure were both normal (photo: R. Grant Morshedi MD)

Conjunctival Foreign Bodies

These may cause similar symptoms to corneal foreign bodies, but to a lesser degree due to decreased sensory innervation compared to the cornea. Careful evaluation of the palpebral conjunctiva through lid eversion may lead to discovery of an innocuous retained foreign body. Ophthalmology consultation is indicated for patients with foreign bodies which are deeply embedded, subconjunctival, or present in the context of a conjunctival laceration.[20] A conjunctival foreign body may be removed, similar to how a corneal foreign body is removed. After removal, the patient should receive an antibiotic ointment (Table 9.6) and be referred to ophthalmology in 1–3 days.

Conjunctival Abrasions

Conjunctival abrasions may occur from blunt injuries and mild chemical or thermal burns. They may present as epithelial irregularities that fluoresce under cobalt blue light with fluorescein staining and may be associated with corneal defects as well. A detailed ocular examination should be performed to rule out other injuries. Isolated conjunctival abrasions are treated with antibiotic ointment (Table 9.6). Referral to an ophthalmologist for a complete eye examination within 1–3 days of injury is a reasonable precaution in patients who are contact lens wearers or for all other patients if symptoms are not resolving. These injuries typically heal in 1–3 days.[20]

Orbital Fractures

Orbital fractures typically occur due to blunt trauma. They are often associated with other significant facial trauma or intracranial injury. Initial evaluation should focus on airway, breathing, and circulation. In addition to other facial or intracranial injury, there is often associated significant intraocular injury, such as ruptured globe, hyphema, or retinal injury. The most common location of an isolated orbital fracture is the floor (known as a blow-out fracture) medial to the infra-orbital nerve (CN V2). The next most common location is the medial wall. The lateral wall and lateral floor are not typically found in isolation. Rather, they are associated findings with zygomaticomaxillary complex fractures (ZMC fracture).

After evaluating for life-threatening conditions, the ophthalmic exam should evaluate for periocular or craniofacial injuries. Start by assessing the visual acuity of each eye. The patient may have a complaint of diplopia, which is multifactorial (edema, ocular muscle injury, nerve damage, hemorrhage). Then perform an external exam of the periocular

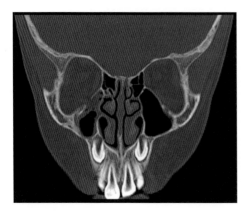

Figure 9.12 Coronal CT orbits showing blowout fracture of right orbital floor, with inferior rectus muscle incarceration in the relatively small fracture (courtesy: Crimson House Publishing LLC)

tissues. Assess for widened intercanthal distance and limited extraocular motility. In the setting of orbital floor fracture, the inferior rectus may be entrapped, leading to limited upward gaze on the affected side (Figure 9.12). In the setting of medial orbital wall fracture, the medial rectus may be entrapped, leading to limited lateral gaze on the affected side. There may be decreased sensation (hypesthesia) to the forehead or the cheek from injury to the supraorbital (CN V1) or infraorbital nerves (CN V2), respectively, as a result of a fracture. Most common is the V2 dermatomal distribution. The pupils should be evaluated for afferent pupillary defect. The ocular motility is then assessed. Limitation may be evidence of orbital fracture, periorbital swelling, orbital hemorrhage, or extraocular muscle defect (laceration or hematoma).

NOTE: If rupture globe is suspected and the eyelid is obscuring the eye, it is recommended to defer for urgent ophthalmology consult, as any pressure on the eye or eyelid can expulse the intra-ocular contents. Place a vaulted cover over the eye and contact an ophthalmologist for urgent consult or transfer.

Evaluation of the globe should focus on quickly identifying any vision-threatening conditions, such as ruptured globe, orbital compartment syndrome, retinal detachment, or hyphema. Evaluation of the globe may reveal exophthalmos due to periorbital swelling and hemorrhage, or enophthalmos as the result of a large medial wall and floor fracture. However, enophthalmos is typically masked in the acute setting due to swelling. Assess for signs of a ruptured globe, such as extrusion of intraocular contents, severe conjunctival hemorrhage, or a misshapen pupil. Finally, perform a detailed slit-lamp examination assessing for conjunctival lacerations, scleral lacerations, exposed uvea, corneal abrasions, corneal lacerations, hyphema, iritis, iris tears, iris deformities, or lens dislocation. Lastly, perform a fundoscopic examination, assessing for vitreous hemorrhage or retinal injury.

CT scan should be performed for a patient with orbital trauma and any of the following: periocular ecchymosis and swelling, lateral canthal displacement, proptosis, enophthalmos, limited ocular motility, cranial nerve V1/V2 hypesthesia, decreased visual acuity, severe periorbital pain, or inadequate examination in conditions such as excessive soft tissue swelling or altered mental status.[22] Figure 9.12 demonstrates inferior rectus muscle entrapment in an orbital floor fracture.

Management of orbital fractures should first focus on life-threatening conditions, followed by vision-threatening conditions. Obtain an emergent ophthalmology consultation if the patient is found to have any globe injuries, suspected ruptured globe, or severe

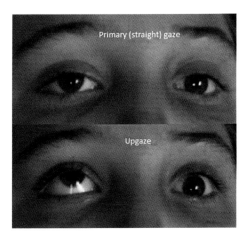

Figure 9.13a "White-eyed fracture." Demonstration of upgaze deficit on right eye (courtesy: Dr. Alice Behrens)

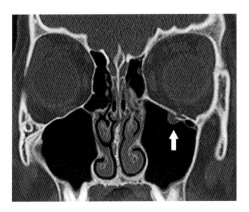

Figure 9.13b "White-eyed fracture." In same patient as Figure 9.13a, the corresponding CT image showing orbital floor fracture and inferior rectus entrapment (courtesy: Dr. Josh Hardin)

vagal symptoms as a result of the oculocardiac reflex. The latter is typically seen in younger patients (under 18) who have an extraocular muscle not only trapped within a fracture, but also being compressed (causing ischemia). Younger patients' orbital bones are more pliable and tend to fracture as a trapped-door. Additionally, orbital fractures in younger patients have less swelling and can appear completely normal, the so-called white-eyed fracture. However, when assessing ocular motility, the eye will not move, and the heart rate becomes bradycardic. These types of fractures are easily overlooked and harbor grave consequences (permanent damage to the ocular muscle and diplopia). In this setting, an orbital surgeon should be consulted immediately and the fracture repaired as soon as medically possible.[23] Figure 9.13a demonstrates the upgaze deficit and Figure 9.13b demonstrates the corresponding CT image showing the orbital floor fracture and the inferior rectus entrapment.

The emergency physician may need to initially manage these conditions through protection of the globe, elevation of the head, intravenous fluids, antiemetics, and pain control. A patient with orbital hematomas exhibiting signs of orbital compartment syndrome may require emergent lateral canthotomy to decompress the orbit.

All orbital wall fractures with no other associated injuries and normal initial eye examination in the ED should be referred to an ophthalmologist for an outpatient dilated examination to rule out any unidentified retinal tears or detachments.[7] For patients with a history of chronic sinus infections, or for the isolated medial wall, start oral antibiotics (i.e. cephalexin or clindamycin for 7–10 days).[7] Instruct the patient to not blow his/her nose for at least 4–5 weeks from date of injury. Isolated orbital wall fractures with or without entrapment and without any eye injury do not require immediate surgery and can be referred within 1–4 days to an ophthalmic plastic surgeon (oculoplastics); or to both an ophthalmologist and either an oral maxillofacial surgeon, or an otolaryngologist (depending on the local referral patterns). Most repairs are performed between 10–14 days after initial injury. The only orbital fracture emergency is the white-eye fracture discussed above (normal external exam, but has limited ocular motility, and bradycardia/nausea with ocular movement).[23]

Pitfalls in ED evaluation and management

- While eye protection decreases the risk of eye trauma, it does not completely prevent it. Just because a patient states he/she was wearing eye protection, the emergency physician should still be diligent in performing a complete eye physical examination to evaluate for injuries if the patient has a complaint.
- The emergency physician should have a high index of suspicion for associated injuries with eye trauma. Be aware of the increased risk for additional facial trauma, intracranial or cervical spine injury, or cranial nerve injury.
- Most patients with eye trauma can be appropriately managed in the ED and safely discharged home with close outpatient ophthalmology follow up. However, the emergency physician should know which conditions described in this chapter require emergent ophthalmology consultation vs. urgent or routine outpatient ophthalmology follow up.
- If an open globe injury is suspected, do not place any drops in the eye (i.e. topical anesthetic, fluorescein, etc.) and do not place excessive pressure on the globe through use of examination maneuvers (i.e. ocular ultrasound, prying lids open, tonometry, etc.). Simply cover the eye with a shield and provide supportive care while arranging emergent ophthalmology consultation.
- While most orbital wall fractures are benign and can be followed up as an outpatient, special attention should be paid for evaluation of the more serious and occult "white-eyed fracture" in younger patients, where the eye appears normal on straight gaze, but will demonstrate deficits in ocular motility with associated bradycardia.

References

1. United States Eye Injury Registry. Available at: https://useir.org/epidemiology/. Accessed January 27, 2018.

2. Pandita A, Merriman M. Ocular trauma epidemiology: 10-year retrospective study. N Z Med J. 2012;125:61.

3. Kanoff JM, Turalba AV, Andreoli MT, Andreoli CM. Characteristics and outcomes of work-related open globe injuries. Am J Ophthalmol. 2010;150:265.

4. Kuhn F, Morris R, Witherspoon CD, Mann L. Epidemiology of blinding trauma in the United States Eye Injury Registry. Ophthalmic Epidemiol. 2006;13:209.

5. Gardiner MF. Approach to eye injuries in the ED. 2017. www.uptodate.com. Accessed December 14, 2017.

6. Harlan JB Jr, Pieramici DJ. Evaluation of patients with ocular trauma. *Ophthalmol Clin North Am*. 2002;15:153.

7. Tintinalli, JE. *Tintinalli's Emergency Medicine: A Comprehensive Study Guide*, 8th ed. New York: McGraw Hill Education; 2016.

8. Gardiner, MF. (August 25). Overview of eye injuries in the ED. 2017. www.uptodate.com. Accessed December 14, 2017.

9. Bennett JL, Gonzalez MO. Carotid-cavernous fistulas. 2017. www.uptodate.com. Accessed January 2,2018.

10. Liang W, Xiaofeng Y, Weiguo L, et al. Traumatic carotid cavernous fistula accompanying basilar skull fracture: a study on the incidence of traumatic carotid cavernous fistula in the patients with basilar skull fracture and the prognostic analysis about traumatic carotid cavernous fistula. *J Trauma*. 2007;63:1014.

11. Lewis AI, Tomsick TA, Tew JM Jr. Management of 100 consecutive direct carotid-cavernous fistulas: results of treatment with detachable balloons. *Neurosurgery*. 1995;36:239.

12. Gupta AK, Purkayastha S, Krishnamoorthy T, et al. Endovascular treatment of direct carotid cavernous fistulae: a pictorial review. *Neuroradiology*. 2006;48:831.

13. Wang W, Li YD, Li MH, et al. Endovascular treatment of post-traumatic direct carotid-cavernous fistulas: a single-center experience. *J Clin Neurosci*. 2011;18:24.

14. de Keizer R. Carotid-cavernous and orbital arteriovenous fistulas: ocular features, diagnostic and hemodynamic considerations in relation to visual impairment and morbidity. *Orbit*. 2003;22:121.

15. Brandt MT, Haug RH. Traumatic hyphema: a comprehensive review. *J Oral Maxillofac Surg*. 2001;59:1462.

16. Deibel JP, Cowling K. Ocular inflammation and infection. *Emerg Med Clin North Am*. 2013;31(2):387–97.

17. Alotaibi AG, Osman EA, Allam KH, et al. One month outcome of ocular related emergencies in a tertiary hospital in Central Saudi Arabia. *Saudi Med J*. 2011;32:1256.

18. Swaminathan A, Otterness K, Milne K, Rezaie S. The safety of topical anesthetics in the treatment of corneal abrasions: a review. *J Emerg Med*. 2015;49(5):810–15.

19. Ball IM, Seabrook J, Desai N, Allen L, Anderson S. Dilute proparacaine for the management of acute corneal injuries in the emergency department. *CJEM*. 2010;12(5):389–96.

20. Gardiner MF, Kloek CE. Conjunctival injury. 2017. www.uptodate.com. Accessed December 28, 2107.

21. Bord SP, Linden J. Trauma to the globe and orbit. *Emerg Med Clin N Am*. 2008;26:97.

22. Neuman MI, Bachur RG. Orbital fractures. 2017. www.uptodate.com. Accessed December 29, 2017.

23. Yew C, Shaari R, Rahman SA, et al. White-eyed blowout fracture: diagnostic pitfalls and review of literature. *Injury*. 2015;46:1856–59.

Cervical Spine Trauma

Katja Goldflam

Injury of the cervical spine occurs most commonly due to high impact blunt trauma.[1-3] It is the most commonly injured portion of the spine as it is not as well protected as the lower thoracic and lumbar spine. The most commonly injured vertebrae are C2 and C5-7, and injuries are more common in males than females.[1,2,4]

Anatomy

The cervical spine consists of seven vertebrae, including the atlas and axis (C1 and C2, respectively), that permit rotation of the head on the spinal column. Multiple ligaments hold the bony components in place, giving rise to the three columns of the cervical spine described by Denis[5] (Table 10.1). Any single column injury may be considered stable, while two-column injuries result in greater mobility, and three-column injuries are always unstable.

History and Physical Examination

- Patients most often have a known history of trauma, with high energy blunt trauma being the most common etiology.[1,2]
- Unconscious or altered patients who are unable to provide a reliable history or physical examination should raise suspicion for cervical spine injury in the appropriate clinical setting.
- Pain with or without range of motion of the neck is common.
- Paresthesias, focal weakness, and other focal neurologic deficits may occur.
- A rectal examination should be performed to assess for rectal tone.
- Patients may have external signs of trauma, tenderness to palpation over the midline, or step-offs on examination of the cervical spine.

Table 10.1 Spinal columns

Anterior column	Anterior longitudinal ligament, anterior annulus fibrosus, as well as anterior half of vertebral body, and adjacent intervertebral disk
Middle column	Posterior longitudinal ligament and posterior annulus fibrosus, as well as posterior half of vertebral body, and adjacent intervertebral disk
Posterior column	Posterior ligamentous complex, transverse and spinous processes, pedicles, laminae, and facet joints

- Though used in validated clinical guidelines and part of the current EAST practice management guidelines,[6] the reliability of the physical examination has been questioned. One study found the clinical examination, defined as neck pain, external trauma, neurologic deficit, or tenderness or other palpable abnormalities over the cervical spine to be 76.9% sensitive with a negative predictive value 95.7% when compared to CT findings.[7]

Immobilization

- When suspicion for injury exists, the cervical spine should be immobilized with in-line stabilization in a rigid collar until imaging is obtained.[8]
- Alternatively, the collar may be cleared clinically using the NEXUS or Canadian C-spine criteria, as detailed in the next section.[9-11]
- Patients that have persistent symptoms, such as midline tenderness to palpation, should remain immobilized in a cervical collar until an MRI can be performed to evaluate for ligamentous injury or appropriate follow up is arranged.[12,13]
- Recent debate has focused on the possible harms of cervical spine immobilization, including raised intracranial pressure in patients with head injury, delays in resuscitation, and complications of airway management,[14,15] however it remains the current standard of care.

Decision to Image

- Two commonly used criteria to help decide when imaging is appropriate are the NEXUS and Canadian Cervical Spine Rule.
- *NEXUS:*[9]
  - These five criteria have been validated with a 100% sensitivity of excluding cervical spine fractures, with original studies utilizing C-spine radiographs and not CT.
  - If absence of all five criteria are met, the cervical collar can be removed safely without any imaging (Box 10.1).
- *Canadian C-spine Rule:*[10,11,16]
  - This rule allows for clearance of a greater number of patients when compared to NEXUS (Table 10.2).

Exclusion criteria:
- Non-trauma patients
- GCS <15
- Unstable vital signs
- Age <16 years
- Acute paralysis

Box 10.1 NEXUS Criteria[9]
- Midline tenderness
- Neurologic deficits
- Altered mental status
- Intoxication
- Distracting injury

Table 10.2 Canadian C-spine rule

High-risk criteria	Age >65, paresthesias in any extremities, dangerous mechanism
Low-risk criteria	Sitting position in the ED, ambulatory at any time, delayed onset of neck pain, no midline tenderness

- Known vertebral disease
- Previous cervical spine surgery

Application of the rule:

- Patients with ANY high-risk criteria should be imaged.
- Patients without high risk criteria but who DO NOT MEET ANY low risk criteria should be imaged.
- Patients who have NO high-risk criteria and AT LEAST ONE low-risk criteria should be asked to range their neck 45° left and right; if unable to do so, they should be imaged (some pain is acceptable as long as the range of motion is not limited).

There is some evidence to suggest that, in patients older than 55 years, midline tenderness of the cervical spine may not be a good enough indicator of injury, and that more liberal use of imaging should be considered.[17]

Imaging

- Patients who meet the above criteria or are in some other way considered high-risk should undergo imaging.
- Plain radiographs have largely been replaced by CT as the preferred imaging modality.[6]
- Certain patients with low suspicion for injury and expected normal anatomy (i.e. no history of arthritis, osteoporosis, etc.) may be considered for evaluation by plain radiographs, but the sensitivity for acute fractures is limited.[4,18,19]
- One such meta-analysis by Holmes and Akkinepalli[18] in 2005 showed a pooled sensitivity for plain radiographs of 52% and 98% for CT.
- Plain radiographs include three views:
  - Lateral
  - Anteroposterior
  - Odontoid

- CT scans should visualize the entire cervical spine from the occiput of the skull to the junction of C7 and T1 for complete imaging.
- In patients with fractures found on CT completion, imaging of the entire spine should be performed, as up to 19% of patients may have additional non-contiguous vertebral fractures in the cervical, thoracic, or lumbar spine.[3,20]
- MRI should be obtained in patients with concern for ligamentous or spinal cord injury, including patients with normal CT scans with persistent pain or neurologic findings.[12,13]
- Flexion/extension views should not be used in obtunded patients. While they may be considered in alert patients if MRI is not available,[21,22] a recent review by Oh et al.[23] in 2016 shows their diagnostic value is likely limited and that they add little further information to a negative CT scan.

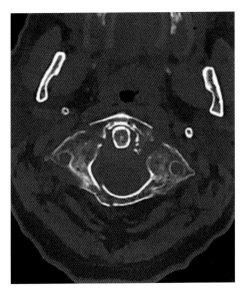

Figure 10.1 Jefferson burst fracture of C1 (image courtesy of Hellerhoff, reproduced here under CC BY-SA 3.0 license https://creativecommons.org/licenses/by-sa/3.0/)

- Vascular imaging with CTA or MRA should be considered in patients where there is concern for injury to the vessels, including with fractures to the skull base or foramina.[24–26]

Types of Fractures/Patterns

- These depend on the location of injury, as well as the mechanism of trauma.
- Injuries to the atlas (C1) and axis (C2) are often unstable, which include:
  - Occipital condyle fracture
  - Atlanto-occipital dislocation
  - Atlanto-axial dislocation
  - Jefferson (burst) fracture of C1 (Figure 10.1)
  - Odontoid/dens fracture of C2 (Figure 10.2)
  - Hangman's fracture of C2 (Figure 10.3)
- Fractures of the C3–7 vertebrae vary in stability and are classified by the pattern of injury:[5,27–29]
  - Compression-flexion
  - Compression-extension
  - Vertical compression (axial loading)
  - Distraction-flexion
  - Distraction-extension
  - Lateral flexion

General ED Management

- Immobilization should be maintained in all patients with known fractures; a padded collar should be used to prevent pressure sores and discomfort with long-term wear.[30]
- Adequate pain control should be ensured.

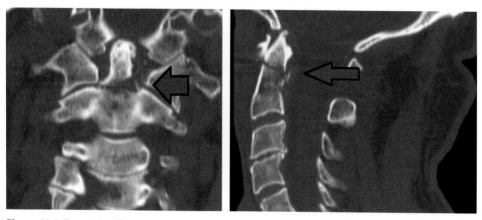

Figure 10.2 Type 2 dens fracture (images courtesy of James Heilman, MD, reproduced here under CC BY-SA 4.0 license https://creativecommons.org/licenses/by-sa/4.0/)

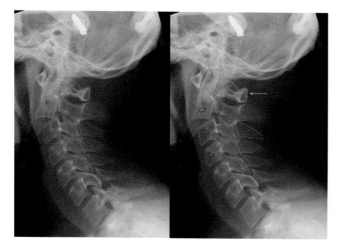

Figure 10.3 Hangman's fracture of C2 (images courtesy of Lucien Monfils, reproduced here under CC BY-SA 3.0 license https://creativecommons.org/licenses/by-sa/3.0/)

- Neurologic checks should be performed periodically to recognize any deterioration in neurologic status early.
- Need for surgical intervention will depend on the fracture pattern, (specifically stability vs instability), evidence of neurologic compromise (e.g. from nerve impingement, edema, or hematoma), as well as patient characteristics and suitability for operative repair.
  - This should be determined by a consultant spine surgeon.
- Reasons for admission include:
  - Unstable fracture patterns
  - Planned surgical intervention
  - Neurologic deficits
  - Concern for possible progressive decompensation
  - Additional significant injuries requiring monitoring or intervention
  - Lack of a safe disposition plan

- Patients with stable fractures, clear follow up plans, and no safety concerns may be considered for discharge.
- Strict return precautions should include any change in or worsening of symptoms, including pain and neurologic complaints.

Airway Management

- High cervical spine neurologic injuries likely result in respiratory compromise.
- Trauma to the C1–3 vertebrae and adjacent spinal cord is most likely to cause phrenic nerve injury, though patients with injury up to C5 are at risk.
- Phrenic nerve injury will result in paralysis of the diaphragm and respiratory depression.
- Additional trauma around the area of the cervical spine may be indicative of proximal airway injury, including airway edema, soft tissue swelling, or expanding hematomas, and a low threshold for intubation should be maintained.
- In emergent cases, rapid sequence intubation should be performed while strict in-line stabilization is maintained.[31]
- When the clinical situation permits and intubation is performed on a more elective basis, awake fiberoptic intubation allows for minimal movement and exacerbation of injury.

Steroids

Based on current data, steroids are not recommended in patients with spinal cord injury.[32]

- No conclusive Class I or II evidence of beneficial effects exists, and Class III data is methodologically limited or inconsistent.
- Harmful side-effects reported included wound infections and other infectious complications, hyperglycemia, and GI hemorrhage, as well as higher mortality unrelated to severity of injuries.

Complications

- *Additional traumatic injuries* may be present, including trauma to lower parts of the spine, and should be evaluated appropriately.[3,20]
  - In one series, 57% of patients had additional extra-spinal injuries, and 19% had non-contiguous spinal trauma.[20]

- *Neurological findings* may be suggestive of complete or partial spinal cord injury.
  - Complete spinal cord injury: complete loss of motor and sensory function below the level of injury.
  - Partial spinal cord syndromes are shown in Table 10.3.[33,34]

- *Spinal cord injury without radiographic abnormality* (SCIWORA) is a rare but important clinical entity, the definition of which is changing in the era of MRI.[33,35]
  - Strong evidence-based recommendations for management are missing due to the diversity of patients included in this definition.
  - Recently developed MRI classifications are being used for prognostication based on imaging patterns.[35]

Table 10.3 Partial spinal cord syndromes

Central cord syndrome	Cervical motor weakness of upper extremities greater than lower extremities
Hemisection (Brown-Sequard) syndrome	Ipsilateral motor and proprioception/light touch loss; contralateral pain and temperature sensation loss
Anterior cord syndrome	Motor function and pain/temperature sensation loss; sparing of light touch and proprioception

- *Hypotension*:
  - Hemorrhagic shock should be considered as the etiology in any trauma patient.
  - Neurogenic shock may occur secondary to decreased sympathetic output after injury to the upper spinal cord; the resultant unopposed vagal tone causes vasodilation and hypotension without the expected reflexive tachycardia (i.e. a relative bradycardia).[33,36]
  - In patients unresponsive to resuscitation with fluids or blood, vasopressors should be initiated for presumed neurogenic shock. A mean arterial pressure goal of 80 mm Hg is recommended.

- *Spinal shock* describes the neurologic findings that accompany the acute period of injury to the spinal cord.
  - The deficits may be temporary, and permanent deficits can only be confirmed once the shock period has passed.
  - Absent bulbocavernosus and cremasteric reflexes confirm the diagnosis.[33]

- *Vascular injuries* are most common in patients with hyperextension or hyperflexion mechanisms, fractures at the base of the skull or of the vascular foraminae, and especially in patients with C1–3 injuries.[24–26]

Clinical Clearance of Cervical Spine

In patients with negative imaging, the collar should be opened anteriorly, and the posterior midline should be re-examined for tenderness to palpation. Patients with persistent pain or tenderness should remain with the collar in place. When no midline tenderness is found, patients should be asked to range their neck left and right 45° in each direction, as well as up and down; if this does not elicit any discomfort the collar can be safely removed.[10,37]

Consultation Indications

Any patient with evidence of cervical spine fracture or neurologic injury should be evaluated by an appropriate consultant, either a neurologic or orthopedic spine surgeon. Involvement of social work or a care management team may be beneficial when any long-term safety or disposition concerns exist.

Pitfalls in ED Management

- Not maintaining appropriate cervical spine immobilization
- Not managing airway early

- Not considering additional traumatic injuries
- Not imaging the remainder of the spine[3,20]
- Not considering vascular injury, especially in higher cervical spine lesions (C3 and above)

Key Points

- Immobilization prior to imaging in any patient with concern for cervical spine injury is recommended.
- CT scans should be the first line of imaging.
- MRI (or appropriate follow up if not available) should be obtained if concern for ligamentous injury remains after negative CT imaging.
- Use the NEXUS or Canadian C-Spine Rule when considering imaging.
- Consider complications including neurologic injury without bony trauma, spinal shock, vascular injuries, and SCIWORA.
- Clinically clear the cervical spine when appropriate.
- Ensure appropriate consultation and follow up when indicated.

References

1. Oliver M, Inaba K, Tang A, et al. The changing epidemiology of spinal trauma: a 13-year review from a Level I trauma centre. *Injury.* 2012;43(8):1296–300.

2. Hasler RM, Exadaktylos AK, Bouamra O, et al. Epidemiology and predictors of cervical spine injury in adult major trauma patients: a multicenter cohort study. *J Trauma Acute Care Surg.* 2012;72(4):975–81.

3. Nelson DW, Martin MJ, Martin ND, Beekley A. Evaluation of the risk of noncontiguous fractures of the spine in blunt trauma. *J Trauma Acute Care Surg.* 2013;75(1):135–39.

4. Greenbaum J, Walters N, Levy PD. An evidenced-based approach to radiographic assessment of cervical spine injuries in the emergency department. *J Emerg Med.* 2009;36(1):64–71.

5. Denis F. Spinal instability as defined by the three-column spine concept in acute spinal trauma. *Clin Orthop Relat Res.* 1984; (189):65–76.

6. Como JJ, Diaz JJ, Dunham CM, et al. Practice management guidelines for identification of cervical spine injuries following trauma: update from the Eastern Association for the Surgery of Trauma Practice Management Guidelines Committee. *J Trauma.* 2009;67(3):651–59.

7. Duane TM, Dechert T, Wolfe LG, et al. Clinical examination and its reliability in identifying cervical spine fractures. *J Trauma.* 2007;62(6):1405–8, discussion 1408–10.

8. ATLS Subcommittee; American College of Surgeons' Committee on Trauma; International ATLS working group. Advanced trauma life support (ATLS®): the ninth edition. *J Trauma Acute Care Surg.* 2013;74(5):1363–66.

9. Hoffman JR, Mower WR, Wolfson AB, Todd KH, Zucker MI. Validity of a set of clinical criteria to rule out injury to the cervical spine in patients with blunt trauma. National Emergency X-Radiography Utilization Study Group. *N Engl J Med.* 2000;343(2):94–99.

10. Stiell IG, Wells GA, Vandemheen KL, et al. The Canadian C-spine rule for radiography in alert and stable trauma patients. *JAMA.* 2001;286(15):1841–48.

11. Stiell IG, Clement CM, McKnight RD, et al. The Canadian C-spine rule versus the

NEXUS low-risk criteria in patients with trauma. *N Engl J Med.* 2003;349(26):2510–18.

12. Goldberg AL, Kershah SM. Advances in imaging of vertebral and spinal cord injury. *J Spinal Cord Med.* 2010;33(2):105–16.

13. Ackland HM, Cameron PA, Varma DK et al. Cervical spine magnetic resonance imaging in alert, neurologically intact trauma patients with persistent midline tenderness and negative computed tomography results. *Ann Emerg Med.* 2011;58(6):521–30.

14. Abram S, Bulstrode C. Routine spinal immobilization in trauma patients: what are the advantages and disadvantages? *Surgeon.* 2010;8(4):218–22.

15. Deasy C, Cameron P. Routine application of cervical collars – what is the evidence? *Injury.* 2011;42(9):841–42.

16. Bandiera G, Stiell IG, Wells GA, et al. The Canadian C-spine rule performs better than unstructured physician judgment. *Ann Emerg Med.* 2003;42(3):395–402.

17. Healey CD, Spilman SK, King BD, Sherrill JE 2nd, Pelaez CA. Asymptomatic cervical spine fractures: current guidelines can fail older patients. *J Trauma Acute Care Surg.* 2017;83(1):119–25.

18. Holmes JF, Akkinepalli R. Computed tomography versus plain radiography to screen for cervical spine injury: A meta-analysis. *J Trauma.* 2005;58(5):902–5.

19. Mathen R, Inaba K, Munera F, et al. Prospective evaluation of multislice computed tomography versus plain radiographic cervical spine clearance in trauma patients. *J Trauma.* 2007;62(6):1427–31.

20. Miller CP, Brubacher JW, Biswas D, et al. The incidence of noncontiguous spinal fractures and other traumatic injuries associated with cervical spine fractures: a 10-year experience at an academic medical center. *Spine.* 2011;36(19):1532–40.

21. Crim JR, Moore K, Brodke D. Clearance of the cervical spine in multitrauma patients: the role of advanced imaging. *Semin Ultrasound CT MR.* 2001;22(4):283–305.

22. Pollack CV Jr, Hendey GW, Martin DR, Hoffman JR, Mower WR; NEXUS Group. Use of flexion-extension radiographs of the cervical spine in blunt trauma. *Ann Emerg Med.* 2001;38(1):8–11.

23. Oh JJ, Asha SE, Curtis K. Diagnostic accuracy of flexion-extension radiography for the detection of ligamentous cervical spine injury following a normal cervical spine computed tomography. *Emerg Med Australas.* 2016;28(4):450–55.

24. Biffl WL, Moore EE, Offner PJ, Burch JM. Blunt carotid and vertebral arterial injuries. *World J Surg.* 2001;25(8):1036–43.

25. Miller PR, Fabian TC, Croce MA, et al. Prospective screening for blunt cerebrovascular injuries: analysis of diagnostic modalities and outcomes. *Ann Surg.* 2002; 236(3):386–93.

26. Kopelman TR, Leeds S, Beradordoni NE, et al. Incidence of blunt cerebrovascular injury in low-risk cervical spine fractures. *Am J Surg.* 2011;202(6):684–88.

27. Allen BL, Ferguson RL, Lehmann TR, O'Brien RP. A mechanistic classification of closed, indirect fractures and dislocations of the lower cervical spine. *Spine.* 1982;7(1):1–27.

28. Vaccaro AR, Hurlbert RJ, Fisher CG, et al. The sub-axial cervical spine injury classification system (SLIC): a novel approach to recognize the importance of morphology, neurology and integrity of the disco-ligamentous complex. *Spine.* 2007;32(21):2365–74.

29. Vaccaro AR, Koerner JD, Radcliff KE, et al. AOSpine subaxial cervical spine injury classification system. *Eur Spine J.* 2016;25(7):2173–84.

30. Tescher AN, Rindflesch AB, Youdas JW, et al. Comparison of cervical range-of-motion restriction and craniofacial tissue-interface pressure with 2 adjustable and 2 standard cervical collars. *Spine.* 2016;41(6):E304–12.

31. Crosby ET. Airway management in adults after cervical spine trauma. *Anesthesiology.* 2006;104(6):1293–318.

32. Hurlbert RJ, Hadley MN, Walters BC, et al. Pharmacological therapy for acute spinal cord injury. *Neurosurgery.* 2015;76(Suppl 1):S71–83.

33. Eckert MJ, Martin MJ. Trauma: Spinal cord injury. *Surg Clin North Am.* 2017;97 (5):1031–45.

34. Stein DM, Knight WA 4th. Emergency neurological life support: traumatic spine injury. *Neurocrit Care.* 2017;27(Suppl 1): 170–80.

35. Boese CK, Lechler P. Spinal cord injury without radiologic abnormalities in adults: a systematic review. *J Trauma Acute Care Surg.* 2013;75(2):320–30.

36. Licinia P, Nowitzke AM. Approach and considerations regarding the patient with spinal injury. *Injury.* 2005;36(Suppl 2): B2–12.

37. Duane TM, Young AJ, Vanguri P, et al. Defining the cervical spine clearance algorithm: a single-institution prospective study of more than 9,000 patients. *J Trauma Acute Care Surg.* 2016;81 (3):541–47.

Thoracolumbar Trauma

Terren Trott

11

Thoracolumbar trauma involves a spectrum of injuries, from stable and unstable bony injury to spinal cord compression and spinal cord lesions. Thoracolumbar trauma most often results from motor vehicle collisions; however, falls and violent crimes also constitute a modest proportion. The general population experiences up to 64 cases of thoracolumbar injury per 100,000 people, though only a minor portion of these injuries lead to serious neurological deficit.[1]

Anatomy

The thoracolumbar spine is composed of 12 thoracic vertebrae and 5 lumbar vertebrae. The sacrum is formed by five fused vertebrae, and the coccyx by four fused vertebrae. The upper thoracic spine (T1–T10) is more rigid, owing to rib cage stabilization, and the structure of the vertebrae limit rotation, flexion, and extension. Injury in this area is associated with a substantial mechanism. The spinal canal in the thoracic spine is also narrower, leading to a higher proportion of complete spinal cord injury when injury does occur. The thoraco-lumbar junction (T11–L2) is a transitional zone between the thoracic and lumbar vertebral anatomy that is highly flexible and constitutes approximately 50% of thoracolumbar injuries.[1,2] The lower lumbar spine (L3–L5) is wider, owing to its weight bearing role, and the lumbar canal is also wider with less frequent spinal cord injury.

- The thoracic spine is least likely to have injury but will have the highest proportion of complete spinal cord injury.
- The transitional zone (T11–L2) is most susceptible to injury.
- The lower lumbar spine has the lowest proportion of complete spinal cord injury.

The spinal cord exits the skull through the foramen magnum and terminates in the *conus medulla*, at approximately the L1 level. The nerve roots of the corresponding vertebra exit below the vertebra. The final filament of the spinal cord is the *filum terminale* and attaches to the sacrum to anchor the spinal cord. The filum terminale and remainder of nerves ending past the conus medulla constitute the *cauda equina*.[2]

Spinal cord injury can be described as complete and incomplete lesions. Complete spinal cord injury is defined as the complete loss of motor and sensory function below the injury. Incomplete spinal cord injury will have partial deficits of sensory or motor function. The American Spinal Injury Association (ASIA) defines these terms in greater detail:[3]

A. Complete: No sensory or motor function is preserved in sacral segments S4–S5
B. Incomplete: Sensory, but not motor, function is preserved below the neurologic level and extends through sacral segments S4–S5

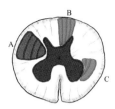

Figure 11.1 Spinal tracts

– *Corticospinal lesions (A)* are upper motor lesions with ipsilateral muscle weakness, spasticity, increased deep tendon reflexes at the level of the lesion .
– *Spinothalamic lesions (C)* involve the loss of pain and temperature contralateral to the lesion and one to two levels below the injury.
– *Dorsal column lesions (B)* involve ipsilateral loss of vibratory and positional sense at the level of the lesion.

Box 11.1 Signs and Symptoms Concerning For Spinal Injury

Suspect injury in:
- Back pain
- Neurological deficits
- Altered mental status
- Intoxication
- Concerning mechanism
- Symptoms of neurogenic shock

C. Incomplete: Motor function is preserved below the neurologic level, and most key muscles below the neurologic level have a muscle grade of less than 3

D. Incomplete: Motor function is preserved below the neurologic level, and most key muscles below the neurologic level have a muscle grade that is greater than or equal to 3

E. Normal: Sensory and motor functions are normal

Three principle spinal tracts are involved in partial and complete spinal cord injuries: corticospinal lesions, spinothalamic lesions, and dorsal column lesions (Figure 11.1).

- *Corticospinal lesions* (A) are upper motor lesions with ipsilateral muscle weakness, spasticity, and increased deep tendon reflexes at the level of the lesion.
- *Spinothalamic lesions* (C) involve the loss of pain and temperature contralateral to the lesion and one to two levels below the injury.
- *Dorsal column lesions* (B) involve ipsilateral loss of vibratory and positional sense at the level of the lesion.

Pre-Hospital Management

Despite a lack of strong evidence, any patient with suspected thoracolumbar injury should be transported with a long backboard.

- Patients should be considered at risk for injury with complaints of pain in the spine, neurologic deficits, altered mental status or intoxication, or with a concerning mechanism (Box 11.1).
- Prolonged backboard use is known to cause bedsores, induce respiratory compromise, and cause patient discomfort, thus removal should be prompt once in the emergency department.[4]
- With continued concern for thoracolumbar trauma, strict log roll precautions should be maintained.

Table 11.1 Motor groups and correlating muscle function

Motor Level	Muscle Groups	Motor Function
T1	Intrinsic hand muscles	Hand grasp
T2–T8	Chest muscles	
T9–T12	Abdominal muscles	
L1–L3	Iliopsoas	Hip flexion
L2–L4	Quadriceps	Knee extension
L4–S2	Hamstrings	Knee flexion
L4, L5	Tibialis Anterior	Ankle dorsiflexion
L5, S1	Extensor Hallucis Longus	Great toe extension
S1, S2	Gastrocnemius	Ankle plantar flexion
S2–S4	Bladder and anal sphincter	Voluntary rectal tone

Examination of Suspected Thoracolumbar Trauma

After initial stabilization of a trauma patient, a thorough secondary physical exam should be obtained. This should include palpation of the spine for step offs and deformities, motor function of all major muscle groups, sensory testing, and a digital rectal exam (Table 11.1). Examination of the perineum may demonstrate decreased sensation, loss of rectal tone, or priapism, all suggesting spinal cord involvement.[5]

It is important to note the physical exam alone may not have high sensitivity and specificity for identifying injury. One study found that 52% of known thoracolumbar injuries demonstrated abnormal clinical exam findings, including tenderness to palpation. Furthermore, when pain was elicited, it was in an inaccurate location almost 40% of the time. Injuries of higher severity were more likely to have positive exam findings, with the highest sensitivity and specificity reported at 79% and 84%, respectively.[6]

Muscle strength can be graded on a scale from 0 to 5, as defined by ASIA,[3] and reflexes should be assessed (Tables 11.2 and 11.3). Loss of reflexes or tendon jerks implies a complete spinal cord lesion, whereas spasticity or increased tone may suggest a partial cord lesion.

Imaging Thoracolumbar Trauma

Imaging the spine is indicated in patients with severe pain, bony tenderness, palpable subluxations, neurologic deficits, or a concerning mechanism of injury. Concomitant injury and mechanism of injury are important because physical exam alone, including tenderness to palpation, may be normal in up to 40% of patients.[5]

- The modality of choice is computed tomography.[5,7] This modality has the highest resolution of bony abnormalities and should be the initial form of imaging.

Table 11.2 Muscle grading[3]

	Muscle Strength
0	No movement or contractions
1	Minimal movement
2	Active movement but unable to resist gravity
3	Active movement against gravity
4	Active movement against light resistance
5	Active movement against full resistance

Table 11.3 Reflex grading[3]

	Reflexes
0	Absent
1	Hypoactive
2	Normal
3	Hyperactive without sustained clonus
4	Sustained clonus

- Plain films have a lower sensitivity and are liable to miss injury.[5] Furthermore, plain films are unable to fully visualize the middle and posterior columns and have even lower sensitivity in obese patients.
- If any spinal injury is found, a low threshold should be had to image the entire spine; up to 15% of injuries will have additional injuries.[7–9]
- While CT is the modality of choice for bony injury, if ligamentous or neural injury is suspected, an MR should be ordered. This is typically done in consultation with a spine specialist.

Classification

The most common way to describe fractures of the spine is with the three-column system (Figure 11.2). This system assumes stability of a fracture when only one column is involved; however, clinical judgment should be used.[10–14]

- *Anterior column*: from the anterior longitudinal ligament through the anterior two thirds of the vertebral body.
- *Middle column*: from the posterior third of the vertebral bodies through the posterior longitudinal ligament.
- *Posterior column*: from the facets through the spinous ligament.

Table 11.4 Fracture classification

Fracture	Mechanism	Stability	Management
Compression fracture	Flexion or compression	Stable if <50% and no neuro symptoms	Pain management, possible bracing, possible consultation
Burst fracture	Compression	Unstable	Spinal precautions, spine consultation
Chance fracture	Flexion-distraction	Unstable	Spinal precautions, spine consultation
Translational injuries	Shearing forces	Unstable	Spinal precautions, spine consultation
Transverse process fracture	Multiple mechanisms	Stable	Pain control
Spinous process fracture	Multiple mechanisms	Stable	Pain control
Pars interarticularis fracture	Multiple mechanisms	Stable	Pain control

– *Anterior column:* from the anterior longitudinal ligament through the anterior two thirds of the vertebral body.
– *Middle column:* from the posterior third of the vertebral bodies through the posterior longitudinal ligament.
– *Posterior column:* from the facets through the spinous ligament.

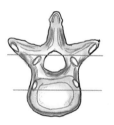

Figure 11.2 The three column classification system

Injury Patterns (Table 11.4)

Compression Fractures

These are the most common form of fracture and are most often due to flexion of the spine or axial compression. This pattern also represents the most common elderly fragility fracture, affecting 50% of patients over 80 years old (Figure 11.3).

- Fractures most commonly occurs in the anterior column and may result in the failure of the anterior longitudinal ligament. These fractures are almost always stable unless there is a loss of height greater than 50% or loss of integrity of the posterior longitudinal ligament.[11–14]

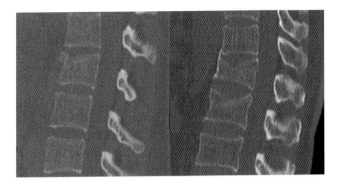

Figure 11.3 The first image shows a superior end-plate fracture of L2 with minimal loss of height in a 20-year-old after an MVC. The second image shows compression fractures of T12 and L1 after a fall in a 70-year-old man

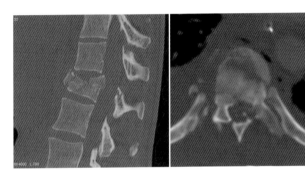

Figure 11.4 This image demonstrates a burst fracture of T12 with involvement of all three columns with retropulsion of fragments into the spinal column

- Management of smaller deformities (20–30% compression) typically involves pain control, increasing levels of activity, and physical therapy. Some practices may involve a spinal surgeon for bracing recommendations.[13,14]
- Injuries with greater degrees of compression or any neurological symptoms require consultation with a spinal specialist.

Burst Fractures

Burst fractures compose 15% of all thoracolumbar fractures and are most commonly caused by axial compression of the spine (Figure 11.4).

- These fractures may involve all three columns and are considered unstable. Retropulsion of bony fragments into the spinal column may lead to neurologic deficits.[11]
- Management includes strict spinal precautions, consultation with a spinal specialist, and frequent neuro checks.[15,16]

Chance Fractures

Chance fractures represent a flexion-distraction injury pattern with a focal point of the anterior longitudinal ligament. This often results in a loss of height of the anterior column with an apparent increase in height and transverse fracture line through the middle and posterior columns. This injury pattern was more prevalent when lap belt only seatbelts were in use (Figure 11.5).

- These injuries are considered unstable, since there is failure of all three columns.[11]

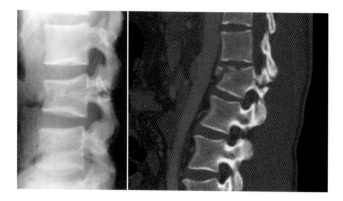

Figure 11.5 This image shows a chance fracture of L1. There is compression of the anterior column with a horizontal fracture line though the second and third columns

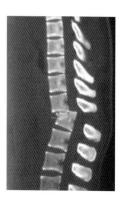

Figure 11.6 This image shows a translational injury of T12 with retropulsion of the vertebra into the spinal canal. There is an additional compressional deformity of T12

- They are frequently associated with intra-abdominal injuries, and abdominal imaging is recommended with CT.[17,18]
- Management consists of strict spinal precautions, frequent neurologic checks, and consultation with a spine specialist.[17]

Translational/Fracture-Dislocation Injuries

This injury pattern is infrequent and constitutes less than 2% of spinal fractures. Translational injuries are caused by a shearing mechanism, such as rapid acceleration or deceleration or direct trauma to the back (Figure 11.6).

- These are considered unstable and are almost always associated with neurological injury.[11]
- Management consists of strict spinal precautions, frequent neuro checks, and consultation with a spine specialist. The majority of these injuries will be operatively managed.[11,14]

Transverse Process, Spinous Process, Pars Interarticularis Fractures

These fractures are common, but rarely cause any form of neurological injury. Management consists of pain control and outpatient referral (Figure 11.7).

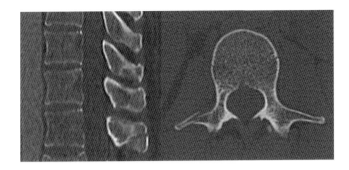

Figure 11.7 The first image shows a spinous process fracture through T12. The second image shows a right transverse process fracture at T10

Incomplete Spinal Cord Syndromes

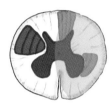

Brown-Sequard Syndrome
Typically, this syndrome is the result of penetrating trauma causing hemi-section of the cord via direct injury. Findings include loss of ipsilateral position and vibratory sense, ipsilateral motor loss,and contralateral loss of pain and temperatureone to two levels below the lesion(Figure 11.8).

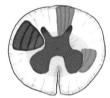

Central Cord Syndrome
This injury pattern is most often found in cervical hyperflexion, as may result from motor vehicle collisions. Findings include loss of motor function, typically greater in the upper extremities than the lower. However, complete quadriplegia may result. Typically, the spinothalamic tracts are spared or minimally involved (Figure 11.8).

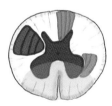

Anterior Cord Syndrome
Often the results of cervical hyperextension, this results in the loss of motor, pain, and temperature function bilaterally below the lesion while vibratory and position sense remain intact. This syndrome may also result from thrombosis of the anterior vertebral artery or direct anterior trauma (Figure 11.8).

Figure 11.8 From top to bottom: Brown-Sequard Syndrome, Central Cord Syndrome, Anterior Cord Syndrome

Incomplete Spinal Cord Syndromes

Brown-Sequard Syndrome

Typically, this syndrome is the result of penetrating trauma causing hemi-section of the cord via direct injury. Findings include loss of ipsilateral position and vibratory sense, ipsilateral motor loss, and contralateral loss of pain and temperature one to two levels below the lesion (Figure 11.8).

Central Cord Syndrome

This injury pattern is most often found in cervical hyperflexion, as may result from motor vehicle collisions. Findings include loss of motor function, typically greater in the upper extremities than the lower. However, complete quadriplegia may result. Typically, the spinothalamic tracts are spared or minimally involved (Figure 11.8).

Anterior Cord Syndrome

Often due to cervical hyperextension, this results in the loss of motor, pain, and temperature function bilaterally below the lesion, while vibratory and position sense remain intact. This syndrome may also result from thrombosis of the anterior vertebral artery or direct anterior trauma (Figure 11.8).

Pitfalls

- A thorough physical exam, including motor and sensory throughout all dermatomes, is necessary to reduce the risk of a missed spinal injury.
- However, relying solely on clinical exam demonstrates a low sensitivity and specificity.
- Not working up additional spinal injury, thoracic or abdominal injury, once a spinal injury is identified.
- Utilizing plain films in suspected thoracolumbar trauma will miss injuries, especially in the obese, elderly, or in injury to the second and third columns.

Key Points

- There are no validated spinal clearance rules for the thoracolumbar spine. Using a combination of motor and sensory exam, mechanism, and concomitant injuries guides the provider in appropriate work up.
- Any spinal injury with neurologic deficits is considered unstable and requires strict logroll precautions, neurological checks, and timely spinal consultation.
- CT scan demonstrates the highest sensitivity for thoracolumbar trauma and should always follow any abnormal x-ray, if x-ray was ordered.
- MR is the modality of choice for suspected spinal cord injury or ligamentous injury.
- Burst fractures, Chance fractures, and Translational injuries have the highest incidence of neurological injury. Compression, spinous process, and facet fractures are the least likely to have spinal cord injury.

References

1. van den Berg ME, Castellote JM, Mahillo-Fernandez I, de Pedro-Cuesta J. Incidence of spinal cord injury worldwide: a systematic review. *Neuroepidemiology.* 2010;34:184.

2. Holmes JF, Miller PQ, Panacek EA, et al. Epidemiology of thoracolumbar spine injury in blunt trauma. *Acad Emerg Med.* 2001;8:866.

3. American Spinal Injury Association. *International Standards for Neurological Classifications of Spinal Cord Injury.* revised ed. Chicago, IL: American Spinal Injury Association; 2000, pp. 1–23.

4. Gardner A, Grannum S, Porter K. Thoracic and lumbar spine fractures. *Trauma.* 2005;7:77.

5. Linares HA, Mawson AR, Suarez E, Biundo JJ. Association between pressure sores and immobilization in the immediate post-injury period. *Orthopedics*. 1987;10:571.

6. Inaba K, DuBose J, Barmparas G, et al. Clinical examination is insufficient to rule out thoracolumbar spine injuries. *J Trauma*. 2010;70:174–79.

7. Hsu JM, Joseph T, Ellis AM. Thoracolumbar fracture in blunt trauma patients: guidelines for diagnosis and imaging. *Injury*. 2003;34:426.

8. Berry GE, Adams S, Harris MB, et al. Are plain radiographs of the spine necessary during evaluation after blunt trauma? Accuracy of screening torso computed tomography in thoracic/lumbar spine fracture diagnosis. *J Trauma*. 2005;59:1410.

9. Krueger MA, Green DA, Hoyt D, Garfin SR. Overlooked spine injuries associated with lumbar transverse process fractures. *Clin Orthop Relat Res*. 1996;(327):191–95.

10. Winslow JE 3rd, Hensberry R, Bozeman WP, et al. Risk of thoracolumbar fractures doubled in victims of motor vehicle collisions with cervical spine fractures. *J Trauma*. 2006;61:686.

11. Vaccaro AR, Lehman RA Jr, Hurlbert RJ, et al. A new classification of thoracolumbar injuries: the importance of injury morphology, the integrity of the posterior ligamentous complex, and neurologic status. *Spine (Phila Pa 1976)*. 2005;30:2325.

12. Vollmer DG, Gegg C. Classification and acute management of thoracolumbar fractures. *Neurosurg Clin N Am*. 1997;8:499.

13. Chapman JR, Anderson PA. Thoracolumbar spine fractures with neurologic deficit. *Orthop Clin North Am*. 1994;25:595.

14. Campbell SE, Phillips CD, Dubovsky E, et al. The value of CT in determining potential instability of simple wedge-compression fractures of the lumbar spine. *AJNR Am J Neuroradiol*. 1995;16:1385.

15. Patel AA, Dailey A, Brodke DS, et al. Thoracolumbar spine trauma classification: the thoracolumbar injury classification and severity score system and case examples. *J Neurosurg Spine*. 2009;10:201.

16. Ballock RT, Mackersie R, Abitbol JJ, et al. Can burst fractures be predicted from plain radiographs? *J Bone Joint Surg Br*. 1992;74:147.

17. Dai LY. Imaging diagnosis of thoracolumbar burst fractures. *Chin Med Sci J*. 2004;19:142.

18. Anderson PA, Rivara FP, Maier RV, Drake C. The epidemiology of seatbelt-associated injuries. *J Trauma*. 1991;31:60.

Chapter 12

Neck Trauma

Christopher B. Colwell

Injury to the neck can have significant consequences. Given the number of vital structures confined to a relatively small space, it is not surprising that trauma to the neck accounts for some of the highest rates of mortality in trauma patients.[1] The three categories of neck trauma include blunt, penetrating, and strangulation or hanging, each with different associated injuries.

Anatomy

The neck contains a number of vital structures condensed into a relatively small area. Areas of greatest concern include vascular injuries, neurologic injuries, and injuries to the aerodigestive tract.

- The anterior triangle of the neck is bordered superiorly by the inferior border of the mandible and posteriorly by the medial aspect of the sternocleidomastoid muscle. The common carotid artery bifurcates into the external and internal carotid arteries in the anterior triangle, which also contains the aerodigestive tract and cranial nerves VII, IX, X, XI, and XII. The internal jugular vein, as well as the vagus and hypoglossal nerves, are contained within the anterior triangle.

- The posterior triangle is bordered by the sternocleidomastoid anteriorly, the clavicle inferiorly, and the anterior border of the trapezius muscle posteriorly. The spinal cord is the most significant structure in the posterior triangle of the neck.

- For the management of penetrating trauma, the anatomy of the neck has historically been divided into three zones, which will be described in the section on penetrating injuries.

- The neck can also be divided anatomically into facial planes. The platysma muscle stretches from the facial muscles to the thorax, and anatomically divides superficial from deep wounds. Wounds that do not penetrate the platysma do not generally lead to significant morbidity or mortality. The superficial fascia lies anterior to the platysma, while the deep fascia lies posteriorly.

Penetrating Injuries

Penetrating injuries are most commonly stab wounds or gunshot wounds but can be other types of projectile injuries as well. Historically, penetrating injuries to the neck have been described in one of three zones (Figures 12.1–12.4). While the particular zone involved no longer guides the management to the same degree, understanding the zones is still useful when communicating these injuries to consultants.

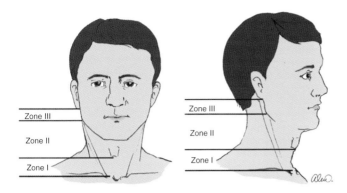

Figure 12.1 Anatomical zones of the neck. Zone I is confined between the clavicle and the cricoid cartilage, zone II between the cricoid and the angle of the mandible, and zone III between the angle of the mandible and the base of the skull (illustration by Alexis Demetriades, reproduced with permission from *Color Atlas of Emergency Trauma, Second Edition*)

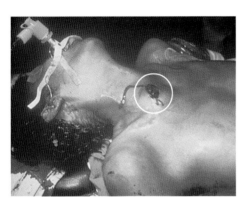

Figure 12.2 Zone I penetrating injury (reproduced with permission from *Color Atlas of Emergency Trauma, Second Edition*)

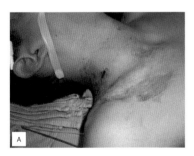
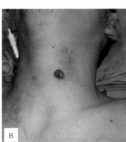

Figure 12.3 Zone II penetrating injuries. (A) Knife wound. (B) Gunshot wound (reproduced with permission from *Color Atlas of Emergency Trauma, Second Edition*)

- Zone I begins at the sternal notch and clavicles and extends superiorly to the cricoid cartilage.
- Zone II involves the area between the cricoid cartilage and the angle of the mandible.
- Zone III extends from the angle of the mandible to the base of the skull.

These zones have been used to help guide management, as injuries in zone II are most accessible to surgical intervention. In what has been called the "selective approach," zone II injuries underwent surgical exploration in the operating room, while patients with injuries in zone I and zone II underwent endoscopy and angiography. More current technology

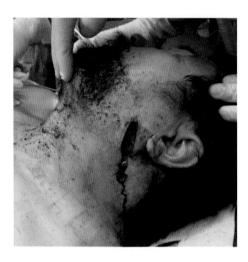

Figure 12.4 Zone III stab wound to the neck (reproduced with permission from *Color Atlas of Emergency Trauma, Second Edition*)

using Multi-Detector Computed Tomographic Angiography (MDCTA) has allowed the safe and non-invasive evaluation of the critical neck structures and is now the gold standard for evaluating stable injuries in any zone that are causing symptoms.[2]

- In unstable patients or those who have clear evidence (hard signs) of vascular or aerodigestive injuries, surgical exploration is indicated. Hard signs of vascular or aerodigestive injury include:
  - Active hemorrhage
  - Expanding or pulsatile hematoma
  - Bruit or thrill in the area of injury
  - Massive hemoptysis
  - Stridor or airway compromise
  - Hematemesis
  - Air bubbling through the injury site.

- Soft signs of penetrating neck trauma include:
  - Minor hemoptysis
  - Dysphonia
  - Dysphagia
  - Subcutaneous or mediastinal air
  - Non-expanding hematoma

In stable patients with penetrating neck trauma, a reasonable approach is to perform a complete physical exam including an evaluation of the neck. Stable patients exhibiting soft signs of neck injury should undergo MDCTA (64 slice or higher). Stable patients with no hard or soft signs of neck injury can be managed with observation.[3]

Blunt Injuries

Blunt injuries to the neck will commonly occur from motor vehicle accidents but can occur from assaults or falls as well. The primary concerns in blunt injury to the neck include spinal fracture, spinal cord injury, and blunt cerebrovascular injury (BCVI). Cervical spine injuries have a reported incidence of 2% to 15%, with 10% to 20% of those incidents including injury to the spinal cord.[4] Failure to diagnose unstable fractures and/or ligamentous injury may result in permanent neurologic damage; therefore, a great deal of effort has gone into determining the most effective way to evaluate blunt trauma patients for cervical spine injury.[5]

- Two decision rules have been described and validated for determining the need for radiographic evaluation of the cervical spine in victims of blunt trauma. The National Emergency X-Radiography Utilization Study (NEXUS) has demonstrated that clinical evaluation can be sufficient to rule out injury.[6] The NEXUS criteria for clearing the cervical spine include:
  - No midline spinal tenderness
  - No focal neurologic deficit
  - No altered level of consciousness
  - No intoxication
  - No painful distracting injury

- An alternative decision rule is the Canadian Cervical Spine Rule, which involves a 3-step process.[7] The process is as follows:
  - Step 1: Is there any high risk factor that mandates radiography?
    - Age over 65
    - Mechanism of injury considered dangerous
    - Numbness or tingling present in the extremities

    Dangerous mechanisms include a fall from an elevation of 3 feet or higher; a bicycle collision; an axial load to the head; or a motor vehicle collision involving high speed, rollover, or ejection. If the answer is no to the existence of a high risk factor, then proceed to step 2.

  - Step 2: Are there any low risk factors that indicate safe assessment of range of motion? Low risk factors include:
    - Simple rear-end motor vehicle collision
    - Patient was ambulatory at any time since the injury
    - Delayed onset of neck pain
    - Patient is in a sitting position in the emergency department
    - Absence of midline cervical spine tenderness

    If any low risk factors are present, proceed to Step 3.

  - Step 3
    - Is the patient able to actively rotate his or her neck 45° left and right?

    If yes, radiography is not performed.

In patients who do not meet criteria for clearance, imaging is indicated. Some patients may need a period of observation to allow metabolization of alcohol or other intoxicants before they can be clinically cleared. There are over 3 million patients with spinal trauma every year, with an imaging cost of over $3.4 billion.[8] In patients where radiographic evaluation is needed, there is some debate over the best modality.

- While some have argued there is still a role for plain x-rays in the evaluation of neck trauma patients,[8,9] others say the superiority of multislice CT scan makes it the modality of choice for all patients.[10,11]
- In high risk patients, such as those with neurologic symptoms, significant midline tenderness, or the elderly, CT is clearly superior to plain radiographs.
- For patients with an abnormal neurologic exam, there is a small but clinically significant incidence of missed injury with CT scans, and, in these patients, magnetic resonance imaging (MRI) is warranted.[12] Based on the current literature, a reasonable algorithm would be:

  . No risk: Nothing
  . Low risk: Plain radiographs and re-evaluate
  . Higher risk (unable to evaluate [altered], concerning exam, elderly): CT scan
  . Persistent or progressive neurologic deficit not completely explained on the CT: MRI

Alcohol and drug intoxication are common in trauma patients and can result in significant delays to cervical spine clearance. In these patients, CT scans are highly reliable for identifying all clinically significant cervical spine injuries. Spine clearance based on a normal CT scan among intoxicated patients with no gross motor deficits appears to be a safe option that avoids prolonged observation and unnecessary immobilization.[4] Computed tomography also appears to be effective in ruling out other injuries, including ligamentous injuries, in blunt trauma patients.[13]

One of the most widely accepted strategies when evaluating patients with possible cervical spine injuries involves cervical spine immobilization using a hard cervical collar. It is important to note that, like immobilization on a hard board, this practice is not based on randomized, controlled trials. Like long boards, hard cervical collars may cause harm. They can result in abnormal distraction within the upper cervical in the presence of a severe injury.[14] Motion is generated when cervical collars are applied and removed,[15] and they do not effectively reduce motion in the unstable cervical spine.[16] The cervical collar may not result in any decrease in motion during extrication.[17] In fact, self-extrication without a collar may result in less deviation of the cervical spine from the neutral position than extrication using the cervical collar.[18] While not providing adequate protection from motion, the hard cervical collar may also cause harm. There is a high incidence of category 1 pressure ulcers and indentation marks associated with hard cervical collars, and the pain due to the application of the cervical collar and head blocks may cause undesirable movement and bias the clinical examination.[19,20] Application of the cervical collar raises intracranial pressure (ICP) in head injured patients,[21] reduces venous return,[22] and complicates airway management.[23] While still considered standard, the current practice of cervical spine immobilization needs to be re-evaluated and revised to ensure the proper care of blunt trauma patients.

While once considered rare, BCVI has been found in 1% to 2% of blunt trauma patients.[24] The diagnosis of this injury is important as the incidence of stroke is 25% and mortality is as high as 13% if left untreated.[25] The internal carotid artery is the most frequently injured artery, followed by the vertebral artery (Figures 12.5 and 12.6). The Western Trauma Association recommends screening for BCVI in patients who have experienced a high-energy transfer mechanism with:

- Displaced mid-face fracture (LeFort II or III)
- Basilar skull fracture with carotid canal involvement

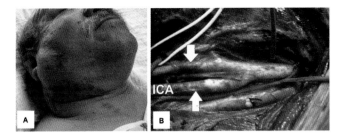

Figure 12.5 Patient with seatbelt sign on the right side of the neck and unexplained hemiplegia. (A) A "seatbelt" sign on the neck should increase suspicion for vascular injury. (B) The intraoperative findings show the carotid contusion and underlying thrombosis of the internal and external carotid arteries (arrows) (reproduced with permission from *Color Atlas of Emergency Trauma, Second Edition*)

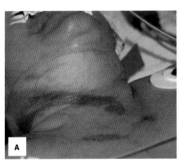
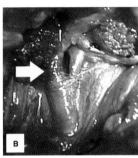

Figure 12.6 Patient with seatbelt sign on the neck (A). Surgical exploration shows bruising and underlying thrombosis of the internal carotid artery (arrow) (B) (reproduced with permission from *Color Atlas of Emergency Trauma, Second Edition*)

- Closed head injury consistent with diffuse axonal injury and GCS <6
- Cervical vertebral body or transverse foramen fracture, subluxation, or ligamentous injury at any level
- Any fracture at C1–C2
- Near hanging with anoxia
- Clothesline type injury or seatbelt abrasion with significant swelling, pain, or altered mental status[26]

Screening for BCVI should be done with 64 slice or greater MDCTA.[27] Treatment of BCVI will depend on the type and location of the injury, as well as the presence of other injuries. Treatment options include observation, anticoagulation, and surgery. Anticoagulation with either heparin or antiplatelet agents have comparable outcomes.[28] Surgical treatment may include ligation, resection, or endovascular stent therapy. Endovascular stents have typically been used for higher grade lesions, while low grade lesions are often managed with anticoagulation and/or antiplatelet therapy.[29] Appropriate treatment reduces the stroke rate from about 25% to just under 4%.[30]

Laryngotracheal injuries are rare but can result in significant morbidity or mortality (Figure 12.7). Most laryngotracheal injuries occur as a result of motor vehicle accidents where an inadequately restrained driver's neck contacts the steering wheel.[31] Other mechanisms include clothesline injuries and assaults. A quiescent phase has been described with progressive subclinical airway edema or hematoma that can result in delayed airway obstruction.[32] Computed tomography of the neck is the imaging modality of choice when there is concern for laryngotracheal injuries.[33] Airway compromise is the greatest concern in patients with laryngotracheal trauma, and these patients should be closely monitored.

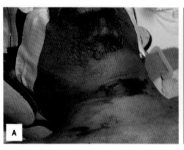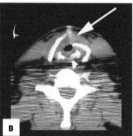

Figure 12.7 (A) Patient with blunt force trauma to the anterior neck. (B) CT scan showing fracture of the larynx (reproduced with permission from *Color Atlas of Emergency Trauma, Second Edition*)

Awake fiberoptic intubation is likely the best route for securing the airway when available. Paralysis could precipitate a loss of the airway in the event a complete transection of the trachea has occurred and the musculature of the neck is stabilizing the trachea (clothesline injury). A surgical airway may be necessary. While small mucosal injuries and non-displaced fractures can be managed conservatively, more significant injuries require surgical repair.[31]

Strangulation and Hanging

Strangulation refers to external compression of the neck and tends to be either manual (hands) or ligature, but it can be positional.

- The external force causes venous congestion and stasis of cerebral blood flow, resulting in loss of consciousness.
- Once the victim loses consciousness, relaxation of the neck musculature allows complete arterial occlusion that can lead to permanent brain injury or death due to cerebral anoxia and ischemia. Obstruction of cerebral venous return rather than acute airway compromise is the more likely pathophysiologic mechanism.
- Judicial hanging involves a fall distance of at least the height of the victim and results in a forceful distraction of the head from the neck and body.
- These injuries lead to high cervical spine fractures and spinal cord transection. Non-judicial hangings typically involve falls from lesser heights and are often inadequate to injure the cervical spine other than in the elderly.[34]
- Near-hanging typically refers to survivors of attempted hangings. Ten percent of violent deaths in the United States are due to strangulation. Hanging is the second most common means of suicide death, so it is not uncommon to see these injuries in the ED.[35,36]
- External trauma may or may not be evident in victims of strangulations or hangings. Petechial hemorrhages, sometimes referred to as Tardieu spots, can be seen in the conjunctiva, mucous membranes, and skin cephalad to the pressure point, and have been described in asphyxia deaths but can also be seen in otherwise uninjured patients.
- Injuries associated with strangulation include laryngotracheal fractures and carotid artery injuries.[37]
- Dyspnea, dysphonia, or odynophagia is concerning for laryngeal or tracheal injury and should be evaluated with either laryngobronchoscopy or MDCTA of the neck. Any

concern for carotid artery injury, including any neurologic deficit not explained on head CT, should undergo MDCTA.

- Cervical spine fractures are uncommon in strangulation injuries and in hangings involving a fall of less than the patient's height or strangulation injuries.[38] Patients with strangulation and hanging injuries, even when self-inflicted, are at risk for domestic abuse, and evaluation for abuse is warranted.[39]

Airway Management

Airway management remains a critical priority in neck trauma patients. Situations such as hematomas, upper airway hemorrhage, subcutaneous emphysema, and voice changes are indications to consider early endotracheal intubation while the airway is still accessible. Expanding neck hematomas require early intervention.

- Airway management in the setting of a possible unstable cervical spine should be handled with particular attention to avoid unnecessary spinal movement. Although the ideal method of airway management remains the subject of some debate, rapid sequence orotracheal intubation with video laryngoscopy has been shown to be safe and effective and may reduce the number of failed intubations.[40]
- Video laryngoscopy also has the advantage of less need for manipulation of the neck.[41,42]
- When endotracheal intubation cannot be performed or is unsuccessful, surgical cricothyrotomy is indicated.

Pitfalls

- Failure to diagnose unstable fractures and/or ligamentous injury in victims of blunt neck trauma.
- Failure to recognize hard signs of vascular or aerodigestive injuries in victims of penetrating neck trauma.
- Failure to remove patients from cervical spine immobilization in a timely manner when appropriate.
- Failure to consider blunt cerebrovascular injury in appropriate patients.
- Application of a hard cervical collar in penetrating neck trauma.
- Forcing kyphotic elderly patients into a hard cervical collar.
- Failure to recognize potential challenges of airway management in neck trauma and have a backup plan.

Key Points

- Platysma violation defines serious penetrating neck trauma.
- There is less emphasis on the zones of the neck determining management and more emphasis on management being determined by the presentation. Unstable or hard signs should go to the operating room, soft signs should warrant MDCTA of the neck, and no signs can be managed with observation.

- Patients with blunt traumatic injuries warrant concern for the cervical spine. Patients that cannot be cleared by a validated clinical decision rule should undergo radiographic evaluation.
- Blunt vascular injuries can be asymptomatic but can present with either immediate or delayed neurologic sequelae.
- The hard cervical collar is not indicated in penetrating trauma and may not provide a benefit in blunt trauma patients.

References

1. Rodriques-Luna, MR, Guarneros-Zarate, JE, Hernandez-Mendez JR, et al. Defining Zone I of penetrating neck trauma: a surgical controversy in the light of clinical anatomy. *J Trauma Acute Care Surg.* 2016;80(4):670–73.

2. Shiroff AM, Gale SC, Martin ND, et al. Penetrating neck trauma: a review of management strategies and discussion of the 'no zone' approach. *Amer Surg.* 2013;79 (1):23–29.

3. Inaba K, Branco BC, Menaker J, et al. Evaluation of multidetector computed tomography for penetrating neck injury: a prospective multicenter study. *J Trauma.* 2012;72(3):576–84.

4. Bush L, Brookshire R, Roche B, et al. Evaluation of cervical spine clearance by computed tomographic scan alone in intoxicated patients with blunt trauma. *JAMA Surg.* 2016;151 (9):807–13.

5. Vanguri P, Young AJ, Weber WF, et al. Computed tomographic scan: it's not just about the fracture. *J Trauma Acute Care Surg.* 2014;77(4):604–7.

6. Hoffman JR, Mower WR, Wolfson AB, et al. Validity of a set of clinical criteria to rule out injury to the cervical spine in patients with blunt trauma. *N Engl J Med.* 2000;343:94–97.

7. Stiell IG, Wells GA, Vandemheen KL, et al. The Canadian C-spine rule for radiography in alert and stable trauma patients. *JAMA.* 2001;286:1841–48.

8. Munera F, Rivas LA, Nunez DB Jr, Quencer RM. Imaging evaluation of adult spinal injuries: emphasis on multidetector CT in cervical spine trauma. *Radiology.* 2012;263 (3):645–60.

9. Holmes JF, Akkinepalli R. Computed tomography versus plain radiography to screen for cervical spine injury: a meta-analysis. *J Trauma.* 2005;58(5):902–5.

10. Griffen MM, Frykberg ER, Kerwin AJ, et al. Radiographic clearance of blunt cervical spine injury: plain radiograph or computed tomography scan? *J Trauma.* 2003;55 (2):222–26.

11. Mathen R, Inaba K, Munera F, et al. Prospective evaluation of multislice computed tomography versus plain radiographic cervical spine clearance in trauma patients. *J Trauma.* 2007;62 (6):1427–31.

12. Inaba K, Byerly S, Bush LD, et al. Cervical spinal clearance: a prospective Western Trauma Association multi-institutional trial. *J Trauma Acute Care Surg.* 2016;81 (6):1122–30.

13. Vanguri P, Young AJ, Weber WF, et al. Computed tomographic scan: it's not just about the fracture. *J Trauma Acute Care Surg.* 2014;77:604–7.

14. Ben-Galim P, Dreiangle N, Mattox KL, et al. Extrication collars can result in abnormal separation between vertebrae in the presence of a dissociative injury. *J Trauma.* 2010;69(2):447–50.

15. Prasam ML, Conrad B, Del Rossi G, et al. Motion generated in the unstable cervical spine during the application and removal of cervical immobilization collars. *J Trauma Acute Care Surg.* 2012;72 (6):1609–13.

16. Horodyski M, DiPaola CP, Conrad BP, Rechtine GR 2nd. Cervical collars are

insufficient for immobilizing an unstable cervical spine injury. *J Emerg Med.* 2011;41 (5):513–19.

17. Engsberg JR, Standeven JW, Shurtleff TL, et al. Cervical spine motion during extrication. *J Emerg Med.* 2013;44 (1):122–27.

18. Dixon M, O'Halloren A, Hannigan A, et al. Confirmation of suboptimal protocols in spinal immobilization. *Emerg Med J.* 2015;32(12):939–45.

19. Ham WH, Schoonhoven L, Schuurmans MJ, Leenen LP. Pressure ulcers, indentation marks and pain from cervical spine immobilization with extrication collars and head blocks: an observational study. *Injury.* 2016;47(9):1924–31.

20. Ham WH, Schoonhoven L, Schuurmans MJ, Leenen LP. Pressure ulcers from spinal immobilization in trauma patients: a systematic review. *J Trauma Acute Care Surg.* 2014;76(4):1131–41.

21. Mobbs RJ, Stoodley MA, Fuller J. Effect of cervical collar on intracranial pressure after head injury. *ANZ J Surg.* 2002;72 (6):389–91.

22. Sundstrom T, Asbjomsen H, Habiba S, et al. Prehospital use of cervical collars in trauma patients: a critical review. *J Neurotrauma.* 2014;31(6):531–40.

23. Gaither JB, Spaite DW, Stolz U, et al. Prevalence of difficult airway predictors in cases of failed prehospital intubation. *J Emerg Med.* 2014;47(3):294–300.

24. Goodein RB, Beery PR, Dorbish RJ, et al. Computed tomographic angiography versus conventional angiography for the diagnosis of blunt cerebrovascular injury in trauma patients. *J Trauma.* 2009;67 (5):1046–50.

25. Bruns BR, Tesoriero R, Kufera J, et al. Blunt cerebrovascular injury screening guidelines: what are we willing to miss? *J Trauma Acute Care Surg.* 2014;76:691–95.

26. Biffl WL, Cothren CC, Moore EE, et al. Western Trauma Association critical decisions in trauma: screening for and treatment of blunt cerebrovascular injuries. *J Trauma.* 2009;67(6):1150–53.

27. Paulus EM, Fabian TC, Savage SA, et al. Blunt cerebrovascular injury screening with 64-channel multidetector computed tomography: more slices finally cut it. *J Trauma Acute Care Surg.* 2014;76 (2):279–85.

28. Cothren CC, Biffl WL, Moore EE, et al. Treatment for blunt cerebrovascular injuries: equivalence of anticoagulation and antiplatelet agent. *Arch Surg.* 2009;144 (7):685–90.

29. DiCocco JM, Fabian TC, Emmett KP, et al. Optimal outcomes for patients with blunt cerebrovascular injury: tailoring treatment to the lesion. *J Trauma.* 2011;212:549–57.

30. Parks NA, Croce MA. Use of computed tomography in the emergency room to evaluate blunt cerebrovascular injury. *Adv Surg.* 2012;46:205–17.

31. Comer BT, Gal TJ. Recognition and management of the spectrum of acute laryngeal trauma. *J Emerg Med.* 2012;43(5): e289–93.

32. Schaefer SD. The acute management of external laryngeal trauma: a 27-year experience. *Arch Otolaryngol Head Neck Surg.* 1992;118(6):598–604.

33. Schaefer SD. Management of acute blunt and penetrating external laryngeal trauma. *Laryngoscope.* 2014;124(1):233–44.

34. Nikolic S, Zivkovic V. Cervical spine injuries in suicidal hangings without a long-drop – patterns and possible underlying mechanisms of injury: an autopsy study. *Forensic Sci Med Pathol.* 2014;10(2):193–97.

35. McClane GE, Strack GB, Hawley D: A review of 300 attempted strangulation cases part II: clinical evaluation of the surviving victim. *J Emerg Med.* 2001;21 (3):311–15.

36. US Bureau of the Census. *Statistical Abstract of the United States*, 129th ed. Washington DC: US Bureau of the Census; 2010.

37. Salim A, Martin M, Sangthong B, et al. Near-hanging injuries: a 10-year experience. *Injury.* 2006;37(5):435–39.

38. Sep D, Thies K-C. Strangulation injuries in children. *Resuscitation*. 2007;74(2):386–91.

39. Shields LB, Hunsaker DM, Hunsaker JC 3rd. Suicide: a ten-year retrospective review of Kentucky medical examiner cases. *J Forensic Sci*. 2005;50 (3):613–17.

40. Lewis SR, Butler AR, Parker J, et al. Videolaryngoscopy versus direct laryngoscopy for adults requiring tracheal intubation. *Cochrane Database Systematic Review*. 2016;11:CD011136.

41. Carter E, Smally A, Delgado J. Trauma intubation protocol success before and after acquisition of video laryngoscopy. *Ann Emerg Med*. 2013;10:S77.

42. Green-Hopkins I, Nagler J. Endotracheal intubation in pediatric patients using video laryngoscopy: an evidence-based review. *Pediatr Emerg Med Pract*. 2015;12(8):1–22.

Chapter 13

Pulmonary Trauma

Manpreet Singh and Dennis Kim

Chest trauma is present in almost two thirds of all trauma patients, varying in severity from a simple rib fracture to penetrating injury to the heart.[1] Blunt chest trauma accounts for 90% of cases, where less than 10% require surgical intervention.[1] Understanding chest trauma mechanism is key to the approach when evaluating and managing an individual with potential chest trauma.

The primary survey should focus on excluding or treating the life-threatening injuries in Box 13.1.

The secondary survey should focus on excluding or treating the potential life-threatening injuries in Box 13.2.

Box 13.1 Primary Survey

1 – Airway obstruction
2 – Tension pneumothorax
3 – Open pneumothorax
4 – Massive hemothorax
5 – Flail chest
6 – Cardiac tamponade*

*These entities will be discussed in Chapter 14.

Box 13.2 Secondary Survey

7 – Pulmonary contusion
8 – Myocardial contusion*
9 – Aortic disruption*
10 – Traumatic diaphragmatic rupture
11 – Tracheobronchial disruption
12 – Esophageal disruption

  *These entities will be discussed in Chapter 14.

Airway Obstruction

- *Pathophysiology*: Airway obstruction is a major cause of death and morbidity, where the mantra of airway management with in-line cervical spine stabilization is key.
- *Presentation*: Details on airway obstruction presentation discussed in Chapter 2.
- *Treatment*: Details on airway obstruction management discussed in Chapter 2.

Procedure – In-Line Stabilization

This is key to maintain a neutral position so the head is not inadvertently moved due to a concern for cervical spine injury, which may be unstable. There is a 2–12% risk of cervical spine injury in major trauma, where 7–14% may be unstable.[2] Approximately 10% of comatose trauma patients have a cervical spine injury.[2]

To perform in-line stabilization, an assistant crouches at the head of the bed beside the intubator, with the assistant's hands on the patient's trapezius muscles, supporting the patient's head between the forearms. Alternatively, standing beside the patient in the front, the assistant can hold the head with his/her hands while anchoring at the trapezius.

Tension Pneumothorax

- *Pathophysiology*: This injury is associated with the presence of intra-pleural air under positive-pressure from the respiratory cycle. Air enters the chest in a one-way valve type manner, but it cannot leave. As a result, with build-up of intra-pleural air there is reduced blood return to the heart (decreased preload), leading to decreased cardiac output (Figure 13.1).[3]
- *Presentation*: Prompt recognition is key, so always consider this in a rapidly deteriorating patient with signs of pneumothorax, which include worsening tachycardia and respiratory distress, eventually leading to cardiac collapse. Findings such as tracheal deviation, distended neck veins, and displaced PMI are late findings, where there is considerable variability of their presence.[3]
- *Diagnosis*: This can be difficult, as mentioned above, so reliance on history alone may be key in the correct clinical context. It can present in an intubated traumatic patient, where ventilation becomes progressively difficult, leading to high peak airway pressures.[3] Ultrasound can provide rapid diagnosis by demonstrating a lung point due to absent lung sliding.
- *Treatment*: Management requires immediate chest decompression, through either needle decompression or finger thoracostomy followed by chest tube placement.[3]

Procedure – Needle Decompression

Traditional treatment includes placement of a large bore angiocatheter in the second intercostal space at the mid-clavicular line.[4] Incorrect placement can lead to vascular (internal mammary or subclavian) or cardiac damage. However, it may only be effective 20–50% of time due to chest wall thickness.[4]

Longer angiocatheters have been advocated as they tend to increase the success rate, but the risk/benefits should be weighed.[4] Iatrogenic vascular, visceral, and parenchymal injuries have been reported using longer ones. Recently, many have advocated the fifth intercostal space at the mid-axillary line as a location of decompression, where there is a thinner chest wall and no major blood vessels nearby.[4] Though potentially safer, the major downsides of this include dislodgement in transport with movement of the patient arms on the side (Figures 13.2 and 13.3).

Procedure – Pleur-Evac Setup and Troubleshooting

All chest tube collection systems are based on three chambers: (1) Collection Bottle, (2) Water Seal, and (3) Suction Control. Fluid from the chest drains into the first bottle, whether it is serous or sanguineous fluid. The collection chamber is graduated and

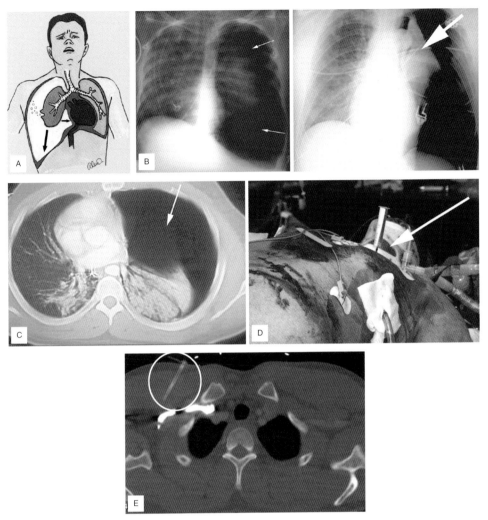

Figure 13.1 Tension pneumothorax. (A) Illustration showing mechanism of tension pneumothorax. Extrapulmonary air under tension collapses the lung, depresses the diaphragm, and pushes the heart toward the opposite side. The normal lung is compressed in the contralateral pleural cavity. These changes cause cardiorespiratory failure. (B) Chest x-rays showing a large tension pneumothorax on the left side, mediastinal shift to the opposite side, and downward displacement of the left hemidiaphragm. Arrows point to tension pneumothorax. (C) Tension pneumothorax on the CT scan (arrow). Note the deviation of the heart to the right. (D) Photograph showing a thoracostomy needle in place, below the middle of the clavicle. (E) CT scan shows that the thoracostomy needle is located into the subcutaneous tissues, outside the pleural cavity. This is a common technical problem (reproduced with permission from *Color Atlas of Emergency Trauma, Second Edition*, illustration at (A) by Alexis Demetriades)

measured.[5] Bottle one is for chest tube fluid control. Bottle two is for chest tube air control. Air from the chest tube bubbles into bottle two, which is the water seal and usually 2 cm. This is called the "air leak" monitor, and it also prevents air from entering back into the chest tube system. The water seal should show bubbling, which should diminish over time once a pneumothorax is resolving. A persistent leak suggests a leak at the insertion site or

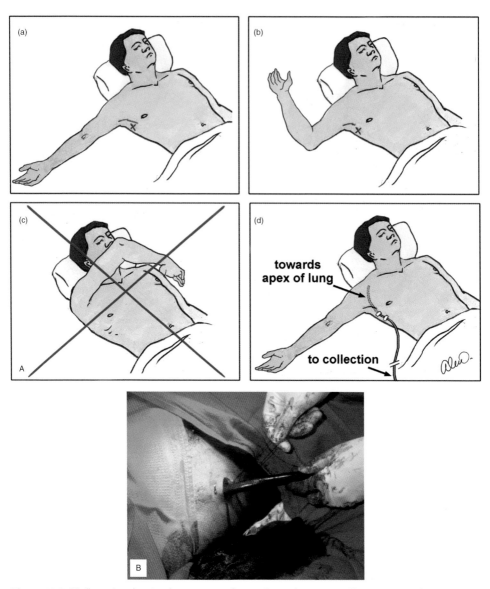

Figure 13.2 (A) Illustration showing the sequence of open chest tube insertion. The patient is in the supine position, and the arm is abducted at 90 degrees (a). The insertion site should be in the midaxillary line, at the fourth or fifth intercostal space (b). Abduction and internal rotation of the arm is a suboptimal position because of the interposition of the latissimus dorsi muscle (c). The tube is directed posteriorly toward the apex (d). (B) Photograph showing thoracostomy tube being secured in place with horizontal mattress suture (reproduced with permission from *Color Atlas of Emergency Trauma, Second Edition*, illustrations by Alexis Demetriades)

bad chest tube, or tracheobronchial injury. Obstruction usually results in no bubbling. When no suction is applied, it is set to water seal.[5] Bottle three is the vacuum or suction control, which allows for precise control on suction. There is an atmospheric vent, which is the safety valve of the system, submerged in 20 cm of water.

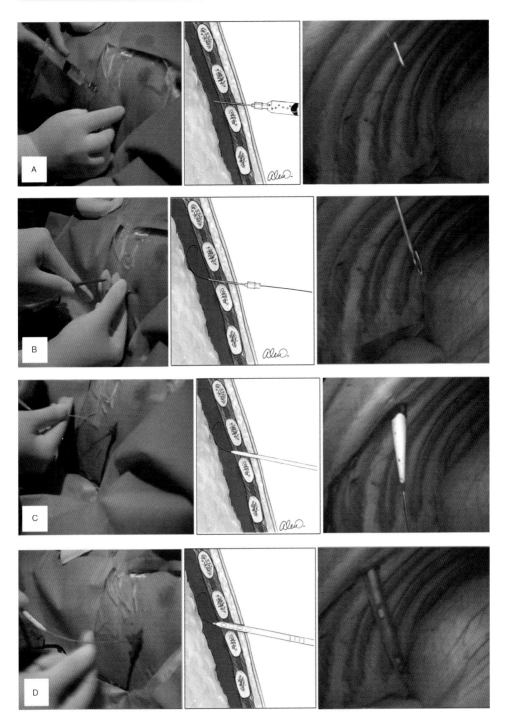

Figure 13.3 Illustration depicting step-by-step the insertion of a chest tube with the percutaneous dilational technique (illustration, photograph of procedure, thoracoscopic view): The needle, attached to a syringe containing sterile water, is inserted through the fourth to fifth intercostal space, close to the superior border of the rib, in order to avoid injury to the intercostal vessels. (A) Aspiration of air or blood confirms the intrathoracic position of the needle. (B) A guidewire is inserted though the needle into the thoracic cavity. Serial dilatation over the wire (C) is followed by insertion of the chest tube over the guidewire (D) (reproduced with permission from *Color Atlas of Emergency Trauma, Second Edition*, illustrations by Alexis Demetriades)

Procedure – Chest Tube Removal

A suture removal set and dressing material should be ready, along with proper dressing (glove, gown, mask, and eye shield). Explain to the patient the procedure. The goal is to pull the tube before any air can enter the thorax and have the patient increase intra-thoracic pressure by holding his/her breath and bearing down doing a valsalva maneuver. If the patient is ventilated, perform an inspiratory pause. Pull the chest tube and put a dressing on the site. Keep this on for 48 hours, and keep dry and clean.[1]

Open Pneumothorax

- *Pathophysiology*: This is described as a "sucking chest wound," which occurs when the wound is greater than two thirds of the diameter of the trachea. At a wound this size, air will enter a chest wall wound, preferentially leading to pneumothorax.[6]
- *Presentation*: Besides visible "sucking" of air into the wound, there is rapid, shallow, and labored breathing with reduced hemithorax expansion accompanied by decreased breath sounds and hyperresonance on physical exam.[6]
- *Diagnosis*: Visible "sucking" of air or dressing overlying the wound is often visible on exam cueing the diagnosis.
- *Treatment*: Cover the wound with an occlusive 3-sided dressing that acts as a flutter valve to allow air out, but prevents "sucking in."[6] After this, a formal tube thoracostomy is placed, while the wound is formally explored at another time.

Massive Hemothorax

- *Pathophysiology*: This condition may result in exsanguination from blunt or penetrating injury, originating from major vessels, intercostal vessels, heart, or lungs (Figures 13.4 and 13.5).[1]
- *Presentation*: Signs of hemorrhagic shock based on vitals and physical exam may be present, where the patient may become anxious or agitated. Massive hemothorax that meets the following indications may need thoracotomy urgently:[1,7]

  - Initial output >1500 cc (approximately 1/3rd blood volume)
  - Output >200 cc/h for 2–4 hours

- *Diagnosis*: Though diagnosis is partly based on chest tube output, always consider it with a large volume hemothorax diagnosed on exam (difficult to appreciate) or imaging (i.e. CXR or ultrasound) in a dyspneic, hemodynamically unstable patient.[1]
- *Treatment*: Resuscitation is key to rapidly restore blood volume lost while definitive management is taken by the trauma surgeon. Large bore IV access is recommended through upper extremity peripherals, humeral IO, or central access. Using autotransfusions, as well as activating the massive transfusion protocol, may be required for resuscitation.

Procedure – Autologous Transfusion

Most chest tube collection systems have optional autotransfusion canisters, which are used to collect blood and hung like a bag of blood from the blood bank.[7] It is key to heparinize the collection system prior to this, though some state the blood may be retransfused up to 6 hours. Ultimately, the manufacturer's instructions should be followed (Figure 13.6).

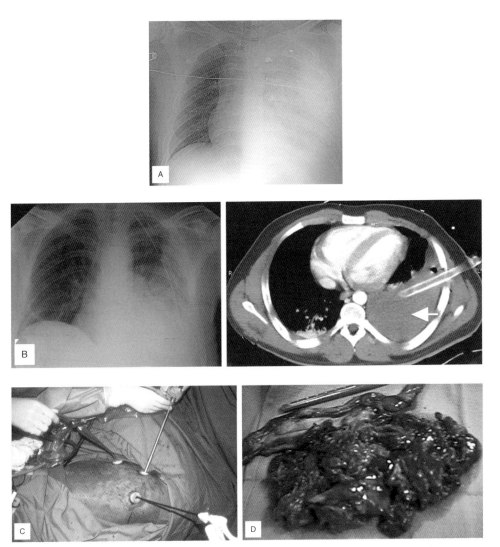

Figure 13.4 Hemothorax. (A) Chest radiograph with extensive opacification of the left hemithorax due to massive hemothorax with mediastinal shift to the opposite side and retained fragments of a missile. (B) Gunshot wound to the left chest with suspected "residual hemothorax" on chest x-ray (left) 2 days after injury. Residual hemothorax is confirmed by CT scan (right). (C) Thoracoscopic evacuation of the residual hemothorax. The procedure should be performed within the first 5 days of injury, before organization of the clot and fibrin encapsulation of the lung. (D) Photograph of material removed during decortication for persistent residual hemothorax and lung entrapment, a few weeks after injury. Delayed evacuation of a clotted hemothorax is difficult and requires thoracotomy and decortication (reproduced with permission from *Color Atlas of Emergency Trauma, Second Edition*)

Though autologous transfusion has been shown to provide immediate blood for resuscitation and pose no serious complications,[8] it is associated with pro-inflammatory cytokines, is depleted of coagulation factors compared to venous blood, and one "unit" of autologous transfused blood is less than one unit of pRBC.[9,10] Further research is required to evaluate patient outcomes with autologous transfusion.

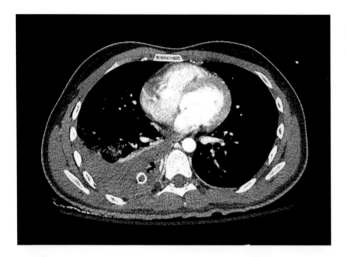

Figure 13.5 Image demonstrating arterial blush in a patient with massive hemothorax following chest tube insertion (image: Dennis Kim, MD)

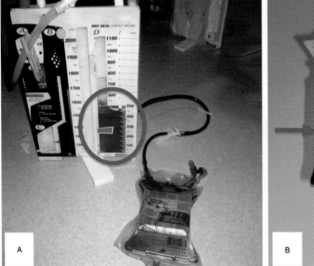
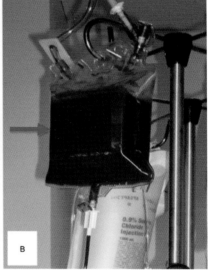

Figure 13.6 Autotransfusion system utilization in hemothorax. The collection chamber of the drainage system (circle) is connected to a negative pressure autotransfusion bag and the blood is actively sucked into the bag (A). (1 mL of citrate per 10 mL of blood is added to the collection system before drainage.) The collected blood is autotransfused using standard techniques (B) (reproduced with permission from *Color Atlas of Emergency Trauma, Second Edition*)

Flail Chest

- *Pathophysiology*: A flail chest includes fractures of two or more adjacent ribs in two or more places, which can result in a flail segment whereby a portion of chest wall is in discontinuity with the chest wall.[11] Paradoxical chest wall movement or respiration may result in significant pain, hypoventilation, and ventilatory failure. Hypoxemia may also result due to atelectasis and shunting.[11] Approximately 25–40% of patients with a flail chest will require mechanical ventilator support (Figure 13.7).[11]

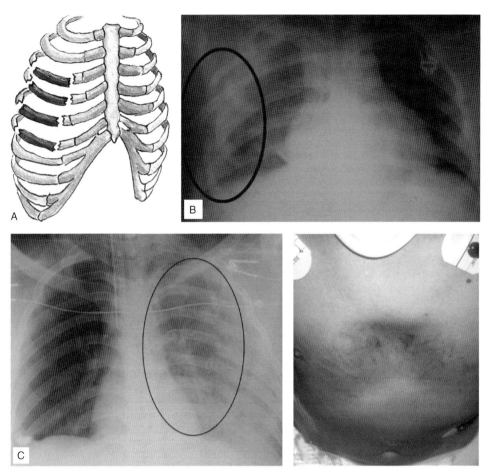

Figure 13.7 Flail chest. (A) Double fractures of at least three adjacent ribs are required in order to produce a flail chest. (B) Chest x-ray showing a left flail chest with underlying lung contusion. (C) Patient with a flail sternal segment; Note the midsternal depression (right) (reproduced with permission from *Color Atlas of Emergency Trauma, Second Edition,* illustration at A by Robert Amaral)

- *Presentation*: Pain is common in patients with rib fractures and a flail chest. Clinical exam may reveal paradoxical chest wall movement on inspection (affected hemithorax moves inward as contralateral unaffected side expands during inspiration).[11] Crepitus and tenderness may be elicited upon palpation of the chest wall. The injury most commonly involves the anterior or anterolateral chest wall.[11]
- *Diagnosis*: Chest x-ray and CT scan are often obtained to further identify the location and number of fractures, in addition to the presence and severity of displacement. However, visual observation in a fair habitus individual often leads to its prompt diagnosis.
- *Treatment*: Patients should be carefully monitored for adequate ventilation and oxygenation, and fluids should be given judiciously in order to minimize potential blossoming of pulmonary contusions, which are often associated with it.[11] Aggressive pain control remains the mainstay of therapy, especially multi-modal

(i.e. NSAIDs, opioids, nerve blocks), in conjunction with supplemental oxygen and pulmonary hygiene.[11] Thoracic epidural insertion is an effective pain control modality. Operative rib fixation has emerged as a potential therapy to decrease the duration of mechanical ventilation in patients requiring invasive ventilation.[11]

Pulmonary Contusion

- *Pathophysiology*: Depending on the size and extent of injury, pulmonary contusions can result in shunt physiology with subsequent hypoxemia. The underlying pathophysiology involves a complex interplay between several possible mechanisms including airway collapse, vasomotor reactivity, and the underlying immune response.[12] Among adults, pulmonary contusions are typically accompanied by rib fractures; in young children with incompletely ossified bones, this may occur in the absence of fractures.[12]
- *Presentation*: In the absence of clinically detectable rib fractures, pulmonary contusions are usually suspected on the basis of the mechanism and presenting vital signs, particularly the presence of unexplained hypoxia.[12]
- *Diagnosis*: Radiographic imaging in the form of chest x-ray and CT scan are better able to delineate the presence and extent of injury. Arterial blood gas analysis may reveal arterial hypoxemia (Figures 13.8 and 13.9).[12]
- *Treatment*: Management is conservative. Supplemental oxygen combined with pulmonary toilet and pain control are the cornerstones of management. Typically, minor contusions will resolve clinically over the course of a week.[12] However, if severe, some patients may require NIPPV or mechanical ventilation for support, which can progress into ARDS 50% of the time.[12]

Traumatic Diaphragmatic Injury

- *Pathophysiology*: This is an uncommon injury, occurring in 3% of all abdominal injuries. Blunt injuries are often associated with large tears vs. penetrating injuries which typically result in smaller defects that may be difficult to detect both clinically and radiographically in the absence of herniation of abdominal viscera. Greater than three-quarters of injuries involve the left side. Following severe blunt thoracoabdominal trauma, the triad of pelvic fracture, diaphragmatic rupture, and blunt thoracic aortic injury may be encountered.[13]
- *Presentation*: The diagnosis is often not readily apparent on clinical exam. In the presence of herniated viscera, absence or diminished breath sounds and the presence of bowel sounds in the chest may be present.[13]
- *Diagnosis*: More commonly, the diagnosis is confirmed via radiographic findings, although the chest x-ray may be normal in up to 50% of patients.[13] The finding of an elevated hemidiaphragm, gastric air bubble, or NG tube in the left hemithorax should raise concern for the presence of a diaphragm injury. CT scans are helpful in the diagnosis provided that visceral herniation is present, where sensitivity ranges from 61–87% and specificity ranges from 72–100%.[13] In patients with penetrating wounds to the thoracoabdominal box, a diagnostic laparoscopy should be performed following a period of observation to evaluate for diaphragm injury (present in 25% of asymptomatic

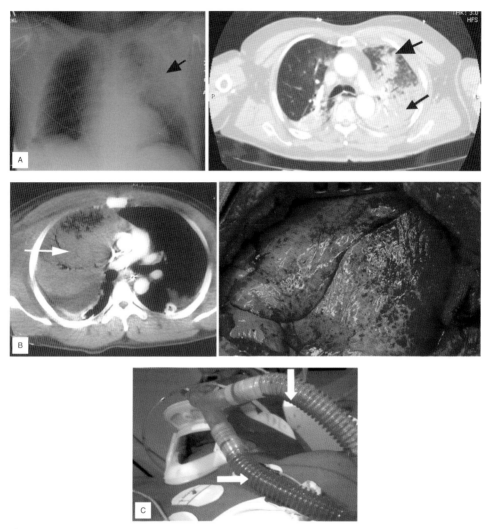

Figure 13.8 (A) Lung contusion: chest x-ray with large opacification in the left lung, highly suspicious for lung contusion (left). Chest CT scan confirms the presence of lung contusion (right). (B) Lung contusion: CT scan appearance of a large contusion (arrow) (left). Intraoperative appearance of the lung contusion (right). (C) Bronchial bleeding in respiratory tubing is a common finding in severe lung contusions. Flooding of the normal lung may result in respiratory failure. Double-lumen endotracheal tube and independent lung ventilation should be considered (reproduced with permission from *Color Atlas of Emergency Trauma, Second Edition*)

patients). Occasionally, a diaphragm injury is discovered at the time of operation for other injuries or indications (Figure 13.10).

- *Treatment*: Diaphragmatic injuries should be repaired, most commonly via a transabdominal approach. Depending upon associated injuries, this may be approached either laparoscopically or open. Right sided diaphragmatic injuries may be managed conservatively or non-operatively as the liver will often buttress the injury, with a lower risk of herniation and strangulation of intra-abdominal contents as a result of this (Figure 13.10).[1,13]

Tracheobronchial Disruption

- *Pathophysiology*: This is an uncommon injury which may occur in 0.5–2% of blunt trauma patients. The majority of injuries (>80%) are located within 2.5 cm of the carina. For penetrating injuries, the majority involve the cervical trachea or larynx.[14]
- *Presentation*: Blunt tracheobronchial disruption rarely occurs in isolation. On physical exam, dyspnea and respiratory distress may be present. Findings of

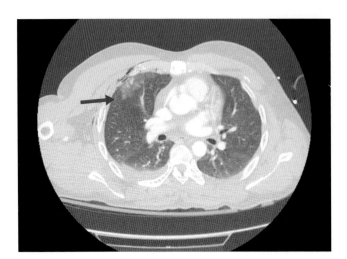

Figure 13.9 Right upper lobe pulmonary contusions, small hemothorax, and subcutaneous emphysema in patient following a high-speed MVC (image: Dennis Kim, MD)

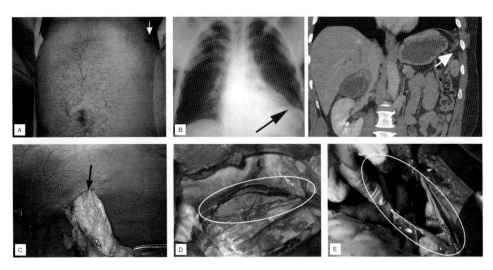

Figure 13.10 (A, B) Penetrating diaphragmatic injuries. (A) Photograph of stab wound to the left thoracoabdominal area (arrow). Penetrating trauma in this area is highly suspicious for diaphragmatic injury. (B) Chest x-ray shows an elevated left diaphragm, which is suspicious for diaphragmatic injury (left). CT scan shows a left diaphragm injury (right). (C) Laparoscopy shows a diaphragmatic perforation with omentum herniating into the left chest. (D) Blunt diaphragmatic rupture: high-speed motor vehicle crash with left diaphragmatic rupture. Note the lung through the tear (left). Post-repair of the injury (right). (E, F) Blunt vs. penetrating diaphragmatic injuries. (E) Appearance of blunt diaphragmatic injuries through a thoracotomy (left) and through a laparotomy (right). Note the large size of the injuries.

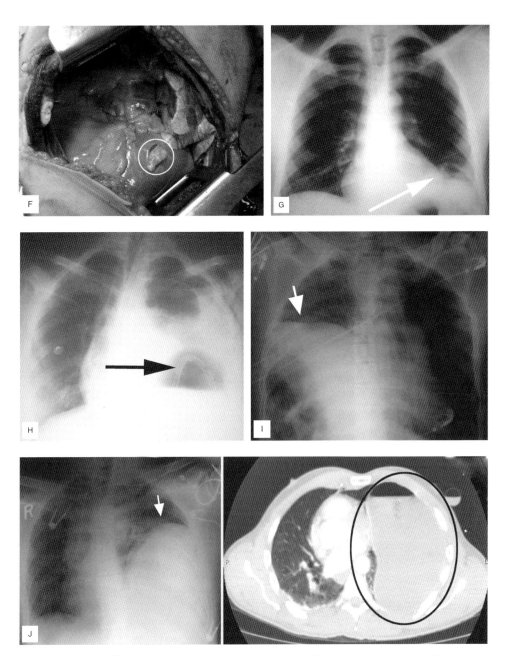

Figure 13.10 (*cont.*) (F) Appearance of a penetrating diaphragmatic injury through a thoracotomy. The injury is usually small (2–3 cm). Note the omentum herniating through the diaphragmatic defect. (G–I) Radiological appearance of traumatic diaphragmatic hernias. (G) Chest x-ray with a suspicious shadow at the base of the left hemithorax following a stab wound many months earlier. Further investigations showed gastric herniation into the chest. (H) Chest x-ray shows the nasogastric tube curling into the left chest (arrow), pathognomonic of gastric herniation. Chest x-ray shows a significantly elevated right diaphragm following a motor vehicle crash two weeks earlier. (I) The entire liver (arrow) and hepatic flexure of the colon were found at laparotomy to be herniated into the right chest. (J) Chest x-ray and CT scan of patient, many months after a stab wound to the left thoracoabdominal area, shows a tension diaphragmatic hernia with significant deviation of the heart to the right chest (left). CT scan showing the stomach herniating into the chest (right).

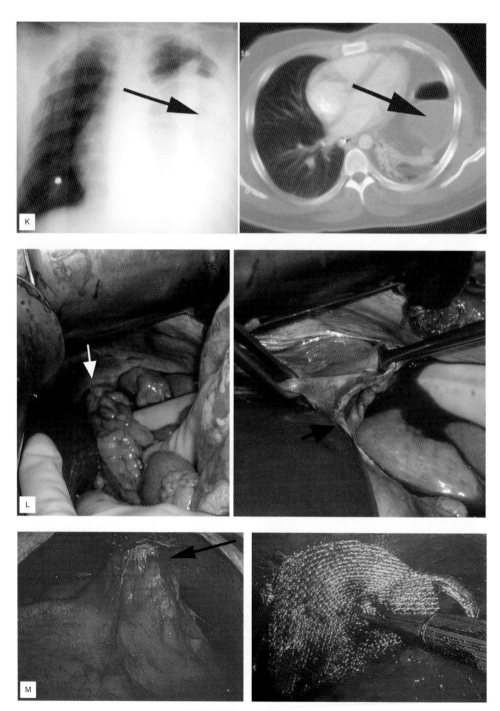

Figure 13.10 (*cont.*) (K) Chest x-ray shows a tension diaphragmatic hernia a few weeks after a stab wound to the left lower chest (left). CT findings confirm the stomach, spleen, and colon herniating into the chest (right). (L) Operative appearance of left diaphragmatic hernia containing colon and omentum (left). Photograph of the diaphragmatic defect after reduction of the hernia contents (right). (M) Laparoscopic appearance of the stomach and omentum herniating into the chest (left) and successful repair with the mesh (right).

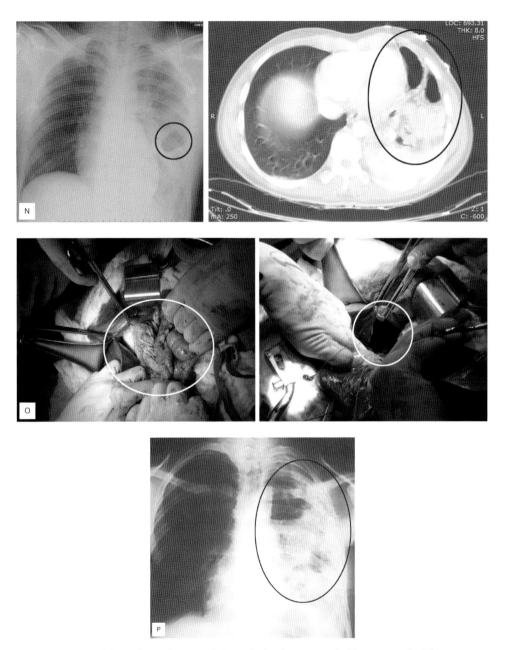

Figure 13.10 (*cont.*) (N) High-speed motor vehicle crash. The chest x-ray is highly suspicious for left traumatic diaphragmatic hernia (left). The CT scan shows herniation of the stomach, spleen, and bowel into the left chest (right). (O) Intraoperative photograph showing a large diaphragmatic hernia with herniation of multiple abdominal contents (left). The photograph on the right shows the diaphragm defect after the reduction of the herniating viscera. (P) Chest x-ray of a large diaphragmatic hernia containing stomach, colon, and small bowel, initially diagnosed and treated as bronchopneumonia. The delay in diagnosis resulted in ischemic necrosis of the colon (reproduced with permission from *Color Atlas of Emergency Trauma, Second Edition*)

massive subcutaneous emphysema, hemoptysis, and pneumothorax are suggestive. Large or massive air leak following chest tube insertion is also suggestive of this injury.[14]

- *Diagnosis*: On chest x-ray, incomplete re-expansion of the lung following chest tube placement or the appearance of a collapsing lung away from the hilum towards the diaphragm (falling lung sign of Kumpe) may be seen. CT thorax may demonstrate non-specific findings such as disruption of the tracheobronchial air column.[1,14] Definitive diagnosis is made via fiberoptic bronchoscopy.
- *Treatment*: Fiberoptic bronchoscopic intubation is the preferred method of securing the airway and serves both therapeutic and diagnostic purposes. Temporary mainstem intubation of the contralateral or unaffected lung may be required. Double-lumen tubes should be inserted with caution in patients with tracheobronchial disruption. A bronchial blocker may be used in patients with more distal bronchial injuries. Timing and extent of operative repair are dictated by the location and size of injury, in addition to the presence of associated injuries.

Esophageal Disruption

- *Pathophysiology*: This is a rare but life-threatening injury which is more common following penetrating vs. blunt trauma. Early recognition is critical to successful outcomes, and delays of >24 hours are associated with increased morbidity and mortality. The condition is more common following a gunshot wound, compared to a stab wound, and the cervical esophagus is more commonly involved than the thoracic esophagus.[15]
- *Presentation*: Blunt trauma, typically a direct blow to the epigastrium or upper abdomen, can result in a tear in the lower esophagus, with a similar clinical picture to patients with esophageal rupture due to Boerhaave's. A high index of suspicion should be maintained in patients with transmediastinal GSWs. Clinical symptoms and signs are not reliably present (i.e. odynophagia, hematemesis, neck pain, dysphagia, etc.), and the mechanism, location of injuries, and proximity of wound tracts to the esophagus on radiographic imaging should increase the index of suspicion for an esophageal injury.
- *Diagnosis*: For patients with a suspected esophageal injury, contrast (Gastrografin) esophagogram (specificity 83%, sensitivity 60–70%) and esophagoscopy (specificity 100%, sensitivity 20%) are the recommended diagnostic procedures of choice (Figure 13.11). CT with IV contrast does not possess 100% sensitivity and specificity but may be utilized, though CT esophagography has better performance.
- *Treatment*: Early recognition and repair with wide drainage are critical for optimal outcomes. This typically involved performing a neck exploration or thoracotomy, depending on whether the location is cervical or thoracic, respectively.[15] The duration of antibiotic therapy is often guided by the patient's clinical status, but broad-spectrum antibiotics covering gram negative and anaerobic species are recommended initially (clindamycin and gentamicin if penicillin allergic, OR piperacillin and tazobactam OR ampicillin/sulbactam or ticarcillin/clavulanate ± clindamycin).[15] More recently, there

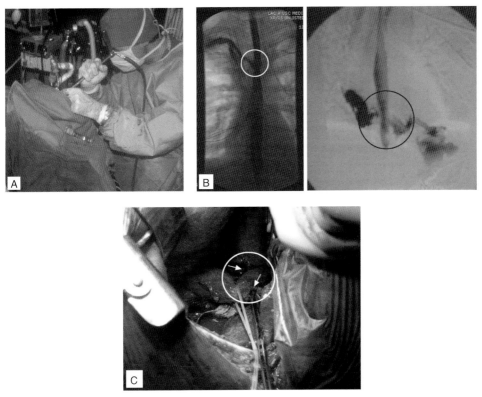

Figure 13.11 (A) Intraoperative rigid esophagoscopy for suspected esophageal injury. (B) Gastric swallow studies showing injuries to the upper thoracic (left) and lower thoracic esophagus (right), following gunshot injuries. (C) Intraoperative photograph showing a through-and-through esophageal wound with suction tip passing through the esophageal perforations (reproduced with permission from *Color Atlas of Emergency Trauma, Second Edition*)

has been an increasing experience with minimally invasive techniques for managing non-traumatic esophageal perforations using covered stents.[15]

Pitfalls in Thoracic Trauma
- Be wary to not mistake a breathing problem with an airway problem.
- Tension pneumothorax is a clinical diagnosis. There is no confirmation needed with x-rays. If unsure based on examination, do a bedside ultrasound.
- Consider autologous transfusion with heparin/citrate for massive hemothorax. Warm blood is better to avoid the lethal triad of trauma (Coagulopathy, Acidosis, Hypothermia).
- Flail chest management involves multimodal approach of analgesia, including opioids, NSAIDs, and nerve blocks.
- Pulmonary contusion can blossom into ARDS quickly, so judicious fluid management is recommended.
- Know the pitfalls of the FAST exam and what can cause false negatives/equivocal exam.

Key Points

- Chest trauma is a common injury seen in many trauma patients, where mechanism sheds light of the type of injuries one can sustain.
- The six deadly chest trauma conditions should always be considered, followed by the potential deadly six causes in the secondary survey as highlighted in the beginning of the chapter.

References

1. Moore E, Feliciano DV, Mattox KL. *Trauma*, 8th ed. New York: McGraw-Hill.

2. Holmes MG, Dagal A, Feinstein BA, et al. Airway management practice in adults with an unstable cervical spine: the Harborview Medical Center experience. *Anesth Analg.* 2018;127(2):450–54.

3. Roberts DJ, Leigh-Smith S, Faris PD, et al. Clinical presentation of patients with tension pneumothorax: a systematic review. *Ann Surg.* 2015;261(6):1068–78.

4. Clemency BM, Tanski CT, Rosenberg M, et al. Sufficient catheter length for pneumothorax needle decompression: a meta-analysis. *Prehosp Disaster Med.* 2015;30(3):249–53.

5. Walker M. The management of thoracic trauma: principles and practice. *Niger J Cardiovasc Thorac Surg.* 2016 1(1):8.

6. Kuhajda I, Zarogoulidis K, Kougiomtzi I, et al. Penetrating trauma. *J Thorac Dis.* 2014;6(Suppl 4):S461–465.

7. Brown C VR, Foulkrod KH, Sadler HT, et al. Autologous blood transfusion during emergency trauma operations. *Arch Surg.* 2010;145(7):690–94.

8. Barriot P, Riou B, Vlars P. Prehospital autotransfusion in life-threatening hemothorax. *Chest.* 1988;93(3):522–26.

9. Salhanick M, Sams V, Pidcoke H, et al. Shed pleural blood from traumatic hemothorax contains elevated levels of pro-inflammatory cytokines. *Shock.* 2016;46(2):144–48.

10. Salhanick M, Corneille M, Higgins R, et al. Autotransfusion of hemothorax blood in trauma patients: is it the same as fresh whole blood? *Am J Surg.* 2011;202 (6):817–21.

11. Dehghan N, de Mestral C, McKee MD, et al. Flail chest injuries: a review of outcomes and treatment practices from the National Trauma Data Bank. *J Trauma Acute Care Surg.* 2014;76 (2):462–68.

12. Pharaon KS, Marasco S, Mayberry J. Rib fractures, flail chest, and pulmonary contusion. *Curr Trauma Rep.* 2015;1 (4):237–42.

13. Fair KA, Gordon NT, Barbosa RR, et al. Traumatic diaphragmatic injury in the American College of Surgeons National Trauma Data Bank: a new examination of a rare diagnosis. *Am J Surg.* 2015;209 (5):864–68.

14. Ludwig C, Koryllos A. Management of chest trauma. *J Thorac Dis.* 2017;9(Suppl 3):S172–177.

15. Dickinson KJ, Blackmon SH. Esophageal perforation. In: Moore LJ, Todd SR, eds. *Common Problems in Acute Care Surgery.* Berlin, Germany: Springer; 2017, pp. 179–84.

Cardiac Trauma

Brit Long

Cardiac trauma is a critical injury, with penetrating cardiothoracic injury accounting for up to a third of traumatic deaths.[1–4] These injuries often involve the heart or great vessels and include traumatic insertion of a foreign body, including invasive iatrogenic injury.[1–8] Blunt cardiac trauma occurs in a wide range of patients, with 8–71% of patients with cardiothoracic trauma demonstrating signs of cardiac injury.[1,2,8] Blunt cardiac injury encompasses all types of injury associated with blunt thoracic trauma to the heart.[8–13] Up to 20% of deaths from motor vehicle collisions (MVCs) are due to this type of injury. Patients with thoracic great vessel injury due to penetrating injury have a high mortality rate (over 90% die at the scene),[14,15] and blunt injury to the thoracic vessels is commonly due to motor vehicle accident.[12,13,16,17] These injuries can result in chest, upper abdominal, back, arm/shoulder, or lower neck pain, as well as hemodynamic instability, nausea/vomiting, and shortness of breath.

Causes

- Penetrating injury most commonly occurs due to guns or knives, often involving only the cardiac wall. The right ventricle (RV) is most commonly affected (40%), followed by the left ventricle (LV) (35%), right atrium (20%), and left atrium (5%) (Figure 14.1).[2,9,17–20] Other structures such as valves, the septum, coronary arteries, or the conduction system may be affected. There are many injuries associated with penetrating injury (Box 14.1).

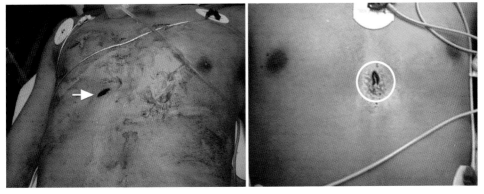

Figure 14.1 Patients with precordial penetrating wounds. Every penetrating injury to the chest, especially in the presence of hypotension, should be considered as a cardiac injury until proven otherwise (reproduced with permission from *Color Atlas of Emergency Trauma, Second Edition*)

Box 14.1 Affected Structures in Cardiac Trauma

Penetrating Cardiac Injury

- Cardiac perforation
- Cardiac laceration
- Pericardial damage
- Retained foreign body
- Structural defect
- Valvular, leaflet, papillary muscle, chorda tendineae injury
- Coronary vessel injury
- Damage to conduction system

Box 14.2 Causes of Blunt Cardiac Injury

Blunt Cardiac Injury

- Crush injury
- Direct thoracic impact
- Blast injury
- Abrupt pressure change in chest and abdomen
- Shearing injury from rapid deceleration
- Injury from rib fracture segment

- Blunt cardiac injury results from a direct blow to the pericardium, often from a sudden deceleration in MVC (Box 14.2). This results in a wide range of symptoms including dysrhythmia to wall rupture (the most devastating injury).[8,9,12,16]
- Great vessel injury is due to penetrating or blunt etiology, both with high mortality rates. Blunt injury of the great vessels is often due to rapid deceleration, with the chest hitting the steering wheel in MVC.[14,21]

Anatomy

- The cardiac box consists of the sternal notch in the superior part, the xiphoid process inferiorly, and the nipples laterally.[1–3,13,22] Knife wounds can directly enter this region, though gunshot wounds can enter the cardiac box through another site due to travel across the mediastinum.
- The heart is surrounded by two layers of pericardium, with the pericardial space containing approximately 5–15 cc of pericardial fluid at baseline.
- The RV is at greatest risk for penetrating and blunt injury due to its exposed surface area to the anterior chest wall, with the atria less affected due to smaller volumes and surface area.[2,18,19]
- The thoracic great vessels include the aorta and brachiocephalic vessels, the left subclavian/left common carotid/pulmonary vessels, the superior and inferior vena cava, and the innominate and azygos veins.[2–4]

Pathophysiology

- Penetrating injuries with knives usually affect one chamber, though gunshot wounds (GSW) may result in multi-chamber perforation.[2,9,17-20] Stab wounds are associated with improved outcomes due to the production of a single slit defect.
- Multichamber and ventricular injuries are associated with worse outcomes.[18-20]
- Blunt injury with myocardial contusion includes subendocardial bleeding with leukocyte migration to the affected area. Coronary blood flow may redistribute due to the injury and release of immune mediators.[4-8]
- Dysrhythmias, acute heart failure, laceration of coronary vessels, and ventricular wall rupture can result in immediate death. Valvular or septal injury can result in regurgitation and shunting, respectively. Vascular spasm from affected coronary vessels may result in presentation similar to myocardial infarction (MI).[4-8]
- Injury, including penetrating and blunt, to the great vessels can result in rapid exsanguination. Vascular injury can lead to dissection, fistula, aneurysm, or pseudoaneurysm formation.
- The proximal descending aorta is the most common injured vessel in the chest (over 80% of cases) at its attachment of the left subclavian artery and ligamentum arteriosum. Branch vessels are involved in 15% of cases (Figure 14.2).[2,23-25]

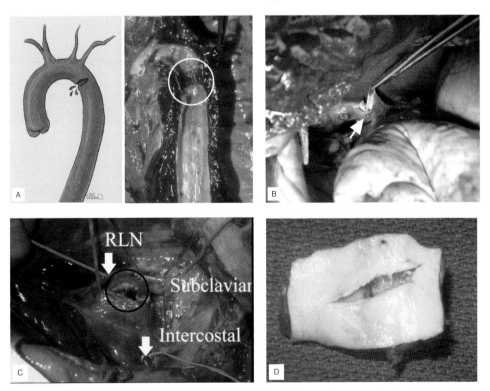

Figure 14.2 Illustration and autopsy specimen of the typical site of blunt aortic rupture, distal to the left subclavian artery (A). Intraoperative photograph of a transected thoracic aorta found at emergency room thoracotomy (B). Intraoperative appearance of thoracic aortic rupture (RLN = Recurrent Laryngeal Nerve) (C). Surgical specimen of a contained aortic rupture. The outside layer of the aorta is intact (D) (reproduced with permission from *Color Atlas of Emergency Trauma, Second Edition*, illustration at A by Alexis Demetriades)

Approach

These patients may demonstrate nonspecific signs and symptoms or present in cardiac arrest. Multisystem injuries and altered sensorium can cloud the picture, and specific signs of cardiac injury such as murmurs may not be detectable in the resuscitation bay due to other patient factors (hypotension) and ambient noise/lighting.[2,9]

History

- Penetrating – Mechanism, vital signs, patient course, suspected injuries, and treatments in the field are valuable. If unstable, history is likely unobtainable. Immediate resuscitation is required for hemodynamic instability.[2,9]
- Blunt – Similar to penetrating trauma, though the quality of chest pain should also be ascertained. Be wary of attributing symptoms to only superficial chest wall injuries, which may hide pericardial/myocardial injury. Dyspnea may be due to a wide range of etiologies, and lightheadedness and palpitations are also common.[2–9,12]
- Great vessel – As discussed, many patients with great vessel injury die at the scene. Patients who arrive in the ED are frequently unstable. They may complain of chest pain, shortness of breath, back pain, limb weakness, and anuria. Mechanism of injury, speed of collision (if MVC), seat belt use, and other injuries should be assessed.[2,12,13,16]

Examination

- Initial vital signs and assessment of ABCs are imperative. Hemodynamic status must be continually monitored, as patients may decompensate quickly. Tachycardia that is unexplained may be the only finding in blunt cardiac trauma.[2,3,9]
- Assessment of breath and heart sounds is difficult and may not be reliable based on patient habitus and ambient noise. Muffled heart sounds with clear lungs may indicate cardiac tamponade.[2,3,9]
- Crackles in the lungs, murmurs, extra heart sounds (S3), and jugular venous distension indicate acute heart failure.
- Vital signs, ABCs, and focused secondary examination are essential, including neurovascular examination of the upper and lower extremities. Deficit may be due to great vessel injury (traumatic dissection). Ultrasound (US) is beneficial as part of the secondary examination to evaluate for cardiac effusion, cardiac tamponade, pulmonary edema, and lung sliding.[2,3,9]
- Most patients with great vessel injury depict outer physical exam signs such as bruising or a wound.
- Hypotension, unequal blood pressures between the upper extremities or upper and lower extremities, thoracic outlet hematoma, seatbelt signs, palpable rib fractures, and flail chest suggest great vessel injury.
- Penetrating wounds should not be probed in the ED, which may worsen bleeding.[2,3,9]

Penetrating Cardiac Trauma

There are several severe injuries associated with death in penetrating injury to the heart.

- Pericardial injury: A large defect in the pericardium can result in sudden bleeding into the thoracic cavity and exsanguination. If the defect is smaller, the injury may result in pericardial tamponade.[2,9]

- Ventricular injuries will often seal themselves due to extensive musculature, as opposed to atrial injuries. Ventricular injuries also seal themselves faster.[9,11]
- Atrial and coronary vessel injuries may be subtle, but injuries can cause rapid decompensation.

Cardiac Tamponade

- This condition results from fluid accumulation under pressure into the pericardial space, found in 2% of penetrating injuries to the chest and abdomen. Up to 80% of stab wounds to the heart result in tamponade. GSWs cause larger pericardial defects and less likely cause tamponade.
- Blood in the pericardial cavity may form a hematoma. Fluid results in elevated pericardial pressures, decreasing RV and LV filling. HR increases to improve RA and RV filling. Even amounts less than 100 mL may result in elevated pericardial pressures.[9,11,19,20]
- RV distension pushes the septum into the LV, decreasing LV filling and cardiac output. This leads to shock and death.[9]
- US is essential in evaluation, as tamponade is difficult to diagnose in trauma patients. Elevated HR and vascular resistance can partially compensate for tamponade, with tachycardia often the first indication. Beck's triad (muffled heart sounds, hypotension, and JVD) is found in less than 10% of patients, and pulsus paradoxus is also not reliable.[10] Narrowed pulse pressure is frequent, and hypotension is an early sign of decompensation.

Cardiac Missile

- This may result from direct injury or embolization. If retained from another site, patients are often stable and observed.
- Treatment of these missiles is dependent on size, mechanism, shape, and location. If symptoms or hemodynamic instability are present, patients should go to the OR for removal of the missile. Others that require removal include those within coronary vessels or those that have embolized.[26–28]

Iatrogenic Injury

- Pericardiocentesis, chest tube placement, coronary catheterization, and electrophysiological and valvular procedures may result in injury.[29]

Blunt Trauma

Several types of blunt cardiac injury are associated with trauma. The most common is myocardial or cardiac contusion, though the term "blunt cardiac injury" has replaced "cardiac contusion" (Figure 14.3). This new term encompasses the following injuries:[2–10,12]

Cardiac Rupture

This is the most severe form of blunt cardiac injury. The right side is at highest risk for rupture, and patients often die at the scene.[2,10,30] Patients who survive may display a murmur. US may immediately diagnose this condition, and if discovered, the patient requires thoracotomy.

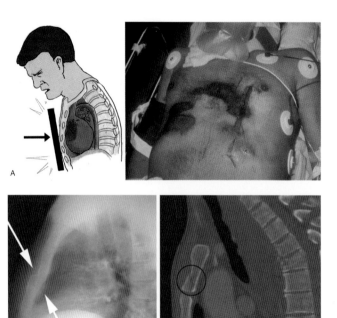

Figure 14.3 (A) Illustration of the mechanism of blunt cardiac injury from steering wheel (left). Photograph of blunt chest trauma to the anterior chest from a steering wheel injury (right). This patient arrived in ventricular tachycardia. (B) Lateral chest radiograph and CT scan showing sternal fractures. This injury is often associated with cardiac trauma. These patients should be evaluated by ECG and serial troponin levels (reproduced with permission from *Color Atlas of Emergency Trauma, Second Edition*, illustration at A by Robert Amaral)

Coronary Vessel Injury/MI

Injury to cardiac vessels is rare. The most common injured vessel is the left anterior descending artery. Coronary vessel dissection and coronary artery disease most often occur in the first 7 days.[31-34] Patients most commonly present with chest pain. Patients require percutaneous intervention, though anticoagulation requires consultation with cardiology and cardiothoracic surgery due to risk of hemorrhage.[2,9,10]

Injury to the Valves, Papillary Muscles, Chordae Tendinae, and Septum

Valvular damage occurs in 10% of cardiac trauma cases, though it usually occurs with other injuries. The aortic valve is the most common valve injured, which may cause aortic regurgitation and pulmonary edema. Injury to the cardiac septum may occur but is rare.[31,32,35] Any new murmur or pulmonary edema in a patient with chest trauma requires US and resuscitation with surgical consultation. Small injuries may heal on their own, but this is not common.

Pericardial Injury

Defects in the pericardium may result from blunt impact, often parallel to the phrenic nerve on the left side of the pericardium.[2,8,9] These defects are often missed, and they may not be associated with symptoms. If herniation occurs, cardiac conduction is often interrupted. Exam can demonstrate pericardial rub, though this is not common. US or CT may demonstrate injury, which requires surgical repair.[2,8-10]

Cardiac Dysfunction

The frequency of this injury is unknown and difficult to determine in the multisystem trauma patient. Patients usually present with chest pain, and patients may also have pulmonary vascular injury, decreasing LV preload, and in combination with RV output, reduced cardiac output may occur. Damage to the myocardial tissue and conduction system can also further harm cardiac output. Monitoring is needed for dysrhythmias, which include tachycardia, bundle branch block, high degree blocks, supraventricular tachycardia, ventricular fibrillation, and premature ventricular contractions, which can occur up to 48 hours after blunt injury.[2,3,13,35]

Commotio Cordis

This injury consists of sudden death associated with blunt injury to the anterior chest wall and is the most common cause of death in young athletes (baseball and lacrosse).[8–10,36] Commotio cordis injury is usually due to a low impact blow that strikes the heart and results in ventricular fibrillation, occurring 10–30 ms before the peak of the T wave. Cardiac anatomy is usually normal. Survival rate is less than 15%. If suspected, immediate compressions and defibrillation are required.[36,37]

Multisystem Trauma

Blunt cardiac injury is associated with many other injuries, often occurring in the setting of multisystem trauma (Table 14.1).[2,9]

Great Vessel Injury

Injury occurs due to direct injury or indirectly through kinetic injury of a passing missile. Great vessel injury can be iatrogenic. Embolization of missiles (such as a bullet) can occur, though this may not result in symptoms.[38–41] As discussed, the most common vessel injured is the aorta. Rupture of the ascending aorta is associated with severe blunt cardiac injury and cardiac rupture.

Table 14.1 Associated injuries in cardiac trauma[2,9]

Injury	Frequency
Head injury	20–73%
Extremity injury	20–66%
Abdominal injury	5–43%
Spinal injury	10–20%
Other thoracic injury	18–92%
Chest pain	18–69%
Rib fracture	4–38%
Flail chest	0–60%
Sternal fracture	7–40%
Pneumothorax	7–64%
Hemothorax	6–58%
Pulmonary contusion	20–40%
Great vessel injury	

Evaluation

- Immediate evaluation of the primary survey is required (ABCDE, FAST), with intravenous access, continuous monitoring, and pulse oximetry.[2,3,9,11]
- Once this is completed, focused secondary examination is needed. A focused neurovascular exam of the extremities should be conducted if possible to evaluate for great vessel injury.

Electrocardiogram (ECG)

An ECG is needed when able. A normal ECG alone is not enough to exclude significant injury, which may miss up to 20% of cases.[13,16,42,43] A significant dysrhythmia can occur within 48 hours of the initial injury (Table 14.2).

- The ECG is more sensitive for left sided rather than right sided injuries. One of the most common findings is persistent tachycardia, which is nonspecific with a variety of etiologies. ST changes, especially elevation, may suggest MI.[9,12,16,44]
- If initial ECG is normal but concern for blunt injury is present, 4–6 hours of continuous cardiac monitoring is needed. If monitoring is normal with no new symptoms, patients may be appropriate for discharge. Any ECG abnormality requires further evaluation.[9,12]
- Pericardial effusion if large may demonstrate low voltage and tachycardia. Electrical alternans, though considered the classic finding for cardiac tamponade, is not 100% sensitive for tamponade.[2,9]

Laboratory Assessment with Cardiac Biomarkers

A great deal of controversy is present concerning biomarkers.

- Creatine kinase (CK)-MB elevates with injuries of other systems such as the liver or intestines. Also, isolated elevation of CK-MB does not predict mortality, and it is not recommended.

Table 14.2 ECG in cardiac trauma[2,9]

Injury	ECG Finding
Myocardial injury	New Q wave ST segment elevation or depression T wave changes
Conduction disorder	Right or left bundle branch block (right more common) Fascicular block (1st, 2nd, or 3rd degree block)
Dysrhythmia	Sinus tachycardia (most common) Sinus bradycardia Atrial, ventricular extra beats Atrial fibrillation/flutter Ventricular tachycardia/fibrillation Atrial tachycardia
Nonspecific	Pericarditis (PR depression, diffuse ST elevation) Prolonged QTc

- Troponin is specific for myocardial injury, though not the etiology.[9,45–47] Troponin sensitivity for cardiac contusion ranges from 12–23%, with specificity over 97% in the setting of trauma.[45–48] Causes of shock other than primary cardiac etiology may also result in troponin elevation.
- Troponin elevation is correlated with decreased ejection fraction, dysrhythmias, and LV dysfunction.[47,48]
- The use of troponin and ECG may improve risk stratification, as negative ECG and troponin are associated with extremely low risk of blunt cardiac injury. Abnormal ECG warrants troponin testing. Any abnormality in ECG and troponin testing strongly suggests blunt cardiac injury.[47–51]

Imaging

Ultrasound

The FAST exam requires cardiac images via the subxiphoid or parasternal long axis view. FAST exam allows evaluation of gross cardiac function and the presence of cardiac effusion (Figure 14.4). US displays a sensitivity and specificity over 99% for detection of pericardial effusion.[2,3,52–56]

- Patients with abnormal cardiac troponin, dysrhythmia, and concern for blunt cardiac injury require US. Transthoracic echocardiogram (TTE) may demonstrate dissection.[9,57]

Transesophageal Echocardiography (TEE)

TEE is portable and fast, with immediate bedside results. This is promising; however, few emergency physicians are trained in this modality. This modality is also useful in the potentially unstable patient.[58] TEE can detect aortic lesions (including full rupture and

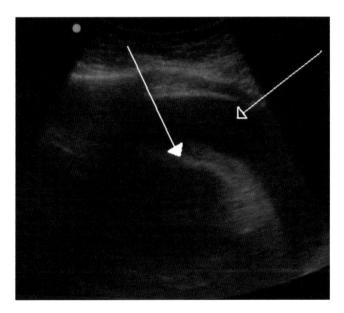

Figure 14.4 Ultrasound with evidence of pericardial tamponade. Solid white arrow is RV, while clear arrow is pericardial effusion (image courtesy of James Heilman, MD, reproduced here under CC BY-SA 3.0 license https://creativecommons.org/licenses/by-sa/3.0/)

Table 14.3 Chest X-ray in great vessel injury[2,9]

Location/Pattern	Finding
Mediastinum	Aortic knob obliteration
	Wide mediastinum
	Left mainstem bronchus depression
	Paravertebral pleural stripe loss
	Aortic knob layering with calcium
	Lateral displacement of the trachea
	Nasogastric tube deviation at T4
Fractures	Sternum
	Scapula
	Multiple ribs
	First rib
	Clavicle
Lateral X-ray	Trachea anterior displacement
	Aortic/pulmonary window absence
Others	Apical pleural hematoma
	Left hemothorax
	Diaphragm injury

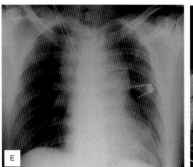 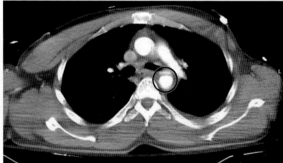

Figure 14.5 Blunt thoracic aortic injury. Chest x-ray shows a widened mediastinum and deviation of the trachea to the right (left). CT image confirms thoracic aortic injury (right) (reproduced with permission from *Color Atlas of Emergency Trauma, Second Edition*)

intimal defects). However, it is contraindicated in patients with potential airway issues (if not already intubated) or cervical spine injury.[54–56]

Chest X-ray

This imaging modality is not sensitive or specific for injury. Cardiomegaly is rare in acute pericardial effusion and tamponade. Widened mediastinum may suggest aortic dissection, with width greater than 8 cm (Figure 14.5, Table 14.3).[2,3,59–62] Other findings include esophageal deviation more than 1 cm to the right of the spine at the T4 level.[62,63] A normal chest X-ray does not rule out aortic injury.

Computed Tomography (CT)

CT of the chest with contrast is the modality of choice for penetrating and blunt chest trauma (Figure 14.6, Table 14.4). Multidetector scanners display sensitivity and specificity approaching 100% for vascular and lung injuries. In penetrating injury, evaluation of injury tract and vascular involvement is essential. However, in blunt cardiac injury, CT may detect wall motion abnormalities.[23–25] CT with IV contrast is definitive for great vessel injury, with defects appearing as irregular vascular contours, vessel lumen abnormalities, dissection, aneurysm/pseudoaneurysm, and acute bleeding. CT also depicts the tract of injury, including knives and missiles.[2,9,23–25]

MRI

This imaging modality is not available in all institutions, and the time required is usually prohibitive. It provides similar information as CT.[2,9]

Management
Penetrating Trauma
Pericardiocentesis

In the setting of penetrating trauma with new pericardial effusion and unstable vital signs, preparation for thoracotomy is required.[2,9,64] Pericardiocentesis may be used to temporize the patient.[2,9,56,64,65]

ED Thoracotomy (EDT)

Unstable patients with cardiac activity and penetrating cardiac injury require the OR emergently. Patients who lose pulses in the ED with penetrating or blunt trauma are eligible for EDT (Table 14.5).[2,3,9,66–68] Others include patients with penetrating thoracic trauma and hemodynamic instability, despite fluid resuscitation or if pulseless less than 15 minutes.[69–72]

- EDT is not recommended if asystole is present with no pericardial effusion, pulselessness >15 minutes, other massive nonsurvivable injuries, no pulse in the field, and blunt cardiac arrest.[2,9]

Table 14.4 CT in great vessel injury[23–25]

Frequency	Injury
Common	Aortic aneurysm/pseudoaneurysm Hemorrhage around the aorta Tracheal and esophageal displacement to the right Luminal intimal flap
Uncommon	Intimal disruption with luminal clot Change in aortic caliber suddenly Diaphragmatic hemorrhage Small aortic caliber in the lower chest and abdomen
Rare	Aortic transection Aortic bleeding

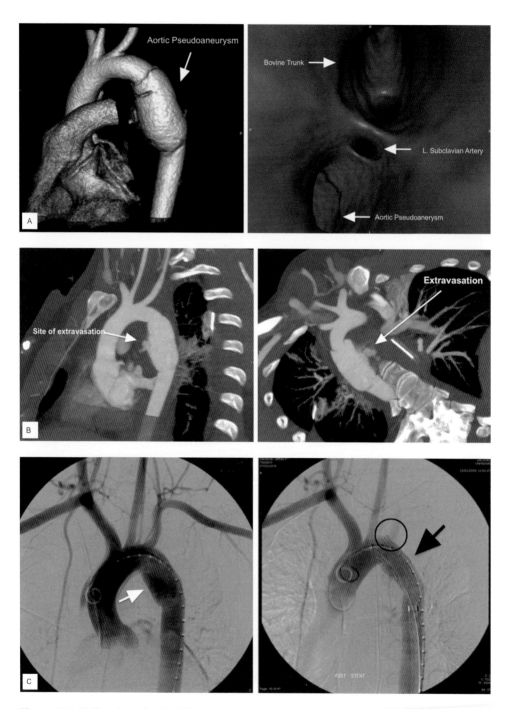

Figure 14.6 (A) CT angiography with 3-D reconstruction shows a contained aortic rupture (left). Endoluminal view of the aortic pseudoaneurysm (right). (B) CT images of a blunt thoracic aortic injury with leak. This patient needs an emergency operation because of the risk of imminent free rupture. (C) Aortogram of traumatic aortic pseudoaneurysm, (left) treated with stent-graft deployment (right). Note the occlusion of the left subclavian artery by the device. (D–F) CT scan showing a rupture of the thoracic aorta (D). CT scan appearance of the deployed stent graft with occlusion of the rupture site (E, F) (reproduced with permission from *Color Atlas of Emergency Trauma, Second Edition*)

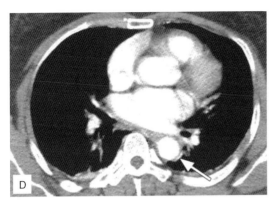
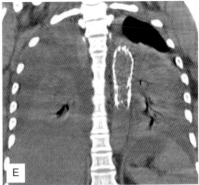
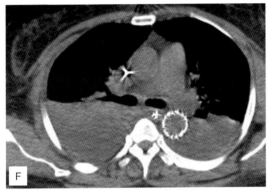

Figure 14.6 *(cont.)*

- Procedure (Figure 14.7): Left anterolateral thoracotomy is the classic procedure. The left sided approach allows exposure of the phrenic nerve, aorta, and left side of the chest cavity.[2,3,66–72]
  - The patient should be intubated with NG/OG placed before the procedure. The left 4th or 5th intercostal space should be identified (the intercostal space below the male's nipple or inframammary fold in a woman), with primary incision at this location.
  - The site should be quickly sterilized and incised with one broad stroke through all layers to the intercostal muscles down to the posterior axillary line. These muscles should be cut with Mayo scissors.
  - A Finochietto retractor is then placed within the chest, with the crank near the bed. The retractor is opened to expose the left chest cavity.
  - Control any hemorrhage with direct pressure. Move the lung to expose the pericardium.
  - Signs of cardiac injury include distended, discolored, and tense pericardial sac. The pericardium should be incised anterior to the phrenic nerve to allow inspection of the heart for injury.
  - Digital occlusion of the wound can be the first maneuver, but a finger should never be inserted into the heart, which can extend the injury.

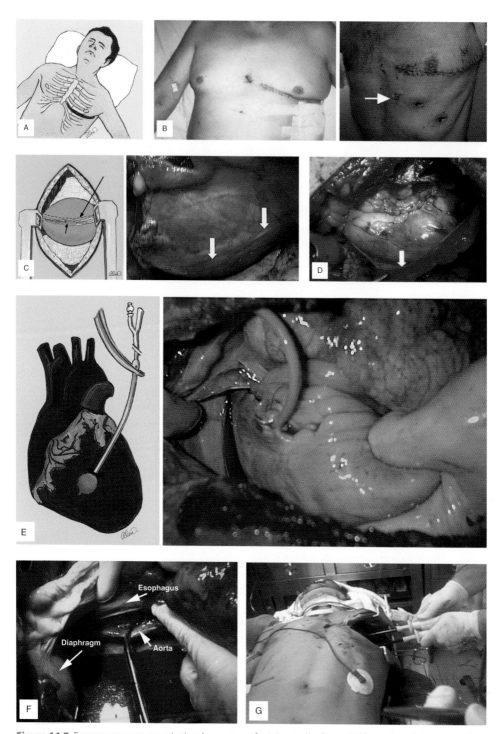

Figure 14.7 Emergency room resuscitative thoracotomy for injury to the heart. (A) Illustration of the incision for a resuscitative emergency department left anterolateral thoracotomy. (B) Photographs showing incisions for

Table 14.5 Trauma association guidelines[71,72]

Eastern Association for the Surgery of Trauma	• EDT is best for patients with penetrating cardiac trauma who arrive to a trauma center with short scene and transport time and witnessed or objectively physiologic signs of life. • EDT should be performed in patients with penetrating noncardiac thoracic injuries, but with low survival rates. EDT may be used to establish the diagnosis of whether the injury is cardiac or noncardiac. • EDT should be rarely performed in patients with cardiac arrest due to blunt trauma with low survival rate and poor neurologic outcomes. EDT should be limited to patients who arrive with vital signs at the trauma center and experience cardiac arrest that is witnessed. • EDT should be performed in patients with exsanguinating abdominal vascular injuries, though with low survival.
Western Trauma Association	• Patients undergoing CPR on arrival to the hospital can be stratified based on injury and transport time. • Indications include: Blunt trauma patients with less than 10 minutes of prehospital CPR, Penetrating torso patients with less than 15 minutes of CPR, patients with penetrating trauma to the neck/extremity with less than 5 minutes of CPR, patients in profound refractory shock. • Following EDT, evaluate the patient's intrinsic cardiac activity. Patients in asystole and no cardiac tamponade should be declared dead.

- Staples via skin stapler is fast and effective. Suturing is also effective but difficult due to cardiac activity. A Foley catheter can be placed within a wound, the balloon inflated and gentle retraction placed on the catheter, and then the catheter sutured into place.
- When suturing, horizontal mattress sutures or interrupted sutures are effective, and pledgets may reinforce the suture and prevent further damage to the heart.
- If cardiac function is absent, internal cardiac massage should be performed. Care should be taken to avoid coronary vessel damage.
- If no left-sided injury is discovered, the thoracotomy should be extended to the right with a clam shell across the sternum and down the right. This may assist with improved exposure to the right side of the heart, as well as the right lung.
- The descending aorta can be cross-clamped.

Figure 14.7 (cont.) resuscitative thoracotomy, in a female and a male patient. (C, D) Illustration and photo of the pericardium at thoracotomy. The phrenic nerve is seen on the lateral aspect of the pericardium. The pericardium should be opened above the nerve (C). The pericardium is opened and the heart exposed (D). (E) Illustration and intraoperative photograph showing the use of a Foley catheter for temporary bleeding control from a cardiac wound. (F) Photograph of a cross-clamping of the thoracic aorta. The clamp should be applied about 3–4 cm above the diaphragm. (G) Photograph of internal cardiac defibrillation during emergency room resuscitative thoracotomy (reproduced with permission from *Color Atlas of Emergency Trauma, Second Edition*, illustrations at A, C and E by Alexis Demetriades)

- If the patient regains pulses or vital signs improve, the patient requires the OR. Survival rate approaches 80% for knife wounds and 40% for gunshot wounds.

A second approach for EDT, perhaps faster with greater exposure, is to perform bilateral finger thoracostomies and then connect these incisions, completing a clamshell.[73-75]

Blunt Trauma

Hypotension in the setting of blunt trauma requires intravascular expansion with IV fluids, preferably blood products. The most common cause of hypotension is injury other than the heart. If the heart is the primary cause of symptoms or hypotension, admission for comprehensive echocardiography and monitoring is required.[9,13] ACLS measures are needed for patients with dysrhythmias. Injuries from blunt trauma such as cardiac rupture, valve injury, papillary muscle/chordae injury, or MI need PCI or surgery.[2,3,9]

Patients with minor ECG changes such as premature atrial/ventricular contractions should be admitted for monitoring and echocardiography. For evaluation of cardiac dysrhythmia or hemodynamic instability, 24–48 hours of monitoring are recommended.[4,5,57]

Great Vessel Injury

Consultation with a trauma surgeon and vascular surgeon is required. Patients with radiographic findings of great vessel injury and hemodynamic instability due to vascular injury will require definitive therapy, though immediate surgical repair is not possible if other injuries such as abdominal or head injuries are present. If aortic dissection is present and surgical repair is not possible, then analgesia and heart rate and blood pressure control are needed. Heart rate around 60 beats/min and systolic blood pressure 110–120 mm Hg is recommended as targets to decrease shearing stress on the aorta. Patients should be counseled to avoid bearing down (such as Valsalva).[2,3,9]

Pitfalls in Cardiac Trauma

- Failure to assess and manage ABCs.
- Failure to consider cardiac trauma in chest trauma.
- Attributing hypotension in trauma is solely due to cardiac trauma.
- Failure to obtain adequate US images of cardiac box, and mistaking pleural effusion for pericardial effusion on US.
- Failure to recognize ECG evidence of blunt cardiac injury.
- Lack of knowledge concerning indications and contraindications for ED thoracotomy.

Key Points

- Cardiac trauma can be penetrating and/or blunt.
- The RV is most at risk for injury, either penetrating or blunt.
- The most common forms of penetrating injury include knife and gunshot wounds, though iatrogenic injury is possible.
- Blunt cardiac injury is associated with cardiac dysfunction, wall rupture, valvular/chordae/papillary muscle injury, coronary vessel injury/MI, and commotio cordis.

- Evaluation includes ABCs, primary, and secondary exam. US is vital in assessment for pericardial effusion, cardiac contractility, pneumothorax, and hemothorax.
- Treatment for unstable patient with penetrating injury, or the patient who loses pulses while in the ED, includes thoracotomy.
- Blunt cardiac injury patients require troponin and ECG. If any abnormality is found, further evaluation with comprehensive echocardiography is needed.

References

1. Liu P, Ren S, Qian S, Wang F. Multiple cardiac perforations following radiofrequency catheter ablation: case report and literature reviews. *Ann Thorac Cardiovasc Surg.* 2012;18:370–74.

2. Ross C, Schwab T. Chapter 262: Cardiac trauma. In Tintinalli JE, Stapczynski JS, Ma J, et al., eds. *Tintinalli's Emergency Medicine: A Comprehensive Study Guide,* 8e. New York: McGraw Hill; 2016. Available at http://accessemergencymedicine.mhmedical.com/content.aspx?bookid=1658&sectionid=109387651. Accessed August 12, 2017.

3. ATLS Subcommittee; American College of Surgeons' Committee on Trauma; International ATLS working group. Advanced trauma life support (ATLS®): the ninth edition. *J Trauma Acute Care Surg.* 2013;74(5):1363–66.

4. Conn A. Chest trauma. In: Legome E, Shockley LW, eds. *Trauma: A Comprehensive Emergency Medicine Approach.* New York: Cambridge University Press; 2011, p. 190.

5. Asensio JA, Garcia-Nunez LM, Patrizio P: Trauma to the heart. In: Feliciano D, Mattox K, Moore E, eds. *Trauma.* New York: McGraw Hill Medical; 2008, p. 569.

6. Marcolini EG, Keegan J. Blunt cardiac injury. *Emerg Med Clin N Am.* 2015;33:519–27.

7. Bamous M, Abdessamad A, Tadili J, et al. Evaluation of penetrating cardiac stab wounds. *Scand J Trauma, Resusc Emerg Med.* 2016;24:6.

8. Schultz JM, Trunkey DD. Blunt cardiac injury. *Crit Care Clin.* 2004;20:57–70.

9. Bernardin B, Troquet JM: Initial management and resuscitation of severe chest trauma. *Emerg Med Clin North Am.* 2012;30:377–400.

10. Bock JS, Benitez RM. Blunt cardiac injury. *Cardiol Clin.* 2012;30:545–55.

11. Brown J, Grover FL. Trauma to the heart. *Chest Surg Clin N Am.* 1997;7:325–41.

12. Elie MC. Blunt cardiac injury. *Mt Sinai J Med.* 2006;73:542–52.

13. Bansal MK, Maraj S, Chewaprooug D, et al. Myocardial contusion injury: redefining the diagnostic algorithm. *Emerg Med J.* 2005;22:465–69.

14. Asaid R, Boyce G, Atkinson N. Endovascular repair of acute traumatic aortic injury: experience of a level-1 trauma center. *Ann Vasc Surg.* 2014;28:1391–95.

15. Rodriguez RM, Anglin D, Langdorf MI, et al. NEXUS chest: validation of a decision instrument for selective chest imaging in blunt trauma. *JAMA Surg.* 2013;148:940–46.

16. Pasquale M, Fabian TC. Practice management guidelines for trauma from the Eastern Association for the Surgery of Trauma. *J Trauma.* 1998;44:941–56.

17. Asensio JA, Berne JD, Demetriades D, et al. One hundred five penetrating cardiac injuries: a 2-year prospective evaluation. *J Trauma.* 1998;44:1073–82.

18. Gunay C, Cingoz F, Kuralay E, et al. Surgical challenges for urgent approach in penetrating heart injuries. *Heart Surg Forum.* 2007;10:E473–77.

19. Reddy D, Muckart DJ. Holes in the heart: an atlas of intracardiac injuries following penetrating trauma. *Interact Cardiovasc Thorac Surg.* 2014;19:56–63.

20. Molina EJ, Gaughan JP, Kulp H, et al. Outcomes after emergency department thoracotomy for penetrating cardiac injuries: a new perspective. *Interact Cardiovasc Thorac Surg.* 2008;7:845–48.

21. Khorsandi M, Skouras C, Shah R. Is there any role for resuscitative emergency department thoracotomy in blunt trauma? *Interact Cardiovasc Thorac Surg.* 2013;16:509–16.

22. Desouza KA, Desouza NA, Pinto RM, et al. Transthoracic echocardiogram is a useful tool in the hemodynamic assessment of patients with chest trauma. *Am J Med Sci.* 2011;34:340–43.

23. Chen MY, Miller PR, McLaughlin CA, et al. The trend of using computed tomography in the detection of acute thoracic aortic and branch vessel injury after blunt thoracic trauma: single-center experience over 13 years. *J Trauma.* 2004;56:783–85.

24. Bruckner BA, DiBardino DJ, Cumbie TC, et al. Critical evaluation of chest computed tomography scans for blunt descending thoracic aortic injury. *Ann Thorac Surg.* 2006:81:1339–46.

25. Mirvis SE: Thoracic vascular injury. *Radiol Clin North Am.* 2006;44:181–97.

26. Lateef Wani M, Ahangar AG, Wani SN, et al. Penetrating cardiac injury: a review. *Trauma Mon.* 2012;17:230–32.

27. Kong VY, Satorius B, Clarke DL. The selective conservative management of penetrating thoracic trauma is still appropriate in the current era. *Injury.* 2015;46:49–53.

28. Bakovic M, Petrovecki V, Strinovic D, et al. Shot through the heart-firepower and potential lethality of air weapons. *J Forensic Sci.* 2014;59:1658–61.

29. Mehrota D, Kejriwal NK. Tricuspid valve repair for torrential tricuspid regurgitation after permanent pacemaker lead extraction. *Tex Heart Inst J.* 2011;38:305–7.

30. Namai A, Sakurai M, Fujiwara H. Five cases of blunt traumatic cardiac rupture: success and failure in surgical management. *Gen Thorac Cardiovsc Surg.* 2007;55:200–4.

31. Shamsi F, Tai JM, Bokhari S. Coronary artery dissection after blunt chest trauma. *BMJ Case Rep.* 2014;2014.

32. Plautz CU, Perron AD, Brady WJ. Electrocardiographic ST segment elevation in the trauma patient: acute myocardial infarction vs myocardial contusion. *Am J Emerg Med.* 2005;23(4):510–6.

33. Foussas SG, Athanasopoulos GD, Cokkinos DV. Myocardial infarction caused by blunt chest injury: possible mechanisms involved – case reports. *Angiology.* 1989;40:313–18.

34. Banzo I, Montero A, Uriarte I, et al. Coronary artery occlusion and myocardial infarction: a seldom encountered complication of blunt chest trauma. *Clin Nucl Med.* 1999;24:94–96.

35. El-Chami MF, Nicholson W, Helmy T. Blunt cardiac trauma. *J Emerg Med.* 2008;35:127–33.

36. Maron BJ, Doerer JJ, Haas TS, et al. Sudden deaths in young competitive athletes: analysis of 1866 deaths in the United States, 1980–2006. *Circulation.* 2009;119 (8):1085–92.

37. Spencer RJ, Sugumar H, Jones E, et al. Commotio cordis: a case of ventricular fibrillation caused by a cricket ball strike to the chest. *Lancet.* 2014;383:1358.

38. Raja AS, Mower WR, Nishijima DK, et al. Prevalence and diagnostic performance of isolated and combined NEXUS chest CT decision criteria. *Acad Emerg Med.* 2016;23:863–69.

39. Rodriguez RM, Langdorf MI, Nishijima D, et al. Derivation and validation of two decision instruments for selective chest CT in blunt trauma: a multicenter prospective observational study (NEXUS Chest CT). *PLoS Med.* 2015;12: e1001883.

40. Arthurs ZM, Starnes BW, Sohn VY, et al. Functional and survival outcomes in traumatic blunt thoracic aortic injuries: an analysis of the National Trauma Databank. *J Vasc Surg.* 2009;49:988–94.

41. McGwin G Jr, Reiff DA, Moran SG, et al. Incidence and characteristics of motor vehicle collision-related blunt thoracic

aortic injury according to age. *J Trauma.* 2002;52:859–65.

42. Skinner DL, Laing GL, Rodseth RN, et al. Blunt cardiac injury in critically ill trauma patients: a single centre experience. *Injury.* 2014;46:66–70.

43. Guild CS, deShazo M, Geraci SA. Negative predictive value of cardiac troponin for predicting adverse cardiac events following blunt chest trauma. *South Med J.* 2014;107:52–56.

44. Fanari Z, Hadid M, Hammami S, et al. Traumatic myocardial infarction in a young athletic patient after a football game. *Del Med J.* 2014;86:213–15.

45. Jackson L, Steward A. Best evidence topic report. Use of troponin for the diagnosis of myocardial contusion after blunt chest trauma. *Emerg Med J.* 2005;22:193–95.

46. van Wijngaarden MH, Karmy-Jones R, Talwar MK, et al. Blunt cardiac injury: a 10 year institutional review. *Injury.* 1997;28:51–55.

47. Jeremias A, Gibson CM. Narrative review: alternative causes for elevated cardiac troponin levels when acute coronary syndromes are excluded. *Ann Intern Med.* 2005;142:786–91.

48. Martin M, Mullenix P, Rhee P, et al. Troponin increases in the critically injured patient: mechanical trauma or physiologic stress? *J Trauma.* 2005;59:1086–91.

49. Barker S, Ghaemmaghami C. Myocardial contusion induced right bundle branch block with ST elevation and troponin elevation. *Am J Emerg Med.* 2009;27:375.

50. Schnuriger B, Exadaktylos E, Sauter T, et al. Highly sensitive cardiac troponin in blunt chest trauma: after the gathering comes the scattering. *J Trauma.* 2011;70:766–67.

51. Rajan GP, Zellweger R. Cardiac troponin I as a predictor of arrhythmia and ventricular dysfunction in trauma patients with myocardial contusion. *J Trauma.* 2014;57:801–8.

52. Ma OJ, Mateer JR, Ogata M, et al. Prospective analysis of a rapid trauma ultrasound examination performed by emergency physicians. *J Trauma.* 1995;38:879–85.

53. Clancy K, Velopulos C, Bilaniuk J, et al. Screening for blunt cardiac injury: an Eastern Association for the Surgery of Trauma practice management guideline. *J Trauma Acute Care.* 2012; 73(5 Suppl 4): S301–6.

54. Chirillo F, Totis O, Cavarzerani A, et al. Usefulness of transthoracic and transoesophageal echocardiography in recognition and management of cardiovascular injuries after blunt chest trauma. *Heart.* 1996;75:301–6.

55. Goarin JP, Cluzel P, Gosgnach M, et al. Evaluation of transesophageal echocardiography for diagnosis of traumatic aortic injury. *Anesthesiology.* 2000;93:1373–77.

56. Vignon P, Boncoeur MP, François B, et al. Comparison of multiplane transesophageal echocardiography and contrast-enhanced helical CT in the diagnosis of blunt traumatic cardiovascular injuries. *Anesthesiology.* 2001;94:615–22.

57. Nagy KK, Krosner SM, Roberts RR, et al. Determining which patients require evaluation for blunt cardiac injury following blunt chest trauma. *World J Surg.* 2001;25:108–11.

58. Ferrada P, Evans D, Wolfe L, et al. Findings of a randomized controlled trial using limited transthoracic echocardiogram as a hemodynamic monitoring tool in the trauma bay. *J Trauma Acute Care Surg.* 2014;76:31–37.

59. Lee WS, Parks NA, Garcia A, et al. Pan computed tomography versus selective computed tomography in stable young adults after blunt trauma with moderate mechanism: A cost-utility analysis. *J Trauma Acute Care Surg.* 2014;77:527–33.

60. Perchinsky MJ, Long WB, Urman S, et al. The broken halo sign: a fractured calcified ring as an unusual sign of traumatic rupture of the thoracic aorta. *Injury.* 1994;25:649–52.

61. Sun X, Hong J, Lowery R, et al. Ascending aortic injuries following blunt trauma. *J Card Surg.* 2013;28:749–55.

62. Ho ML, Gutierrez FR. Chest radiography in thoracic polytrauma. *AJR Am J Roentgenol.* 2009;192:599–612.

63. Marnocha KE, Maglinte DD, Woods J, et al. Blunt chest trauma and suspected aortic rupture: reliability of chest radiograph findings. *Ann Emerg Med.* 1985;14:644–49.

64. Fitzgerald M, Spencer J, Johnson F, et al. Definitive management of acute cardiac tamponade secondary to blunt trauma. *Emerg Med Australas.* 2005;17:494–99.

65. MacFarlane C. Blunt trauma cardiac tamponade: what really counts in management. *Emerg Med Australas.* 2005;17:416–17.

66. Cothren CC, Moore EE. Emergency department thoracotomy for the critically injured patient: objectives, indications, and outcomes. *World J Emerg Surg.* 2006;1:4.

67. Rhee PM, Acosta J, Bridgeman A, et al. Survival after emergency department thoracotomy: review of published data from the past 25 years. *J Am Coll Surg.* 2000;190:288–98.

68. Slessor D, Hunter S. To be blunt: Are we wasting our time? Emergency department thoracotomy following blunt trauma: a systematic review and meta-analysis. *Ann Emerg Med.* 2015;65:297–307.

69. Huber-Wagner S, Lefering R, Qvick M, et al. Outcome in 757 severely injured patients with traumatic cardiorespiratory arrest. *Resuscitation.* 2007;75:276–85.

70. Moore EE, Knudson MM, Burlew CC, et al. Defining the limits of resuscitative emergency department thoracotomy: a contemporary Western Trauma Association perspective. *J Trauma.* 2011;70(2):334–39.

71. Seamon MJ, Haut, ER, Van Arendonk K, et al. An evidence-based approach to patient selection for emergency department thoracotomy: a practice management guideline from the Eastern Association for the Surgery of Trauma. *J Trauma Acute Care Surg.* 2015;79(1):159–73.

72. Burlew CC, Moore EE, Moore FA, et al. Western Trauma Association critical decisions in trauma: resuscitative thoracotomy. *J Trauma Acute Care Surg.* 2012;73(6):1359–63.

73. Lockey D, Crewdsen K, Davies GE. Traumatic cardiac arrest: who are the survivors? *Ann Emerg Med.* 2006;48:240–44.

74. Wise D, Davies GE, Coats T, Lockey D, et al. Emergency thoracotomy: "How to do it." *Emerg Med J.* 2005;22:22–24.

75. Coats TJ, Keogh S, Clark H, Neal M. Prehospital resuscitative thoracotomy for cardiac arrest after penetrating trauma: rational and case series. *J Trauma.* 2001;50:670–73.

Abdominal and Flank Trauma

Michael Gottlieb

Introduction

Abdominal trauma is a significant cause of morbidity and mortality in the United States, with abdominal injuries occurring in approximately 1% of all trauma patients.[1] However, abdominal trauma accounts for over 20% of all trauma-related deaths.[2] Abdominal and flank trauma may result in direct injury to a number of important structures, including the liver, spleen, kidneys, diaphragm, pancreas, and intestines. Unfortunately, the diagnosis may be challenging, as patients often present with multiple other injuries and may not be able to provide a reliable history or examination.[3]

Causes

- Blunt abdominal and flank trauma can occur from a number of causes. One large, multicenter study found that motor vehicle collisions (MVC) were responsible for 81% of cases, followed by falls in 9% of cases, and assault in 7% of cases.[3]
- Penetrating abdominal and flank trauma is divided into two categories: low-energy (i.e. stab wounds) and high-energy (i.e. gunshot wounds). While stab wounds are three times more common, gunshot wounds are responsible for 90% of the mortality from penetrating trauma.[4] Gunshot wounds are further classified into low-velocity (i.e. handgun and low-caliber rifles) and high-velocity (i.e. military and hunting rifles) injuries. High-velocity injuries are associated with more damage. The exception to this is shotgun injuries, which can cause substantial damage at close range, despite being a low-velocity weapon.[5]

Anatomy

- The abdominal compartment extends from the diaphragm to the pelvis and includes both intraperitoneal and retroperitoneal organs. Because the rib cage extends below the diaphragm, upper abdominal organs may overlap with the chest compartment (referred to as the thoraco-abdominal area).
- The flank is the area between the anterior and posterior axillary lines extending from the sixth intercostal space to the iliac crest.
- The most common organs injured include the spleen, liver, kidney, small bowel, and diaphragm.
- The liver, spleen, small bowel, transverse colon, and diaphragm are intraperitoneal, while the kidneys, adrenal glands, ascending colon, and descending colon are located in the retroperitoneum. The pancreas contains both intraperitoneal and retroperitoneal

portions. Injuries that occur within the peritoneal cavity can result in significant blood loss, as the abdomen can store a large amount of blood. The retroperitoneum space is more limited; therefore, injuries within the retroperitoneal compartment are more contained, resulting in decreased blood loss compared with the peritoneum.

Pathophysiology

- Penetrating trauma may remain superficial or traverse multiple tissue planes. While a stab wound follows a relatively direct course, gunshot wounds may alter their trajectory after entering the skin. Therefore, one cannot assume that the trajectory was linear between both skin wounds, and it is important to consider peritoneal involvement in any gunshot wound.
- Blunt trauma occurs from either direct impact to a specific organ or when there is a sudden deceleration which exceeds the elasticity of the organ, resulting in tearing of the organ or supporting structures.
- Children are at increased risk of injury when compared to adults, because their abdomen is less well-protected. Children have thinner abdominal musculature, so it is easier to compress their abdominal organs against their posterior vertebrae. Additionally, their ribs are more elastic, resulting in decreased protection of their liver and spleen.
- Pregnant women are relatively protected from abdominal organ injury by their gravid uterus. However, this is balanced by potential injuries to the uterus (e.g. placental abruption, uterine rupture), as discussed in Chapter 4.
- The risk of injury to a specific organ is related to its size and structure. While the duodenum is smaller than other intraabdominal organs, direct trauma from bicycle handlebars or a misplaced seatbelt can cause significant injury due to its relatively unprotected location. Similarly, injuries to the spleen are more common after blunt trauma because it is less elastic than the other organs. This is particularly problematic in patients with mononucleosis, wherein the spleen becomes enlarged and can have a significant injury despite relatively minimal trauma.

History

- Obtain as much information as possible from the emergency medical services (EMS) personnel. Important information includes the initial vital signs, patient's course, suspected injuries, estimated blood loss at the scene, and any treatments received in transit.
- Additional information from the patient or EMS personnel should include the mechanism, other injuries, allergies, medications, past medical and surgical history, and the last time the patient had anything to eat or drink.
- If the injury was due to an MVC, it is valuable to know the speed of the patient's and other driver's vehicles, condition and drivability of the vehicle, airbag deployment, windshield condition, seatbelt use, and condition of the other passengers and drivers.
- If the injury was due to a fall, the approximate height of the fall, what surface the patient fell on, point of contact on the patient's body, and any areas of contact prior to striking the ground are all useful historical information.

- If the patient was stabbed with an object, it is important to know what type of object, the shape of the object, the length of the object, position of the patient during the injury, and all locations where contact was made, regardless of how significant the injury was felt to be.

Examination

- Blood pressure and heart rate are the most important vital signs when assessing for significant intra-abdominal injury. Hypotension and tachycardia should raise the concern for significant blood loss. However, even transient hypotension is associated with worse outcomes. Importantly, relatively bradycardia may be present in up to 44% of trauma patients and is an independent risk factor for mortality.[6] Additionally, while abnormal vital signs should raise one's concern of intra-abdominal injury, normal vital signs do not exclude significant injury.
- After completion of the primary survey, the secondary survey of the abdomen should include assessment for external abrasions or ecchymoses, as well as abdominal tenderness, guarding, rigidity, or peritoneal signs. Increasing abdominal distension or peritonitis should increase one's concern for ongoing intraperitoneal bleeding.
- Alcohol, drugs, head injury, or significant distracting injuries may reduce the patient's ability to identify abdominal pain or tenderness, with one study suggesting that one-fifth of patients with positive findings on CT for intraabdominal injury did not have tenderness on examination.[3] Additional studies have found that 25–58% of patients with small bowel or mesenteric injury do not have abdominal tenderness.[7,8] A separate study found that 3% of patients with splenic injury had isolated left rib pain without abdominal pain.[9] Therefore, one must be vigilant for intraabdominal injuries and should consider advanced imaging or serial abdominal examinations among patients with concerning symptoms or distracting injuries, despite the absence of abdominal pain.
- It is important to consider the location of the ecchymosis or pain, as this can help suggest the underlying injury. For example, blunt trauma to the right flank should raise one's suspicion of renal or liver injury, while bruising over the epigastric area may suggest potential underlying pancreatic or duodenal injury. Of note, the presence of a "seat belt mark" has been associated with an 8-fold increase in the risk of intra-abdominal injury (Figure 15.1).[10] Cullen's sign (periumbilical ecchymosis) and Turner's sign (flank ecchymosis) may suggest retroperitoneal hemorrhage, but are uncommon and often late findings.[11,12] Kehr's sign (left shoulder pain referred from diaphragmatic irritation) suggests potential splenic injury.[13]
- Patients should be fully exposed, and a thorough skin examination should be performed, including all skin folds, the axillae, and the inguinal area.
- In patients with stab wounds to the anterior abdomen, local wound exploration can be performed to determine whether the injury extends into the peritoneum.[14] However, gunshot wounds or wounds from a sharp and narrow instrument (e.g. icepick) are poor candidates for local exploration (Figure 15.2).
- While gross blood or palpable subcutaneous emphysema on the rectal exam can suggest intra-abdominal injury, these findings are uncommon, and other clinical indicators are typically present prior to these finding. Therefore, many experts recommend deferring or eliminating this examination.[15–17] The exception to this is penetrating trauma to the rectal area or concern for cauda equina syndrome.

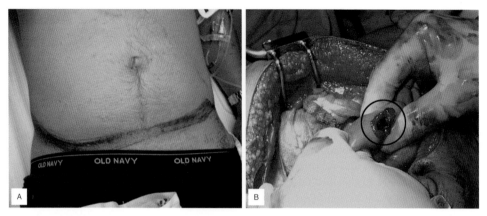

Figure 15.1 Seatbelt mark in a car accident patient. (A) The presence of this sign is a marker of significant intra-abdominal injury. (B) Intraoperative photograph of the same patient showing perforation of the small bowel (reproduced with permission from *Color Atlas of Emergency Trauma, Second Edition*)

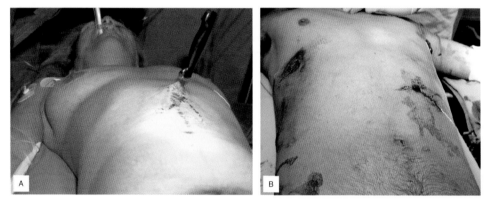

Figure 15.2 (A) Stab wound to the abdomen with impaled knife. These objects should only be removed in the operating room. Only about 50% of anterior abdominal stab wounds have significant injuries requiring surgical repair. (B) Low-velocity gunshot wound. About 75% of these wounds have significant injuries requiring surgical repair (reproduced with permission from *Color Atlas of Emergency Trauma, Second Edition*)

Differential Diagnosis

Penetrating abdominal trauma may result in injury to any intraperitoneal or retroperitoneal structure. The liver, small intestine, and colon are the most common injuries from penetrating trauma.[4] While abdominal vasculature is not commonly injured as a result of stab wounds, it is the fourth most common injury among gunshot wounds. Blunt abdominal trauma can result in injury to the liver, spleen, intestines, pancreas, and diaphragm. Splenic and hepatic injuries represent the majority of intra-abdominal injuries from blunt trauma. Flank trauma can involve the kidney or colon.

Hepatic Injury

Hepatic injury typically presents with right upper quadrant or right flank pain. Stable patients are typically managed non-operatively, while unstable patients require operative

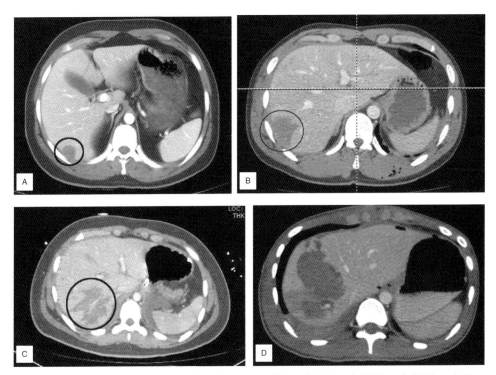

Figure 15.3 CT scans of various grades of blunt liver trauma: (A) grade I, (B) grade II, (C) grade III, (D) grade IV (reproduced with permission from *Color Atlas of Emergency Trauma, Second Edition*)

management. One study of blunt hepatic injury had a 100% salvage rate with non-operative management (Figures 15.3 and 15.4).[18] Table 15.1 includes the American Association of Surgery for Trauma (AAST) grading criteria for liver injury.[19]

Splenic Injury

Splenic injury occurs most commonly with left upper quadrant or left flank trauma but can occur in association with deceleration injuries. Patients present with left upper quadrant pain, which may be associated with left shoulder pain referred from the phrenic nerve. Stable patients may be managed non-operatively with consideration for angiographic embolization, while unstable patients require operative management (Figures 15.5 and 15.6). One study of the non-operative management of blunt splenic injuries had a 90% overall salvage rate, including an 80% salvage rate among grade 4 and 5 injuries.[20] Table 15.2 includes the AAST grading criteria for splenic injury.[19]

Duodenal Injury

These injuries are commonly associated with blunt trauma to the upper abdomen. Patients with duodenal perforations will present with severe abdominal pain and tenderness immediately after the trauma (Figure 15.7). However, patients with duodenal hematoma are often minimally symptomatic for the first several days and may present up to a week later with onset of symptoms. Patients typically present with progressively worsening abdominal pain associated with vomiting and decreased oral intake.

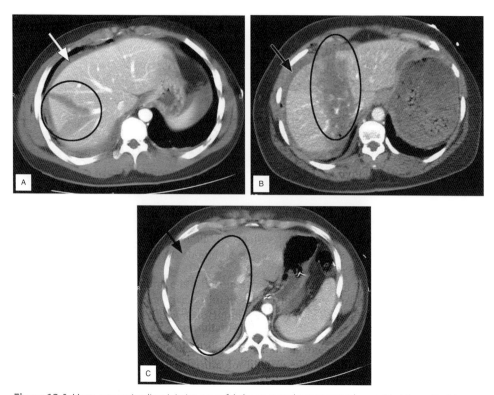

Figure 15.4 Many penetrating liver injuries can safely be managed nonoperatively, provided the patient is hemodynamically stable and has no peritonitis. A CT scan should always be performed: (A) CT scan of stab wound and (B, C) gunshot wounds to the liver successfully managed nonoperatively (reproduced with permission from *Color Atlas of Emergency Trauma, Second Edition*)

Pancreatic Injury

Pancreatic injuries usually present with epigastric pain occurring hours after the initial injury. They may also demonstrate Cullen's or Turner's signs if they are complicated by a significant retroperitoneal hemorrhage (Figure 15.8). Patients are at risk of significant intravascular fluid depletion due to third spacing, thought this is often delayed by hours to days.

Diaphragmatic Injury

Diaphragmatic injuries are most common on the left side because the right hemi-diaphragm is relatively protected by the liver.[21] Diaphragmatic injuries occur in two stages: acute and subacute. Acute injuries may mimic a pneumothorax by presenting with severe, pleuritic, left-sided chest pain associated with absent lung sounds. This is caused by the bowel herniating into the left chest. Subacute diaphragmatic injuries can remain undiagnosed for months to years until the diaphragmatic hernia becomes large enough for bowel to become entrapped. These patients present with symptoms of bowel obstruction. Most

Table 15.1 AAST liver injury grading criteria[19]

Grade	Type	Injury Description
I	Hematoma	Subcapsular, <10% surface area
	Laceration	Capsular tear, <1 cm parenchymal depth
II	Hematoma	Subcapsular, 10–50% surface area intraparenchymal <10 cm in diameter
	Laceration	Capsular tear 1–3 parenchymal depth, <10 cm in length
III	Hematoma	Subcapsular, >50% surface area of ruptured subcapsular or parenchymal hematoma; intraparenchymal hematoma >10 cm or expanding
	Laceration	>3 cm parenchymal depth
IV	Laceration	Parenchymal disruption involving 25–75% hepatic lobe or 1–3 Couinaud's segments
V	Laceration	Parenchymal disruption involving >75% of hepatic lobe or >3 Couinaud's segments within a single lobe
	Vascular	Juxtahepatic venous injuries (i.e. retrohepatic vena cava/central major hepatic veins)
VI	Vascular	Hepatic avulsion

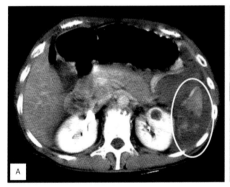 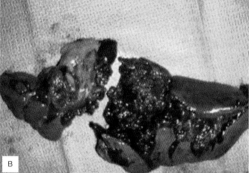

Figure 15.5 (A) Abdominal CT with a grade IV spleen injury. (B) Surgical specimen of the removed ruptured spleen (reproduced with permission from *Color Atlas of Emergency Trauma, Second Edition*)

significant diaphragmatic injuries can be diagnosed by radiography or CT. However, a CT that is negative for diaphragmatic injury cannot rule out the diagnosis.[22] Subtle cases may be missed on imaging but can be found on laparoscopy or laparotomy. Left-sided injuries should be repaired to avoid delayed complications. Right-sided injuries may not need to be repaired because herniation is less likely, due to protection by the liver.

Renal Injury

Renal injury can occur from either a blunt or penetrating mechanism and is associated with flank pain and hematuria. Patients with penetrating injury in this region should receive a

Table 15.2 AAST splenic injury grading criteria[19]

Grade	Type	Injury Description
I	Hematoma	Subcapsular, <10% surface area
	Laceration	Capsular tear, <1 cm parenchymal depth
II	Hematoma	Subcapsular, 10–50% surface area; intraparenchymal, <5 cm in diameter
	Laceration	Capsular tear, 1–3 cm parenchymal depth that does not involve a trabecular vessel
III	Hematoma	Subcapsular, >50% surface area or expanding; ruptured subcapsular or parenchymal hematoma; intraparenchymal hematoma ≥5 cm or expanding
	Laceration	>3 cm parenchymal depth or involving trabecular vessels
IV	Laceration	Laceration involving segmental or hilar vessels producing major devascularization (>25% of spleen)
V	Laceration	Completely shattered spleen
	Vascular	Hilar vascular injury with devascularized spleen

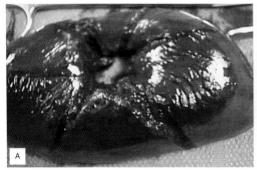
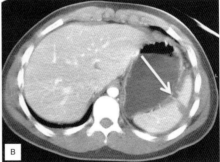

Figure 15.6 (A) Gunshot wound to spleen with extensive damage requiring emergency splenectomy. (B) Low-grade splenic injuries due to a stab wound (reproduced with permission from *Color Atlas of Emergency Trauma, Second Edition*)

CT, while blunt trauma patients should receive a CT if there is gross hematuria or a significant deceleration injury (Figures 15.9 and 15.10).[23,24] Table 15.3 includes the AAST grading criteria for renal injury.[25] Treatment may involve either angiographic or surgical repair. The need for surgical repair and nephrectomy is directly correlated with the grade of renal injury. One large retrospective study found that grade I injuries had 0% risk of surgery or nephrectomy, while 93% of grade V injuries required surgery and 86% required a nephrectomy.[26]

Evaluation

- Initial evaluation should include a primary survey and extended focused assessment with sonography in trauma (E-FAST) examination.[27] Two large-bore intravenous

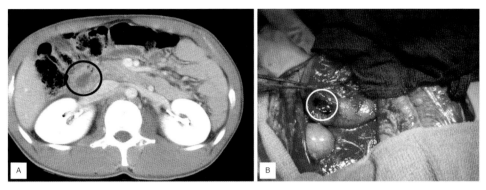

Figure 15.7 Blunt trauma to duodenum. (A) CT demonstrates duodenal wall thickening with intramural air. (B) Intraoperative appearance of duodenal perforation (reproduced with permission from *Color Atlas of Emergency Trauma, Second Edition*)

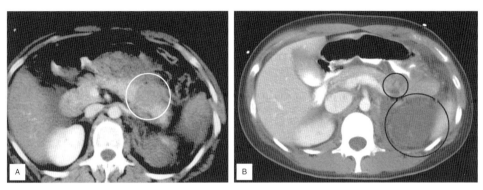

Figure 15.8 (A) CT scan demonstrating distal pancreatic transection (circle). (B) CT scan shows distal pancreatic injury (small circle) and no contrast uptake by the left kidney, due to thrombosis of the left renal artery (large circle) (reproduced with permission from *Color Atlas of Emergency Trauma, Second Edition*)

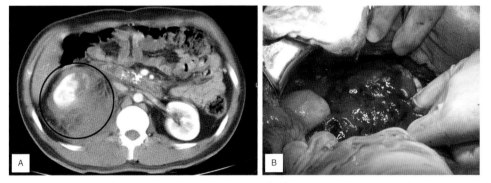

Figure 15.9 (A) CT scan shows a severe right kidney injury with a large surrounding hematoma. (B) Intraoperative appearance of the renal hematoma (reproduced with permission from *Color Atlas of Emergency Trauma, Second Edition*)

catheters should be inserted, and the patient should be placed on a cardiorespiratory monitor with continuous pulse oximetry.
- Once this has been completed, a focused secondary examination should be performed as outlined above.

Table 15.3 AAST renal injury grading criteria[25]

Grade	Type	Injury Description
I	Contusion	Microscopic or gross hematuria, urologic studies normal
	Hematoma	Subcapsular, nonexpanding without parenchymal laceration
II	Hematoma	Nonexpanding perirenal hematoma confirmed to renal retroperitoneum
	Laceration	<1.0 cm parenchymal depth of renal cortex without urinary extravasation
III	Laceration	>1.0 cm parenchymal depth of renal cortex without collecting system rupture or urinary extravasation
IV	Laceration	Parenchymal laceration extending through renal cortex, medulla, and collecting system
	Vascular	Main renal artery or vein injury with contained hemorrhage
V	Laceration	Completely shattered kidney
	Vascular	Avulsion of renal hilum which devascularizes kidney

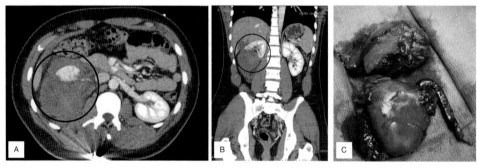

Figure 15.10 Gunshot injury to kidney. (A, B) CT scan shows severe injury and a large perinephric hematoma. A nephrectomy was performed. (C) Note the complete transection of the kidney (reproduced with permission from *Color Atlas of Emergency Trauma, Second Edition*)

Laboratory Testing

- Routine laboratory testing is rarely helpful in the initial evaluation of trauma patients.[28] As a result, some experts have recommended ordering laboratory testing only when a specific clinical need is present.[29–32] Multiple studies have demonstrated a significant cost saving without adverse events by following this strategy.[31,32]
- All patients should receive a bedside glucose test, and all women of childbearing potential should receive a pregnancy test. All pregnant women with abdominal trauma should also have their Rh antibody status determined.
- If additional laboratory testing is indicated, it will often include a complete blood count, basic metabolic panel, liver function testing, lipase, coagulation profile, lactate, and blood type and screen.
- Urinalysis should be obtained in all patients with blunt trauma to the abdomen or flank.[33] Gross hematuria suggests an injury to the genitourinary tract and warrants

further evaluation.[23,33,34] Microscopic hematuria is a sign of mild renal injury and does not require further treatment in a stable patient without a significant deceleration injury.[23,33,34] Because deceleration injuries can be associated with injury to the renal pedicle, further imaging or evaluation is recommended in this patient group if only microscopic hematuria is present.[33]

Imaging

Ultrasound (US)

- The E-FAST examination is recommended for all trauma patients with a significant mechanism of injury as an initial screening test. Studies have demonstrated that it is highly accurate for intraperitoneal fluid and can be completed in 2–3 minutes.[35,36]
- The E-FAST examination contains six views: right upper quadrant (i.e. Morison's pouch), left upper quadrant, suprapubic (i.e. pouch of Douglas), subxiphoid, and bilateral lung fields. Because the bladder provides the sonographic window for the suprapubic view, it is important to perform this prior to Foley placement. If a Foley catheter is already in place, sterile saline may be instilled into the bladder to facilitate visualization.
- The presence of intraperitoneal fluid in an unstable patient is an indication for operative intervention (Figure 15.11). Importantly, in patients with major pelvic trauma and potential bladder rupture, diagnostic peritoneal aspiration may be needed to determine whether the fluid is blood or urine.[37]
- The presence of free fluid in a stable trauma patient should be followed immediately by a CT to identify the type of injury and the need for operative intervention. However, the absence of free fluid does not preclude the need for additional imaging or evaluation, and this should be made on a case-by-case basis in conjunction with the clinical examination.
- The major limitation of ultrasound is its inability to evaluate solid organ injury. While US demonstrates excellent accuracy for hemoperitoneum, it has limited accuracy for hepatic or splenic injury and is not able to diagnose diaphragmatic or intestinal injury.[38] Additionally, US is not recommended as the primary imaging modality for renal injuries, as it has been demonstrated to miss up to 78% of renal injuries.[33,39]

Radiography

- Plain radiographs may be obtained to evaluate for retained foreign bodies but are often of low diagnostic yield for penetrating trauma. If a foreign body is not accounted for, one must consider that the foreign body may be intraluminal or intravascular with the potential for embolization.
- Plain radiographs cannot rule out intraperitoneal injury after blunt trauma. Free air under the diaphragm in an upright chest radiograph indicates hollow viscus injury, but this is a rare finding. Rigler's sign (i.e. clearly defined bowel walls due to free intraperitoneal air) may be seen in the supine radiograph, but this is also an uncommon finding.[40,41]

(A)

(B)

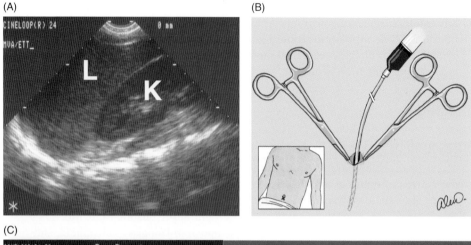

(C)

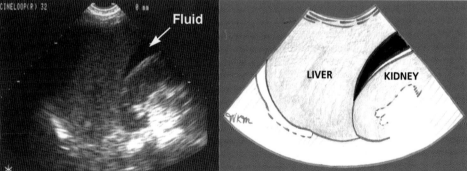

Figure 15.11 (A) Normal FAST: right upper quadrant window depicts liver and right kidney with no free fluid (K, kidney; L, liver). (B) Open diagnostic peritoneal lavage/aspiration technique. This technique is rarely used. (C) FAST exam with free fluid between liver and kidney (arrow) (reproduced with permission from *Color Atlas of Emergency Trauma, Second Edition*, illustration in (B) by Alexis Demetriades)

- Chest radiography may identify a diaphragmatic hernia, but it is only 33–46% accurate.[42,43]
- Chance fractures (i.e. flexion-distraction injuries) of the lumbar spine should raise one's concern for concomitant intra-abdominal injury. Studies have identified associated intra-abdominal injuries in 33–89% of patients with chance fractures, with the majority composed of hollow viscus injuries.[8,44,45]

Computed Tomography (CT)

- Stable trauma patients with concern for intra-abdominal injury should receive a CT of the abdomen and pelvis with intravenous contrast. CT can allow for identification and grading of solid organ injuries, evaluation of hollow viscus injuries, and three-dimensional reconstruction to evaluate the thoracic and lumbar spine. Additionally, CT can allow the provider to determine the trajectory of the knife or missile in penetrating injuries, as well as identify indirect signs of bowel injury, such as free air or edema. However, patients who are unstable should not receive a CT scan, but rather go directly to the operating room.

- CT may also be indicated among patients with an unreliable examination, distracting injury, or who will undergo surgery for an extra-abdominal injury. However, only 1% of patients receiving a CT prior to emergent extra-abdominal surgery were found to have an intra-abdominal injury, and only one patient (0.3%) required a surgical intervention.[46,47] Several clinical decision tools have been developed to reduce CT usage while avoiding complications.[48] One study included the following criteria: Glasgow coma scale (GCS) score less than 14, costal margin tenderness, abdominal tenderness, femur fracture, hematuria level $\geq$25 red blood cells/high powered field, hematocrit level <30%, and abnormal chest radiograph result (defined as pneumothorax or rib fracture). Absence of all of these findings was able to reduce CT use with a negative predictive value of 99%.[49]
- CT is highly accurate for solid organ injury, as well as thoracolumbar spinal injury.[50] However, CT is less sensitive for diaphragmatic (67–84%),[51–53] pancreatic (48–76%),[54–56] or hollow viscus injuries (64–92%).[51,57–59] Therefore, if significant concern is present for one of the above injuries (e.g. seatbelt sign to the upper abdomen, persistent vomiting), the CT should be followed by serial abdominal examinations, diagnostic peritoneal lavage, laparoscopy, or laparotomy.
- If there is concern for retroperitoneal injury, a triple-contrast (i.e. intravenous, oral, and rectal) study is recommended.[60–62]

Diagnostic Peritoneal Lavage (DPL)

- While DPL was previously a common technique in the evaluation of trauma patients (Figure 15.12), it has become less common as CT imaging quality has improved and US is increasingly available in most EDs.
- DPL is highly accurate for the diagnosis of hemoperitoneum and organ injury in blunt trauma.[63–65] For penetrating wounds, DPL is highly accurate for peritoneal penetration, but is unfortunately less accurate for organ injury in the absence of gross blood or enteric contents. One multicenter study found that DPL performed as well as admission and serial examinations in a population with penetrating abdominal wounds.[66]

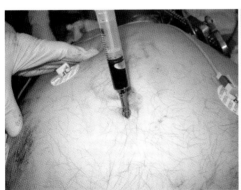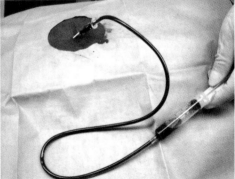

Figure 15.12 Aspiration of gross blood from catheter during DPA (reproduced with permission from *Color Atlas of Emergency Trauma, Second Edition*)

- DPL has several disadvantages, which include that it is invasive, does not identify which organ is injured, and cannot evaluate the retroperitoneum. Additionally, the non-therapeutic laparotomy rate for blunt abdominal trauma has been reported to be as high as 35%.[67]
- The following DPL findings are suggestive of intraperitoneal injury: 10 mL gross blood on initial aspiration, $>500/mm^3$ white blood cells, $>100,000/mm^3$ red blood cells, or the presence of enteric or vegetable matter.[68]

Management

- Hypotensive patients should receive intravenous fluids followed by packed red blood cells (PRBCs) when available. Women of child-bearing potential should receive type O-negative blood, while all other patients should receive type O-positive blood. For patients who require massive transfusion (defined as 10 or more units of PRBCs in 24 hours), it is recommended that they receive plasma, platelets, and PRBCs in a 1:1:1 ratio (see Chapter 3).[69,70]
- For patients with penetrating trauma, one should consider permissive hypotension (i.e. restricted fluid resuscitation) until source control is performed (see Chapter 3).[71,72]
- Patients with evidence of significant intra-abdominal injury (e.g. evisceration, gross blood per rectum, hematemesis), as well as unstable patients with evidence of significant intraperitoneal injury by CT or ultrasound, should be taken directly to the operating room for surgical repair. Delay in operative repair is associated with worse outcomes, with one study finding that a 10-minute delay to the operating room for gunshot wounds was associated with a three-fold increase in mortality.[73]
- Stable patients with stab wounds or low-velocity gunshot wounds to the abdomen should receive a CT of the abdomen and pelvis. If the small bowel or diaphragm is involved, the patient should undergo operative repair. However, isolated peritoneal injury may be managed non-operatively with serial abdominal examinations.[74–77]
- Stable patients with blunt abdominal trauma and concern for intra-abdominal injury should receive a CT of the abdomen and pelvis or serial abdominal examinations.
- Patients with open wounds or lacerations should receive tetanus vaccination if their immunizations are not up-to-date.

Pitfalls in Abdominal and Flank Trauma

- Do not underestimate the mechanism of injury. Patients can have significant intraperitoneal injury despite normal vital signs.
- Patients must be undressed and the skin fully examined to identify any and all potential injuries.
- It is important to account for all bullets in penetrating trauma and consider intravascular migration if not accounted for.
- The absence of abdominal pain does not exclude intra-abdominal injury.
- CT may miss injuries to the diaphragm, small bowel, or pancreas.
- Unstable patients should not be sent to CT.

Key Points

- The most common causes of blunt trauma are MVC, falls, and assault, while penetrating trauma is most commonly caused by stab wounds or gunshot wounds.
- Gunshot wounds are associated with higher mortality than stab wounds.
- The spleen is the most commonly affected organ in blunt trauma, while the small intestines and colon are most commonly affected in penetrating trauma.
- A thorough evaluation is important to identify all associated injuries. This includes a full skin examination for all patients with penetrating wounds.
- Most isolated hepatic and splenic injuries in stable patients can be managed non-operatively.
- CT may miss some diaphragmatic injuries. Therefore, it is important to maintain a high index of suspicion for these injuries in trauma patients.
- Unstable patients should not leave the ED for imaging.
- Unstable patients with evidence of significant abdominal injury, renal injury, or a positive E-FAST examination should undergo operative repair.

References

1. Rutledge R, Hunt JP, Lentz CW, et al. A statewide, population-based time-series analysis of the increasing frequency of nonoperative management of abdominal solid organ injury. *Ann Surg.* 1995;222 (3):311–22.

2. Demetriades D, Murray J, Charalambides K, et al. Trauma fatalities: time and location of hospital deaths. *J Am Coll Surg.* 2004;198 (1):20–6.

3. Livingston DH, Lavery RF, Passannante MR, et al. Admission or observation is not necessary after a negative abdominal computed tomographic scan in patients with suspected blunt abdominal trauma: results of a prospective, multi-institutional trial. *J Trauma.* 1998;44(2):273–80.

4. Nicholas JM, Rix EP, Easley KA, et al. Changing patterns in the management of penetrating abdominal trauma: the more things change, the more they stay the same. *J Trauma.* 2003;55(6):1095–108.

5. Cairns BA, Oller DW, Meyer AA, et al. Management and outcome of abdominal shotgun wounds. Trauma score and the role of exploratory laparotomy. *Ann Surg.* 1995;221(3):272–77.

6. Ley EJ, Salim A, Kohanzadeh S, Mirocha J, Margulies DR. Relative bradycardia in hypotensive trauma patients: a reappraisal. *J Trauma.* 2009;67(5):1051–54.

7. Pikoulis E, Delis S, Psalidas N, et al. Presentation of blunt small intestinal and mesenteric injuries. *Ann R Coll Surg Engl.* 2000;82(2):103–6.

8. Fakhry SM, Watts DD, Luchette FA; EAST Multi-Institutional Hollow Viscus Injury Research Group. Current diagnostic approaches lack sensitivity in the diagnosis of perforated blunt small bowel injury: analysis from 275,557 trauma admissions from the EAST multi-institutional HVI trial. *J Trauma.* 2003;54(2):295–306.

9. Holmes JF, Ngyuen H, Jacoby RC, et al. Do all patients with left costal margin injuries require radiographic evaluation for intraabdominal injury? *Ann Emerg Med.* 2005;46(3):232–36.

10. Velmahos GC, Tatevossian R, Demetriades D. The "seat belt mark" sign: a call for increased vigilance among physicians treating victims of motor vehicle accidents. *Am Surg.* 1999;65(2):181–85.

11. Meyers MA, Feldberg MA, Oliphant M. Grey Turner's sign and Cullen's sign in acute pancreatitis. *Gastrointest Radiol.* 1989;14(1):31–37.

12. Rahbour G, Ullah MR, Yassin N, Thomas GP. Cullen's sign – case report with a

review of the literature. *Int J Surg Case Rep.* 2012;3(5):143–46.

13. Lowenfels AB. Kehr's sign – a neglected aid in rupture of the spleen. *N Engl J Med.* 1966;274(18):1019.

14. Sugrue M, Balogh Z, Lynch J, et al. Guidelines for the management of haemodynamically stable patients with stab wounds to the anterior abdomen. *ANZ J Surg.* 2007;77(8):614–20.

15. Esposito TJ, Ingraham A, Luchette FA, et al. Reasons to omit digital rectal exam in trauma patients: no fingers, no rectum, no useful additional information. *J Trauma.* 2005;59(6):1314–19.

16. Shlamovitz GZ, Mower WR, Bergman J, et al. Poor test characteristics for the digital rectal examination in trauma patients. *Ann Emerg Med.* 2007;50(1):25–33.

17. Ball CG, Jafri SM, Kirkpatrick AW, et al. Traumatic urethral injuries: does the digital rectal examination really help us? *Injury.* 2009;40(9):984–86.

18. Velmahos GC, Toutouzas K, Radin R, et al. High success with nonoperative management of blunt hepatic trauma: the liver is a sturdy organ. *Arch Surg.* 2003;138(5):475–80.

19. Moore EE, Cogbill TH, Jurkovich GJ, et al. Organ injury scaling: spleen and liver (1994 revision). *J Trauma.* 1995;38(3):323–24.

20. Haan JM, Bochicchio GV, Kramer N, Scalea TM. Nonoperative management of blunt splenic injury: a 5-year experience. *J Trauma.* 2005;58(3):492–98.

21. Muroni M, Provenza G, Conte S, et al. Diaphragmatic rupture with right colon and small intestine herniation after blunt trauma: a case report. *J Med Case Rep.* 2010;4:289.

22. Yucel M, Bas G, Kulali F, et al. Evaluation of diaphragm in penetrating left thoracoabdominal stab injuries: the role of multislice computed tomography. *Injury.* 2015;46(9):1734–37.

23. Mee SL, McAninch JW, Robinson AL, Auerbach PS, Carroll PR. Radiographic assessment of renal trauma: a 10-year

prospective study of patient selection. *J Urol.* 1989;141(5):1095–98.

24. Santucci RA, Wessells H, Bartsch G, et al. Evaluation and management of renal injuries: consensus statement of the renal trauma subcommittee. *BJU Int.* 2004;93(7):937–54.

25. Moore EE, Shackford SR, Pachter HL, et al. Organ injury scaling: spleen, liver, and kidney. *J Trauma.* 1989;29(12):1664–66.

26. Santucci RA, McAninch JW, Safir M, et al. Validation of the American Association for the Surgery of Trauma organ injury severity scale for the kidney. *J Trauma.* 2001;50(2):195–200.

27. ATLS Subcommittee; American College of Surgeons' Committee on Trauma; International ATLS working group. Advanced trauma life support (ATLS®): the ninth edition. *J Trauma Acute Care Surg.* 2013;74(5):1363–66.

28. Asimos AW, Gibbs MA, Marx JA, et al. Value of point-of-care blood testing in emergent trauma management. *Trauma.* 2000;48(6):1101–8.

29. Isaacman DJ, Scarfone RJ, Kost SI, et al. Utility of routine laboratory testing for detecting intra-abdominal injury in the pediatric trauma patient. *Pediatrics.* 1993;92(5):691–94.

30. Capraro AJ, Mooney D, Waltzman ML. The use of routine laboratory studies as screening tools in pediatric abdominal trauma. *Pediatr Emerg Care.* 2006;22(7):480–84.

31. Chu UB, Clevenger FW, Imami ER, et al. The impact of selective laboratory evaluation on utilization of laboratory resources and patient care in a level-I trauma center. *Am J Surg.* 1996;172(5):558–62; discussion 562–63.

32. Keller MS, Coln CE, Trimble JA, Green MC, Weber TR. The utility of routine trauma laboratories in pediatric trauma resuscitations. *Am J Surg.* 2004;188(6):671–78.

33. Alsikafi NF, Rosenstein DI. Staging, evaluation, and nonoperative management

of renal injuries. *Urol Clin North Am.* 2006;33(1):13–19.

34. Nicolaisen GS, McAninch JW, Marshall GA, Bluth RF Jr, Carroll PR. Renal trauma: re-evaluation of the indications for radiographic assessment. *J Urol.* 1985;133 (2):183–87.

35. Boulanger BR, McLellan BA, Brenneman FD, et al. Emergent abdominal sonography as a screening test in a new diagnostic algorithm for blunt trauma. *J Trauma.* 1996;40(6):867–74.

36. Boulanger BR, Brenneman FD, Kirkpatrick AW, McLellan BA, Nathens AB. The indeterminate abdominal sonogram in multisystem blunt trauma. *J Trauma.* 1998;45(1):52–56.

37. Tayal VS, Nielsen A, Jones AE, et al. Accuracy of trauma ultrasound in major pelvic injury. *J Trauma.* 2006;61 (6):1453–57.

38. Poletti PA, Kinkel K, Vermeulen B, et al. Blunt abdominal trauma:should US be used to detect both free fluid and organ injuries? *Radiology.* 2003;227(1):95–103.

39. Smith JK, Kenney PJ. Imaging of renal trauma. *Radiol Clin North Am.* 2003;41 (5):1019–35.

40. Milanchi S, Wood D. Rigler's sign in a patient with massive pneumoperitoneum. *Emerg Med J.* 2006;23(11):884.

41. Gottlieb M. Abnormal radiographs in a child. *Vis J Emerg Med.* 2016;4:33–34.

42. Gelman R, Mirvis SE, Gens D. Diaphragmatic rupture due to blunt trauma: sensitivity of plain chest radiographs. *AJR Am J Roentgenol.* 1991;156(1):51–57.

43. Shapiro MJ, Heiberg E, Durham RM, Luchtefeld W, Mazuski JE. The unreliability of CT scans and initial chest radiographs in evaluating blunt trauma induced diaphragmatic rupture. *Clin Radiol.* 1996;51(1):27–30.

44. Anderson PA, Rivara FP, Maier RV, Drake C. The epidemiology of seatbelt-associated injuries. *J Trauma.* 1991;31(1):60–67.

45. Tyroch AH, McGuire EL, McLean SF, et al. The association between chance fractures

and intra-abdominal injuries revisited: a multicenter review. *Am Surg.* 2005;71 (5):434–38.

46. Gonzalez RP, Han M, Turk B, Luterman A. Screening for abdominal injury prior to emergent extra-abdominal trauma surgery: a prospective study. *J Trauma.* 2004;57 (4):739–41.

47. Schauer BA, Nguyen H, Wisner DH, Holmes JF. Is definitive abdominal evaluation required in blunt trauma victims undergoing urgent extra-abdominal surgery? *Acad Emerg Med.* 2005;12 (8):707–11.

48. Sharples A, Brohi K. Can clinical prediction tools predict the need for computed tomography in blunt abdominal? *A systematic review.* Injury. 2016;47(8):1811–18.

49. Holmes JF, Wisner DH, McGahan JP, Mower WR, Kuppermann N. Clinical prediction rules for identifying adults at very low risk for intra-abdominal injuries after blunt trauma. *Ann Emerg Med.* 2009;54(4):575–84.

50. Hauser CJ, Visvikis G, Hinrichs C, et al. Prospective validation of computed tomographic screening of the thoracolumbar spine in trauma. *J Trauma.* 2003;55(2):228–34.

51. Killeen KL, Shanmuganathan K, Poletti PA, Cooper C, Mirvis SE. Helical computed tomography of bowel and mesenteric injuries. *J Trauma.* 2001;51(1):26–36.

52. Larici AR, Gotway MB, Litt HI, et al. Helical CT with sagittal and coronal reconstructions: accuracy for detection of diaphragmatic injury. *AJR Am J Roentgenol.* 2002;179(2):451–57.

53. Allen TL, Cummins BF, Bonk RT, et al. Computed tomography without oral contrast solution for blunt diaphragmatic injuries in abdominal trauma. *Am J Emerg Med.* 2005;23(3):253–58.

54. Ilahi O, Bochicchio GV, Scalea TM. Efficacy of computed tomography in the diagnosis of pancreatic injury in adult blunt trauma patients: a single-institutional study. *Am Surg.* 2002;68 (8):704–7.

55. Phelan HA, Velmahos GC, Jurkovich GJ, et al. An evaluation of multidetector computed tomography in detecting pancreatic injury: results of a multicenter AAST study. *J Trauma.* 2009;66(3):641–46.

56. Velmahos GC, Tabbara M, Gross R, et al. Blunt pancreatoduodenal injury: a multicenter study of the Research Consortium of New England Centers for Trauma (ReCONECT). *Arch Surg.* 2009;144(5):413–19.

57. Sherck J, Shatney C, Sensaki K, Selivanov V. The accuracy of computed tomography in the diagnosis of blunt small-bowel perforation. *Am J Surg.* 1994;168 (6):670–75.

58. Janzen DL1, Zwirewich CV, Breen DJ, Nagy A. Diagnostic accuracy of helical CT for detection of blunt bowel and mesenteric injuries. *Clin Radiol.* 1998;53(3):193–97.

59. Butela ST, Federle MP, Chang PJ, et al. Performance of CT in detection of bowel injury. *AJR Am J Roentgenol.* 2001;176 (1):129–35.

60. Shanmuganathan K, Mirvis SE, Chiu WC, Killeen KL, Scalea TM. Triple-contrast helical CT in penetrating torso trauma: a prospective study to determine peritoneal violation and the need for laparotomy. *AJR Am J Roentgenol.* 2001;177(6):1247–56.

61. Chiu WC, Shanmuganathan K, Mirvis SE, Scalea TM. Determining the need for laparotomy in penetrating torso trauma: a prospective study using triple-contrast enhanced abdominopelvic computed tomography. *J Trauma.* 2001;51(5):860–68.

62. Dissanaike S, Griswold JA, Frezza EE. Treatment of isolated penetrating flank trauma. *Am Surg.* 2005;71(6):493–96.

63. Bilge A, Sahin M. Diagnostic peritoneal lavage in blunt abdominal trauma. *Eur J Surg.* 1991;157(8):449–51.

64. Liu M, Lee CH, P'eng FK. Prospective comparison of diagnostic peritoneal lavage, computed tomographic scanning, and ultrasonography for the diagnosis of blunt abdominal trauma. *J Trauma.* 1993;35 (2):267–70.

65. Otomo Y, Henmi H, Mashiko K, et al. New diagnostic peritoneal lavage criteria for diagnosis of intestinal injury. *J Trauma.* 1998;44(6):991–97.

66. Biffl WL, Kaups KL, Cothren CC, et al. Management of patients with anterior abdominal stab wounds: a Western Trauma Association multicenter trial. *J Trauma.* 2009;66(5):1294–301.

67. Fryer JP, Graham TL, Fong HM, Burns CM. Diagnostic peritoneal lavage as an indicator for therapeutic surgery. *Can J Surg.* 1991;34(5):471–76.

68. Whitehouse JS, Weigelt JA. Diagnostic peritoneal lavage: a review of indications, technique, and interpretation. *Scand J Trauma Resusc Emerg Med.* 2009;17:13.

69. Borgman MA, Spinella PC, Perkins JG, et al. The ratio of blood products transfused affects mortality in patients receiving massive transfusions at a combat support hospital. *J Trauma.* 2007;63 (4):805–13.

70. Zink KA, Sambasivan CN, Holcomb JB, Chisholm G, Schreiber MA. A high ratio of plasma and platelets to packed red blood cells in the first 6 hours of massive transfusion improves outcomes in a large multicenter study. *Am J Surg.* 2009;197 (5):565–70.

71. Bickell WH, Wall MJ Jr, Pepe PE, et al. Immediate versus delayed fluid resuscitation for hypotensive patients with penetrating torso injuries. *N Engl J Med.* 1994;331(17):1105–9.

72. Dutton RP, Mackenzie CF, Scalea TM. Hypotensive resuscitation during active hemorrhage: impact on in-hospital mortality. *J Trauma.* 2002;52(6):1141–46.

73. Meizoso JP, Ray JJ, Karcutskie CA 4th, et al. Effect of time to operation on mortality for hypotensive patients with gunshot wounds to the torso: the golden 10 minutes. *J Trauma Acute Care Surg.* 2016;81(4):685–91.

74. Zubowski R, Nallathambi M, Ivatury R, Stahl W. Selective conservatism in abdominal stab wounds: the efficacy of serial physical examination. *J Trauma.* 1988;28(12):1665–68.

75. van Haarst EP, van Bezooijen BP, Coene PP, Luitse JS. The efficacy of serial physical

examination in penetrating abdominal trauma. *Injury*. 1999;30(9):599–604.

76. Ertekin C, Yanar H, Taviloglu K, Güloglu R, Alimoglu O. Unnecessary laparotomy by using physical examination and different diagnostic modalities for penetrating abdominal stab wounds. *Emerg Med J*. 2005;22(11):790–94.

77. Navsaria PH, Berli JU, Edu S, Nicol AJ. Non-operative management of abdominal stab wounds – an analysis of 186 patients. *S Afr J Surg*. 2007;45(4):128–30, 132.

Genitourinary Trauma

16

E. Liang Liu

The genitourinary (GU) system includes the kidneys, ureters, bladder, urethra, penis, scrotum, and female genitalia. Of the 27.7 million patients per year presenting to emergency departments (ED) for traumatic injury, about 10% of these traumas primarily involve the GU system, and another 10–15% of patients with abdominal trauma will have GU injuries as well.[1] GU trauma patients are predominantly young (80% less than the age of 45 years) and male (85% of all patients).[2] Delays or missed diagnosis of GU trauma can result in increased morbidity and mortality due to preventable complications with long term consequences.[3]

Overview

- Injury can be a result of penetrating or blunt trauma involving the chest, abdomen, and/ or back.
  - Non-iatrogenic blunt trauma mechanisms, most commonly motor vehicle collisions, account for approximately 90% of injuries to the GU system.[4]
  - GU injuries in sports-related events most commonly involve the external genitalia.[5]
  - Only 1–3% of penetrating trauma involves the GU system.[2]
- The most commonly injured urological organ is the kidney, followed by the testicles and bladder.[2]
- Delays in diagnosis are common as GU injuries rarely occur in isolation.
  - 20–25% of all bladder and urethral injuries associated with pelvic fractures are initially missed.[2]

Signs and Symptoms

- For any trauma, make sure to undress the patient to evaluate for subtle signs such as perineal ecchymosis that may indicate deeper injuries.
- Though more often absent, Grey-Turner's sign, abdominal or flank tenderness or pain, hematuria, and potentially a palpable mass can suggest GU trauma.
  - Hematuria is absent in 5–36% of patients.[1]
  - Even severe injuries such as renal artery injury or ureteropelvic disruption can present without hematuria.
- Suspect bladder injury in the patient who is oliguric despite adequate fluid replacement and in patients who are unable to void but are not hypovolemic.

- Though classic examination findings for ureteral and bladder injuries include blood at the meatus, perineal or scrotal hematoma, and high riding prostate, these findings are uncommon.
- A history of pre-existing renal structural or functional disorders is important to note, which increases the risk for injury and also increases trauma-associated acute kidney injury from insults such as hypotension, rhabdomyolysis, and contrast-induced nephropathy.[6]
- Pre-existing urologic pathology that alter bladder sensation, such as neurogenic bladder disorder, places patients at greater risk of missed injury.[2]

Diagnostic Studies

- *Baseline renal function*: Initial creatinine performed after traumatic injury likely reflects pre-existing renal insufficiency rather than impact of renal or GU injury.[2]
  - Rising urea and creatinine in a patient with isolated GU trauma can suggest renal impairment due to traumatic injury, reabsorption of extravasated urine, or contrast induced nephropathy following diagnostic imaging.

- *Urinalysis* should be performed on all abdominal trauma patients.
  - The first spontaneously voided sample of urine is essential to identify hematuria, as this has the highest sensitivity before fluid administration or diuresis obscures its presence.[2]
  - Hematuria can be gross (i.e. visible) or microscopic (more than five red blood cells per high-power field).[7]
  - Gross hematuria is more suggestive of a bladder or ureter injury.
  - Generally speaking, the greater the degree of hematuria, the greater the risk of significant intra-abdominal injury.
    - 50% of patients with macroscopic hematuria in blunt trauma have renal injuries, and a further 15% have injuries to other intra-abdominal organs.[2]
    - No hematuria is seen in 5% of renal injuries or 20% of renovascular injuries.[8]
    - There is no correlation between amount or presence of hematuria and degree of injury.
  - Management of hematuria depends on the mechanism of injury and the clinical picture (Figure 16.1). The EAST guidelines make suggestions for management of traumatic hematuria.[9]

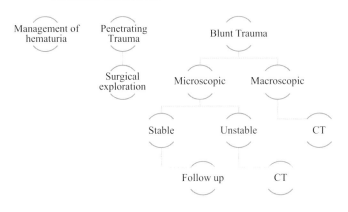

Figure 16.1 Management of hematuria based on EAST guidelines

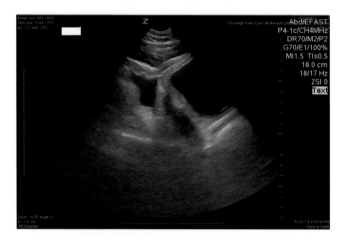

Figure 16.2 Positive FAST exam showing free fluid in the pelvis

- – Penetrating trauma to the abdomen requires surgical exploration.
- – Asymptomatic patients with microscopic hematuria in blunt trauma require no further imaging and can be followed up with repeat urinalysis in 1 week with the primary care provider.
- – In blunt trauma patients with gross hematuria or who are unstable (defined as systolic blood pressure less than 90 mmHg) with microscopic hematuria, a computed tomography (CT) is needed to evaluate for urologic damage.
- – CT is indicated in patients with a significant mechanism of injury including rapid deceleration, significant injury to the flank, rib fracture, significant flank ecchymosis, penetrating injury of abdomen, flank, or lower chest.

- *Bedside ultrasound* is recommended in all abdominal trauma patients.[2]
  - . Ultrasound can identify intraperitoneal fluid but has minimal utility in diagnosing parenchymal trauma or retroperitoneal bleeding.
  - . A focused assessment with sonography in trauma (FAST) exam can be performed at the bedside to evaluate for intraperitoneal bleed (Figure 16.2).
  - . A dedicated bladder view in a patient with or without urinary catheter in place can help evaluate for urinary retention (Figure 16.3).
  - . US can also help detect penile fracture or evaluate for testicular injury and viability and vulnerability of the tissue.

- *CT of the abdomen and pelvis with intravenous (IV) contrast* is the gold standard in assessing renal and GU trauma.[2]
  - . More sensitive and specific than intravenous pyelogram, ultrasound, or angiography.[2]
  - . Better detects, localizes, and characterizes the nature of injuries.
  - . Useful for evaluating other injuries as well as detecting injuries in patients with pre-existing urological structural abnormalities.
  - . Findings that suggest major renal injury include hematoma, urinary extravasation, and lack of contrast enhancement of the renal parenchyma.
  - . Indicated in patients with:[2]

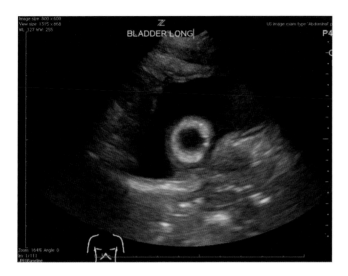

Image size 600 × 600
View size 1315 × 868
WL 127 WW 255
Z
BLADDER LONG
US image exam type 'Abdominal p
P4
-C
Zoom 164% Angle 0
Im 1/111
PEGBaseline

Figure 16.3 Despite the presence of a Foley catheter, this ultrasound of the bladder shows urinary retention

- Blunt abdominal trauma and gross hematuria.
- Blunt abdominal trauma with 5–30 RBCs/HPF when there is hypotension or other signs of shock, or injuries that would require it (such as a positive FAST examination).
- Blunt trauma with injuries known to be associated with renal injury such as rapid deceleration, direct contusion to the flank, flank ecchymosis, or fracture of the lower ribs or thoracolumbar spine, regardless of hematuria.
- Penetrating trauma to upper abdomen or lower thorax regardless of hematuria.

. Conventional CT imaging is obtained before contrast is excreted in the urine and can miss 80% of ureteral injury from blunt trauma.[2]

- 10-minute-delayed CT images of the pelvis should be obtained in the setting of high grade renal injury, ureteropelvic junction injury, or any concern for ureteral injury.[10]
- Findings include extravasation, periureteral urinoma, or a lack of contrast distal to the suspected ureteral injury.

- *CT Cystography*

. Performed by draining the bladder via a Foley catheter or suprapubic catheter, instilling 350 cc of diluted, sterile CT contrast (made with 30 cc of contrast in a 500 cc bag of warmed normal saline) into the bladder by gravity, clamping the catheter, and obtaining CT images of the pelvis.[10]

. Should be added to CT abdomen/pelvis with IV contrast when the patient has:[2]

- Gross hematuria
- Pelvic free fluid without another explanation other than bladder injury
- Any pelvic fracture other than acetabular fractures
- Isolated microhematuria with physician concern
- Difficulty voiding or suprapubic pain and any hematuria
- Penetrating injuries to the buttock, pelvis, or lower abdomen with any hematuria

. Sensitivity for detecting bladder injuries is 78–100%.[11]

- *CT Angiography*: Generally performed perioperatively to localize acute arterial hemorrhage in preparation for surgical repair and/or embolization.
- *Retrograde Urethrogram (RUG)*
  - Should be performed prior to blind insertion of urinary catheter if there is concern for urethral injury, pelvic fracture, the inability to urinate, or significant pelvic swelling or ecchymosis.[12]
  - Performed by gently stretching the penis over the thigh at an oblique angle to radiographically visualize the entire urethra, with x-ray obtained as a scout for comparison before contrast is instilled. Contrast is then instilled into the urethral meatus. Abdominal radiograph is then performed to evaluate for contrast extravasation along the course of the urethra which indicates urethral disruption.[2]
  - This can interfere with contrast used in CT with IV contrast and should be performed in a delayed fashion.
  - A pericatheter RUG can be performed if a urinary catheter has already been placed and urethral injury is suspected.[2]
- *Intravenous Pyelogram (IVP)*: This is an option if CT is unavailable or imaging needs to be carried out in the operating room, though it is less sensitive than CTs and cannot visualize non-urologic injuries.
- *Magnetic Resonance Imaging (MRI)*: While there are some reports citing the use of MRI in evaluation of GU trauma, MRI is never an appropriate imaging study for the unstable patient. Given the more readily available imaging modalities discussed above, its utility in the ED is very limited.[2]

Kidney

Anatomy

- The kidneys and ureters are protected by adjacent anatomic structures but are suspended by the renal pedicle without other firm attachments.
- Damage to these organs usually is secondary to direct flank trauma or rapid deceleration injury: high speed motor vehicle crash, fall from significant height, etc.
  - The kidneys are susceptible to contusions, lacerations (renal fractures), hematomas, avulsions of the renal vasculature, renal artery thrombosis, etc.
  - Fracture of the lower posterior ribs, lower thoracic, or lumbar vertebrae can be associated with renal or urethral injuries.
  - 250,000 traumatic renal injuries occur annually worldwide.[2]
  - The kidneys are often injured in patients with multitrauma and seen in 8–10% of patients hospitalized for abdominal trauma.[2]
- Children are at higher risk of blunt renal injury than adults.[13]
  - Pediatric kidneys are more mobile, larger relative to body size, not as well protected by fat, and more anatomically forward.[13]
- Pre-existing structural urologic pathology such as hydronephrosis, tumors, cysts, strictures, or solitary kidney is highly associated with renal injury after even minor trauma and requires more intensive evaluation. [14]

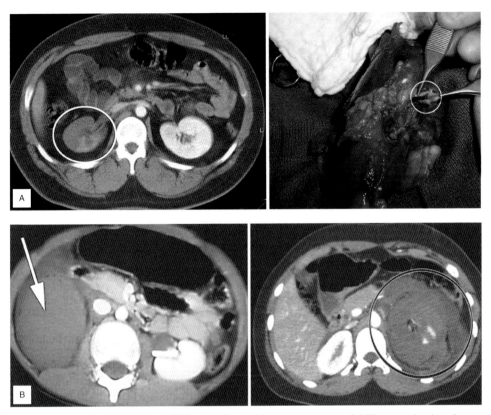

Figure 16.4 (A) CT scan of patient with blunt renal artery injury (no contrast uptake). There is isolated renal artery thrombosis without any parenchymal injury (left). The operative specimen (right) shows a clot in the renal artery. (B) Patients with renal artery thrombosis, associated parenchymal injuries (left), and extensive perirenal hematomas (right). These cases are less likely to be managed successfully with endovascular stenting (reproduced with permission from *Color Atlas of Emergency Trauma, Second Edition*)

Evaluation

- Includes urinalysis, CT abdomen with IV contrast, intravenous pyelogram, and renal angiography if indicated (Figure 16.4).
- Grading of renal injury is important with regard to management and is defined by the American Association for the Surgery of Trauma (Table 16.1).[8]

Management

- Initial management includes fluid resuscitation, bed rest, and serial monitoring of vitals and hemoglobin. Urologic consult should be obtained.
- Most renal injuries (Grades I–III and most grade IV injuries) can be managed conservatively and tend to heal spontaneously.
- Surgical repair is required in the setting of urine extravasation, ongoing bleeding, hemodynamic instability, or suspicion of renovascular injury.[15]
- Renal pedicle injury, most commonly due to deceleration injury involving violent sheering of the kidney on its vascular pedicle, can result in life threatening hemorrhage and renal ischemia.

Table 16.1 Renal injury classification

Grade	Injury
Grade I	• Contusion with microscopic or gross hematuria with normal urologic studies • Nonexpanding subcapsular hematoma without parenchymal laceration
Grade II	• Nonexpanding hematoma confined to the renal retroperitoneum • Laceration less than 1 cm parenchymal depth of the renal cortex without urinary extravasation
Grade III	• Laceration more than 1 cm parenchymal depth of the renal cortex without collecting system rupture or urinary extravasation
Grade IV	• Laceration extending through the renal cortex, medulla, and collecting system • Segmental renal artery or vein injury with contained hemorrhage
Grade V	• Completely shattered kidney • Avulsion of renal hilum that devascularizes the kidney

- . This can lead to thrombosis or complete detachment at the pedicle.
- . Early surgical repair is needed to rescue the kidney, although nephrectomy may result.
- Interventional radiology can also be used to embolize bleeding vessels or stent dissected renal arteries.[2]
- Higher grade renal injuries with anticipated nonoperative management require admission for bed rest, observation, serial hematocrit testing, monitoring of urine output and degree of hematuria, and potentially serial CT scans.

Complications

Complications include uncontrolled hemorrhage, delayed abdominal findings due to retroperitoneal position, thrombosis of renal vein or artery, urine extravasation, infection, abscesses, urinoma formation, secondary hemorrhage, hypertension, "Page" kidney (scarring leading to hypertension), hydronephrosis, calculi, and chronic pyelonephritis.[2]

- Damage to renal vasculature can result in necrosis if left untreated.
- Delayed onset of gross hematuria after injury increases the likelihood for a rare potentially life-threatening complication of renal artery pseudoaneurysm.

Ureter

Anatomy

- Ureters are hollow organs that are highly mobile within the retroperitoneal fat and protected by the psoas muscles. As such, they are rarely injured in blunt trauma.[1]
- Represents less than 1% of GU injuries.[15]
- When injured, they are susceptible to contusion, laceration, transection, and avulsion.
- 95% of ureteral injury is due to gunshot wounds.[15]

- The ureter is injured in approximately 5% of penetrating wounds to the abdomen.[2,7]
- Penetrating trauma involving the ureter often involves simultaneous hollow viscus and vasculature injuries.
- Ureteral injuries due to blunt trauma are seen in conjunction with lumbosacral spine injuries and pelvic fractures, reflecting the extreme force needed to stretch or rupture the walls of the tubular ureter.[16]

Evaluation

- Injury should be expected in the patient with unexplained rise in BUN and creatinine or presence of urinoma on imaging (often delayed).
- Diagnosis requires delayed CT scan images 5–8 minutes after administration of contrast.[15]

Management

Treatment involves operative repair, placement of a ureteral stent, or percutaneous nephrostomy tube placement.[2]

Complications

Complications include urine extravasation with urinoma formation, infection, secondary hemorrhage, and stricture formation leading to hydronephrosis.

Bladder

Anatomy

- Bladder injuries can involve mural contusions, hematoma, laceration, and ruptures.
  - Typically associated with pelvic fractures or penetrating trauma close to the bladder.
- The amount of urine in the bladder at the time of injury is directly related to risk of rupture, as injury often occurs with a distended bladder full of urine.
  - Pregnant women and intoxicated patients (with full bladders) are at higher risk.
- Children are more susceptible to bladder injury as their bladders are an intra-abdominal organ and, thus, less protected by the pelvis.[13]
- Patients can present with lower abdominal pain, hematuria, palpable fullness, azotemia, inability to void, or concomitant pelvic fracture.
  - Only 2% of bladder ruptures are seen in isolation. Assessment should focus on other concomitant injuries.[2]
  - Approximately 80% of bladder injuries occur with pelvic fractures.
- Ruptures are classified as intraperitoneal, extraperitoneal, or combined (Table 16.2).[16]

Evaluation

- Diagnosis is made with a retrograde cystogram or CT cystography in which contrast is injected via urethral catheter.

239

Table 16.2 Bladder rupture classification

Bladder Rupture	Characteristics	Management
Intraperitoneal rupture (25–43% of bladder ruptures)	• Occur at the superior dome of the bladder • Result in urinary extravasation into the peritoneal cavity • Associated with penetrating trauma • Most common type of perforation in children	Laparotomy and surgical repair
Extraperitoneal rupture (50–71% of bladder ruptures)	• Occur along the inferior aspect of the bladder • Result in urinary extravasation into the pelvic cavity • Associated with pelvic fractures	Foley or suprapubic catheter (depending on location of injury) – typically for about 10 days
Combined ruptures (7–14% of bladder ruptures)	• Associated with high mechanisms • 60% mortality rate (compared to overall mortality of bladder injuries of 17–22%) likely due to concomitant injuries	Laparotomy and surgical repair

- Extraperitoneal injuries are characterized by "flame" configuration of extravasation as the contrast infiltrates the paravesical tissues (Figure 16.5).[15]
- In intraperitoneal injuries, contrast can be seen outlining the bowel loops (Figure 16.6).[15]

Management

- Management is typically conservative: patients are treated with Foley or suprapubic catheter depending on location of injury.
- Bladder contusions and hematomas are observed.
- Evaluation for ureteral injury should be performed prior to insertion of indwelling catheter.
- May require endoscopy guided catheter placement, use of a guide wire, or use of a coude tip catheter.
- Injuries to the bladder neck, concomitant rectal injuries, or bony fragments within the bladder may require open surgical management.[15]

Complications

- Typically, bladder injuries heal well without long-term issues.
- Immediate complications include urine extravasation, peritonitis, and infection.
- Rarely, delayed complications include stone formation, fistula, diverticula, and voiding dysfunction.

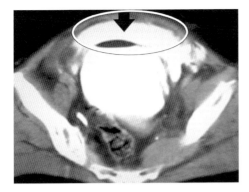

Figure 16.5 CT cystogram showing extraperitoneal rupture. This type of injury can safely be managed with Foley's catheter drainage of the bladder for 10–14 days (reproduced with permission from *Color Atlas of Emergency Trauma, Second Edition*)

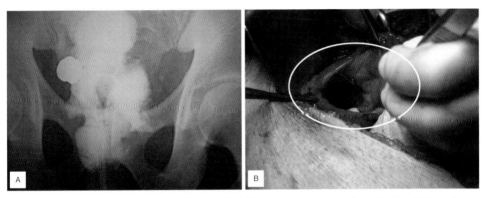

Figure 16.6 Intraperitoneal rupture of the bladder. (A) Voiding cysto-urethrogram shows significant intraperitoneal rupture of the bladder. (B) Intraoperative appearance of the bladder rupture (reproduced with permission from *Color Atlas of Emergency Trauma, Second Edition*)

Urethra

Anatomy

- Men are more likely to suffer injuries to this organ due to the length of the male compared to the female urethra.[12]
- Injury mechanisms include direct blows to the peritoneum, mutilation, and instrumentation.
- Injuries include contusions, stretch injury, partial disruption, complete disruption, or transection.
- Pediatric urethras are less elastic and can result in complete ruptures.[2]
- Classically, urethral trauma is seen in the setting of blood at the urinary meatus, perineal or scrotal hematoma, and a displaced or high-riding prostate on digital rectal exam.
  - Patients can have gross hematuria, edema, ecchymosis, dysuria.
  - Patients may have difficulty with voiding.
  - If blind passage of a Foley catheter is attempted, there may be difficulty with passage.
- The male urethra is divided into the anterior and posterior segments (Table 16.3).[2]

Table 16.3 Male urethral injuries

Segment	Anatomy	Associated Injury
Anterior urethra	Bulbar and penile urethra	More often by straddle injuries and penetrating injuries
Posterior urethra	Prostatic and membranous urethra	Usually result from pelvic fractures and concomitant bladder injuries

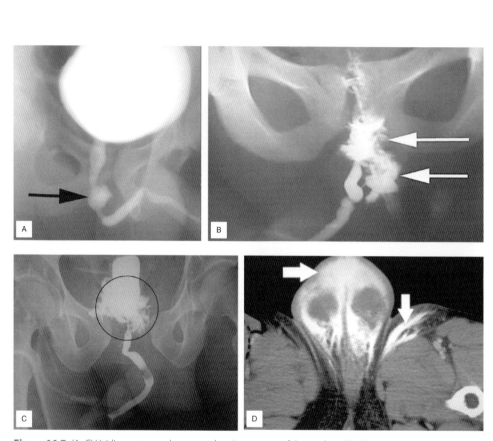

Figure 16.7 (A–C) Voiding cysto-urethrograms showing rupture of the urethra. (D) CT cystogram showing massive extravasation of contrast in the scrotum and extraperitoneal tissues secondary to posterior urethral disruption (reproduced with permission from *Color Atlas of Emergency Trauma, Second Edition*)

Evaluation

Injuries are diagnosed with RUG. Contrast extravasation is pathognomonic for urethral injury (Figure 16.7).[16]

Management

- Urethral injury is a contraindication for blind catheterization.[2]

- A catheter can be placed with the aid of fluoroscopy or flexible endoscopy, though a suprapubic catheter may need to be placed.[15]
- Typically managed with delayed repair, as initial urethral repair is associated with increased risk of hemorrhage, impotence, and infection of pelvic hematoma.

Complications

Complications include stenosis and stricture formation which can result in weakened force of stream, urinary tract infections, dysuria, hematuria, or urinary retention.

Scrotum and Testicle

Anatomy

- Scrotal trauma includes penetrating wounds, burns, or avulsions.
- Clinical exam can review pain, swelling, ecchymosis, and a tender firm scrotal mass that does not transilluminate.[2]
- Occurs due to blunt trauma to the scrotum such as a kick or fall.
- Penetrating injuries can result in lacerations, contusions, avulsions, and even amputation.
- Testicular injuries include contusions or ruptures from blunt trauma. Testicular mass and torsion should also be considered in these patients.
- Testicular rupture occurs when extreme blunt forces cause a rupture of the tunica albuginea that covers the individual testicle, resulting in extrusion of the seminiferous tubules.[17]

Evaluation

Scrotal ultrasound with Doppler can be used to evaluate for testicular torsion, rupture, and fracture.[2]

Management

- External structures are at risk of human and animal bites.[2]
  - Management includes copious irrigation, debridement, broad spectrum antibiotic prophylaxis, tetanus and rabies immunizations if indicated, and early closure of wounds.
  - Recommended antibiotics include beta lactam antibiotics with beta lactamase inhibitor (i.e. amoxicillin-clavulanate), second generation cephalosporins (cefotetan, cefoxitin), or clindamycin with fluoroquinolones.[17]
  - Human bites are contaminated wounds that should never be closed primarily. Empiric antibiotics for these bites include amoxicillin-clavulanate or moxifloxacin.[17]
- Surgical repair is indicated for penetrating injuries, testicular rupture or fracture, expanding hematoma, large hematocele, testicular torsion, non-reducible testicular dislocation, and scrotal degloving.[15]
- Conservative management includes scrotal support via elevation with towels, cold packs, and pain management.[12]

Complications

Complications include testicular pain, atrophy, and impotence.

Penis

Anatomy

- Penile injuries include penetrating trauma, burns, lacerations, contusions, avulsions, sexual trauma, zipper injuries, fractures (rupture of the corpus cavernosum), or strangulations.
- Penile fractures can present with penile ecchymosis, a recognized "pop" or cracking sound, extreme pain, sudden detumescence, and significant swelling with a deformed penis.[2]
  - Occur most often during sexual intercourse as a result of blunt force on an erect penis, causing rupture of the tunica albuginea which covers the corpora cavernosa.
  - Urethral injury occurs with penile factures in roughly 20% of patients.[2]

Evaluation

- Retrograde urethrogram should be performed to evaluate for urethral involvement.

Management

- External structures are at risk of human and animal bites. Bite wounds should be cleaned and the patient given appropriate prophylactic antibiotics.[17]
- Penile fractures require operative management.
- Amputations should be reattached if the amputated part was salvaged and maintained properly.[17]
  - Apply direct pressure to bleeding stump, provide analgesia, and wrap the amputated part in dry sterile gauze before placing on ice.
  - Surgical reimplantation ideally within 6 hours of injury or reconstruction is indicated.[17]
- Zipper injuries should be treated by removing the zipper.
  - One attempt at unzipping the zipper after well lubricating the area with mineral oil is recommended.
  - If unsuccessful, use a sturdy wire cutter (diagonal cutter) to cut the cross bar that goes across the top of the zipper (attaches both sides of the zipper). Once cut, the two places should fall apart, and the teeth will pull away from the skin.[1]
- Burns or avulsion injuries should be treated similarly to that on any other body part.
  - Treatment includes prophylactic antibiotics or tetanus prophylaxis if indicated, appropriate debridement, irrigation, and placement of surgical dressings.
  - Tissue reconstruction is typically performed in a delayed fashion.[15]

Complications

Complications include pain, poor cosmesis, erectile dysfunction, and penile curvature.

Female GU

Anatomy

- Although rare, female GU trauma can result in life threatening bleeding, incontinence, urinary retention, and cosmetic disfigurement.[16]
- Blunt injuries to the vulva and vagina are associated with pelvic trauma in 30%, after consensual intercourse in 25%, sexual assault in 20%, and other blunt trauma in 15% of patients.[18]
- Common injuries include laceration, contusion, hematoma, and swelling or disfigurement.
- Consider injury to the urethra, bladder, rectum, or bowel with genitalia injury.
- In pediatrics, genital injury should prompt a complete examination for other injuries that could be suggestive of sexual abuse.

Evaluation

History and physical examination are often diagnostic.

- Retrograde urethrogram should be performed to evaluate for urethral involvement.

Management

In hemodynamically stable patients, non-steroidal anti-inflammatory medications and ice packs are sufficient for treatment of vulvar injuries, but massive hematomas require surgical management.[16]

Complications

Complications include missed internal injuries, poor cosmesis, stricture, and stenosis.

ED Management

- Maintaining adequate urine output with strict monitoring of intakes and outputs and administration of IV fluids are important.[2]
- Early interventions to divert urine reduce future complications such as infection, ileus, and peritonitis.[2]
- Catheter and urinary diversion
  - Blind insertion of Foley catheter in the trauma patient with potentially undiagnosed urethral injury could potentially further damage an undetected urethral injury.[12]
  - Successful passage of a Foley catheter does not rule out potential urethral injury.
  - If a Foley catheter cannot be easily passed, further attempts are not recommended, and imaging to evaluate urethral injury should be performed.
- Suprapubic catheterization is recommended in cases of severe bladder urethral or genital injury or in selected cases such as prolonged immobilization.
  - Patients with injuries to the anterior urethra are at high risk for a delayed stricture; if a Foley catheter is not possible or contraindicated, a suprapubic catheter is recommended.[19]

- Alternative methods of urinary diversion including ureteral stents and/or percutaneous nephrostomy may be needed depending on the traumatic injury.
- In any penetrating injury, tetanus status of the patient should be assessed, and the patient should receive an update if indicated.
- Notify law enforcement for any traumas including human bites if there is suspicion of criminal activity.
- The use of antibiotics is thought to reduce the incidence of urinary tract infection and perinephric abscesses; they are recommended despite the lack of good evidence supporting their use.[2]
- The majority of injuries to the genitalia including superficial lacerations and zipper injuries do not require emergent urologic evaluation. However, crush injuries to the scrotum or penis should be radiologically evaluated via ultrasound or RUG to evaluate for testicular and/or urethral damage.[12]
- Urology consult is recommended in most GU trauma.
- Gynecology consult should be considered in female external genitalia trauma.

Surgical Indications

- Generally, management of renal and GU injuries have become more conservative and expectant over the years.
- The decision for primary surgical repair vs damage control with delayed surgical management is left to the discretion of the urologist.[2]
- Most grade I, II, or III renal injuries due to blunt trauma are managed nonsurgically, whereas some grade IV and most grade V injuries require intervention.[10]
- Surgery is indicated in renal trauma patients with hypotension, renal pedicle injury, renal artery thrombosis, or urinary extravasation.[20]
- Ureteral injuries are commonly treated primarily with stenting, although debridement and primary anastomosis may be required for severe injuries.[8]
- Intraperitoneal bladder ruptures require operative exploration and repair as they do not heal spontaneously.[12]
- Extraperitoneal ruptures can often be managed nonoperatively with urinary catheter placement.[12]
- Immediate surgical repair of urethral trauma is rarely indicated, but definitive surgical management is needed to minimize risks of erectile dysfunction, incontinence, and stricture formation.[12]
- Testicular dislocation, rupture, traumatic torsion. and penile fracture require operative management.[12]
  - Early intervention in testicular rupture leads to lower rates of testicular necrosis and orchiectomy.
- Large scrotal hematomas, hematoceles, testicular dislocation, scrotal or penile amputation, and female genital injuries are also indications for surgery.[2]
- Interventional radiology can be used diagnostically with angiography to evaluate for continued bleeding and for management with embolization to minimize hemorrhage and stenting of renal arteries or ureteral injuries for repair.[2]

Pitfalls in ED Evaluation and Management

- GU injuries are rarely life threatening and, as a result, diagnosis can often be delayed or even missed. Always have a high index of suspicion for such injuries.
- Avoid blind insertion of a Foley catheter before consideration of urethral injury.
- Make sure to examine the perineum and genitals of patients with traumatic injury to avoid missing key physical exam clues to GU injury.
- Use IV contrast and also consider delayed images to better evaluate the GU system as delayed extravasation of contrast can suggest urinary leak or ongoing hemorrhage.
- Depending on the mechanism of injury, a normal UA may not be sufficient for ruling out GU injuries, especially vascular and penetrating injuries.
- As contrast from a RUG can make interpretation of subsequent CT abdomen/pelvis with IV contrast difficult, make sure to perform CT imaging first prior to RUG.
- Consider GU injury in any patient with trauma to the lower thorax, upper abdomen, or flank.

Key Points

- UA is a helpful screening tool in evaluating a patient with potential GU injury.
- Vaginal, penile, and rectal examinations should be performed in the trauma patient with evidence of GU trauma.
- CT abdomen and pelvis with IV contrast is the gold standard for evaluating GU trauma.
- Consider ultrasound in evaluating for intraperitoneal bleed, urinary retention, and testicular trauma.
- Perform a RUG in any patient with blood at the meatus, pelvic fracture, or suspicious findings on initial CT scan to rule out urethral injury prior to insertion of Foley catheter.
- Any injury of the kidneys, ureter, bladder, or urethral should, at the very least, be discussed with and possibly evaluated by a trauma surgeon and/or urologist while the patient is in the ED.
- If urology or trauma surgery is not available, transfer to a trauma center is appropriate.

References

1. Blair M. Overview of genitourinary trauma. CNE Series 2011. *Urologic Nursing*. 2011;31 (3):139–45.
2. Bryant WK, Shewakramani S. Emergency management of renal and genitourinary trauma: best practice update. *EB Medicine*. 2017;19(8):1–20.
3. Matlock KA, Tyroch AH, Kronfol ZN, McLean SF, Pirela-Cruz MA. Blunt traumatic bladder injury: a 10-year perspective. *Am Surg*. 2013;79(6): 589–93.
4. McGeady JB, Breyer BN. Current epidemiology of genitourinary trauma. *Urol Clin North Am*. 2013;40(3):323–34.
5. Bagga HS, Fisher PB, Tasian GE, et al. Sports-related genitourinary injuries presenting to United States emergency departments. *Urology*. 2015;85(1):239–44.
6. Lynch TH, Martínez-Piñeiro L, Plas E, et al.; European Association of Urology. EAU guidelines on urological trauma. *Eur Urol*. 2005;47(1):1–15.
7. MacDougal DB. Abdominal trauma. In: Newberry L, Criddle LM, eds. *Sheehey's*

Manual of Emergency Care, 6th ed. St Louis: Elsevier Mosby, 2005.

8. Serafetinides E, Kitrey ND, Djakovic N, et al. Review of the current management of upper urinary tract injuries by the EAU trauma guidelines panel. *Eur Assoc Urol.* 2015;67(1):930–36.

9. Holevar M, Ebert J, Luchette F, et al. Practice management guidelines for the management of genitourinary trauma. *Eastern Association for the Surgery of Trauma.* 2004. Available at: www.east.org/education/practice-management-guidelines/genitourinary-trauma-diagnostic-evaluation-of. Accessed August 20, 2018.

10. Chouhan JD, Winer AG, Johnson C, Weiss JP, Hyacinthe LM. Contemporary evaluation and management of renal trauma. *Can J Urol.* 2016;23(2):8191–97.

11. Figler BD, Hoffler CE, Reisman W, et al. Multi-disciplinary update on pelvic fracture associated bladder and urethral injuries. *Injury.* 2012;43(8):1242–49.

12. Lumen N, Kuehhas FE, Djakovic N, et al. Review of the current management of lower urinary tract injuries by the EAU trauma guidelines panel. *Eur Assoc Urol.* 2015;67(1):925–29.

13. Campbell MR. Abdominal and urological trauma. In: Newberry L, Criddle LM, eds.

Sheehey's Manual of Emergency Care, 6th ed. St. Louis, MO: Elsevier Mosby; 2007.

14. Schmidlin FR, Iselin CE, Naimi A, et al. The higher injury risk of abnormal kidneys in blunt renal trauma. *Scand J Urol Nephrol.* 1998;32(6):388–92.

15. Tonkin JB, Tisdale BE, Jordan GH. Assessment and initial management of urologic trauma. *Med Clin N Am.* 2011;95(1):245–51.

16. Schewakramani S, Reed KC. Genitourinary trauma. *Emerg Med Clin N Am.* 2011;29(1):501–18.

17. Chang AJ, Brandes SB. Advances in diagnosis and management of genital injuries. *Urol Clin N Am.* 2013;40(1):427–38.

18. Bryk DJ, Zhao LC. Guideline of guidelines: a review of urological trauma guidelines. *BJU Int.* 2016;117(2):226–34.

19. Morey AF, Brandes S, Dugi DD 3rd, et al. Urotrauma: AUA guideline. *J Urol.* 2014;192(2):327–35.

20. Yeung LL, Brandes SB. Contemporary management of renal trauma: differences between urologist and trauma surgeons. *J Trauma Acute Care Surg.* 2012;72(1):68–75.

Peripheral Vascular Injury

Richard Slama and Mike Jackson

Peripheral vascular injury (PVI) is a major concern in the Emergency Department (ED). According to the CDC, there were 33,594 mortalities related to firearms in 2014.[1] There were 803,007 cases of aggravated assault that occurred in 2016. Nearly 24% of these (190,000) were performed with firearms and 16% (120,000) with cutting instruments.[2] Inevitably, many of these result in damage to the vasculature, leading to blood loss and presentation to the ED. While some forms of injury are immediately life threatening and require emergent intervention, some present asymptomatically, which can lead to delayed or missed diagnoses. Emergency physicians should be well versed in the diagnosis, management, and disposition of these patients. This chapter will focus on the management of penetrating extremity trauma with vascular injury.

Vascular Injury Goals

The first goal of resuscitation and the management of a patient with PVI is hemorrhage control. There are multiple types of vascular injury, which are outlined in Table 17.1. The main focus of this chapter will be extremity hemorrhage/PVI.

- *Extremity Hemorrhage/PVI*, as its name suggests, is any injury to the vasculature of the extremities resulting in hemorrhage. These injuries typically affect smaller vasculature and are more likely to have a better outcome than other types of injuries (Figure 17.1).
- *Junctional Hemorrhage* is defined as hemorrhage where an extremity meets the torso that precludes the effective use of a tourniquet to control bleeding.[5] Examples of junctional hemorrhages include the groin proximal to the inguinal ligament, the buttocks, the gluteal and pelvic areas, the perineum, the axilla and shoulder girdle, and the base of the neck (Figure 17.2).
- *Non Compressible Truncal/Torso Hemorrhage* is defined as trauma to torso vessels, pulmonary parenchyma, solid abdominal organs, and disruption of the bony pelvis.[7] As the name implies, these are injuries not amenable to tourniquets, not amenable to compression, and overall have a very high mortality rate because of the rate of bleeding (Figure 17.3).

Most vascular injuries are obvious in presentation; however, some are subtle, and attention to detail is required.[9] Assessment for both hard and soft signs of injury is vital for injury classification (Table 17.2). This allows the clinician to determine the next best step in managing the patient. In general, patients with hard signs of vascular injury will need immediate intervention, while those with soft signs should receive diagnostic testing to better determine the type of injury. Hard signs of vascular injury are shown in Figure 17.4.

Table 17.1 Vascular injury types

Vascular Injury Type	Examples	Treatment Options
Peripheral	Gunshot to the extremity, partial or complete amputations	Direct pressure, tourniquet, hemostatic dressings, surgical control
Junctional	Groin proximal to the inguinal ligament, the buttocks, the gluteal and pelvic areas, the perineum, the axilla and shoulder girdle, and the base of the neck	Direct pressure, junctional tourniquet, hemostatic dressing, surgical control
Non-compressible truncal hemorrhage	Pulmonary vessels, abdominal aorta, thoracic aorta, heart	Thoracotomy with aortic cross clamping, REBOA, surgical control

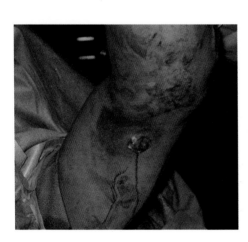

Figure 17.1 Penetrating injury to the upper arm (from *War Surgery in Afghanistan and Iraq*)[3,4]

Physiologic Goals

In an ideal situation, unstable patients with penetrating vascular trauma are transported immediately to the operating room. This is not always the case when caring for trauma patients, as there are many factors than can delay operative intervention (surgical consultant not in house, multiple casualties necessitating triaging, etc.). Because of these factors, it is imperative for the emergency physician to be knowledgeable of how to appropriately resuscitate a patient with active hemorrhage. While Advanced Trauma Life Support (ATLS) provides an excellent basis and systematic approach to trauma patients, there are some aspects of these algorithms that are falling out of favor and less applicable to patients with massive hemorrhage. For example, previous versions of ATLS recommended initial crystalloid resuscitation, which in both military and civilian settings has been associated with poor outcomes including multi-organ failure, death, and abdominal compartment syndrome.[11]

Damage control resuscitation (DCR) is broadly defined as a resuscitative strategy in which hemorrhage is controlled while preventing coagulopathy.[12] Physiologic parameters of DCR are outlined in Box 17.1. The basic underlying principles of DCR include

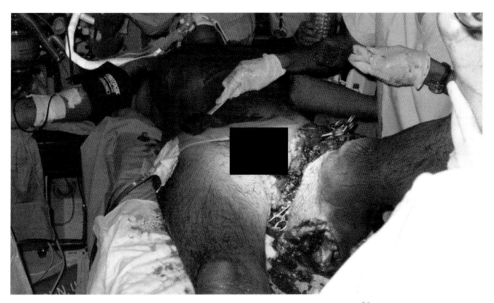

Figure 17.2 Example of junctional injury (from *War Surgery in Afghanistan and Iraq*)[3,6]

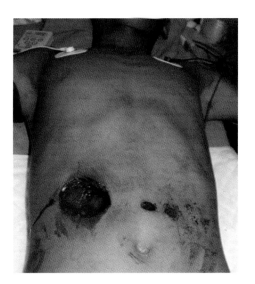

Figure 17.3 Example of NCTH (from *War Surgery in Afghanistan and Iraq*)[3,8]

permissive hypotension, balanced component therapy, and coagulopathy prevention.[13–22] This is further explored in detail in Chapter 3.

Secondary Injuries

While there are numerous complications from penetrating vascular injury, most of these are delayed and occur after initial evaluation and repair. While these are more applicable to the inpatient team, they include limb ischemia, wound infection, and vascular graft/repair thrombosis. There are some complications, though, that the emergency physician should be

Table 17.2 Hard vs. soft signs of vascular injury

Hard Signs	Soft Signs
Absent distal pulse	Subjective reduction in pulse
Expanding or pulsatile hematoma	Large non-pulsatile hematoma
Bruit/thrill	Neural injury
Active hemorrhage	Large hemorrhage on scene
	High risk orthopedic injuries

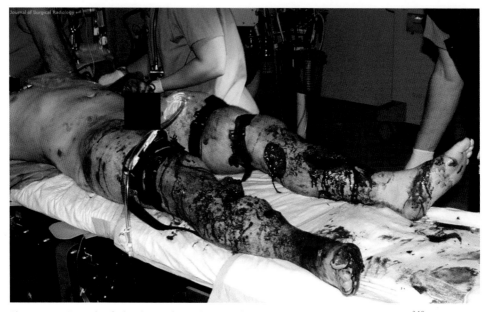

Figure 17.4 Example of a hard sign of vascular injury (from *War Surgery in Afghanistan and Iraq*)[3,10]

Box 17.1 Damage Control Resuscitation Goals

Physiologic parameters for DCR:[23]

- Permissive Hypotension SBP of 80–90 to prevent rebleeding
- Minimal use of crystalloid
- Prevention of coagulopathy
- Temperature >96.8°F
- pH >7.25

---

aware. Most severe penetrating vascular trauma will involve large vessels, and, by the principles of anatomy, these vessels most usually run in neurovascular bundles. It is important to consider concomitant vein and nerve injury when evaluating arterial injury. Although the immediate management may not differ, the importance of performing and documenting a thorough neurovascular is important.

Box 17.2   Control of PVI

Guidelines Control of PVI, Adapted from TCCC Guidelines:[5]

- Identify that patient has sustained a vascular injury.
- Direct pressure over the area of hemorrhage is the first and most important step. This may be performed with or without hemostatic dressings.
- If on an extremity, then it is likely amendable to tourniquet use.
- Apply the tourniquet over the patient's uniform/clothing initially, and if bleeding is not identified, place the tourniquet as "high and tight" as possible.
- If the first tourniquet does not work, then apply a second tourniquet side by side with the first.
- Tourniquet should be converted to a compression dressing as soon as possible if the following are met:

  - No evidence of shock.
  - The wound can be monitored for bleeding.
  - The tourniquet is not being used to control bleeding from an amputated extremity.

- When possible, tourniquets should be converted to compression dressings within 2 hours.
- Tourniquets in place for greater than 6 hours should only be removed if there is adequate monitoring of the patient's vitals, bleeding, and labs.

The documentation and monitoring of the neurovascular exam also becomes important when monitoring for compartment syndrome, which is a mismatch between the volume and contents of a muscular compartment leading to tissue ischemia and necrosis.[24] This can be from many different etiologies, but the basic concepts are increased pressure, decreased volume, or external compression. This pressure overcomes the venous and eventually arterial blood supply leading to extremity pulselessness, paresthesias, pallor, pain, and eventually tissue death. Although management of this condition is ultimately surgical, expeditious diagnosis and treatment is paramount to preventing complications such as contractures.

ED Evaluation and Management

- The most important step in management is hemorrhage control. There are numerous ways to approach this goal, but the Trauma Combat Casualty Care Guidelines summarize this approach (Box 17.2).
- Any patient presenting with life threatening injury should always be evaluated for patency of the airway, work of breathing, and perfusion status. In the best of scenarios this should take place simultaneously while hemorrhage control is being obtained.

While surgery is the definitive answer for most severe penetrating vascular injury, the first principle in the initial management should be hemorrhage control. Direct pressure over the area of bleeding is the first and most important step. After this there are numerous other modalities available for control of bleeding. Other goals of ED resuscitation are listed in Box 17.3.

When acting to control hemorrhage, one must first recognize the type of injury. For most extremity injuries with active hemorrhage, tourniquets are a cheap, readily available, and efficacious method to control bleeding. Tourniquets for the most part had fallen out of favor until their re-emergence in Operation Iraqi Freedom. Multiple studies demonstrate favorable outcomes when tourniquets have been applied in the battlefield setting.[25–27] Tourniquets have become an integral part of Trauma Combat Casualty Care (TCCC). While there are multiple facets to the TCCC guidelines, the basic premise for use is early applications of a tourniquet to a bleeding extremity as "high and tight" as possible until hemorrhage control is obtained.[28]

Tourniquet use in civilian settings was previously limited; however, tourniquets have re-emerged as essential for civilian pre-hospital care. In addition, there are now numerous centers in the United States studying the pre-hospital use of tourniquets.[29] The long standing debate and controversy is whether these devices cause more harm than good.[30] While the injuries incurred during wartime are different than those in the civilian setting, the same principles can still be applied, with appropriate use (Box 17.2). Complications that can occur from tourniquets include compartment syndrome, neuropraxia, nerve paralysis, and limb ischemia.[31] While most complications have been noted at greater than 2 hours, a tourniquet should not be removed if hemorrhage cannot be controlled by other means. In the civilian setting, prolonged tourniquet use should not be as much of an issue as the battlefield, where definitive care is not always immediately available.

For injuries not amendable to tourniquet placement or if a tourniquet is not available, direct pressure over the wound is the next viable option.[32] Clamping and ligation may be performed by a surgeon when indicated, but the initial recommendation for ED management is to avoid these maneuvers when possible, as this may hinder future vessel repair.

Numerous hemostatic agents and dressings are on the market. These agents have been shown to be superior to standard non-hemostatic dressings in numerous studies.[33] However, a recent study that emulated severe penetrating vascular injury in areas not amendable to tourniquet placement showed standard gauze without hemostatic agent compared equally well to hemostatic agents in a swine model.[34] Therefore, while hemostatic agents may confer benefit to some specific types of wounds, the most important aspect of hemorrhage control is direct pressure over the area of vascular injury, regardless of dressing type.

Once hemorrhage control has been accomplished, the next goal is determining those requiring emergent intervention (Figure 17.5).

If the patient has soft signs of vascular injury, the next best step is to perform an Injured Extremity Index (IEI). The IEI is similar to an ankle brachial index, with the exception that this is used to compare opposite extremities, as opposed to upper and lower. The first step is to apply a manual blood pressure cuff, inflate the cuff until cessation of pulses by Doppler, and then determine the pressure at which the arterial Doppler signal returns in the injured extremity as the cuff is deflated, which is the numerator in the equation. Next, the cuff and Doppler are moved to the uninjured extremity, ideally an uninjured upper extremity, and again the pressure at which the arterial Doppler signal returns as the cuff is deflated is recorded as the denominator in the ratio. An IEI >0.90 is normal and has high sensitivity

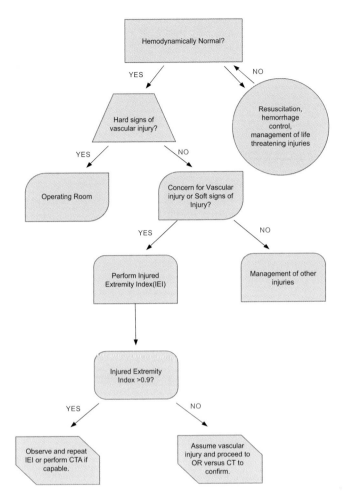

Figure 17.5 PVI Algorithm (from *War Surgery in Afghanistan and Iraq*)[3,8,32]

for excluding major extremity vascular injury.[10] The negative predictive value of an IEI >0.90 approximates 96%.[11] Due to IEI's ease of use, rapidity, and noninvasiveness, it is an ideal test that emergency physicians should use in the care of patients with suspected vascular injury.

CT angiography remains the gold standard for the diagnosis of vascular injuries because of its accuracy, cost, and rapidity.[35,36]

Duplex ultrasound has been evaluated in the diagnosis of this condition but does not have high enough sensitivity to exclude these injuries.[37,38] In formally performed ultrasounds that are interpreted/performed by a vascular technologist or vascular surgeon, a finding of arterial injury by ultrasound may obviate the need for CTA in the correct circumstance. While this test may be useful to rule in arterial injury, it should never be used to exclude arterial injury.[39] To the author's knowledge, there have been no randomized studies on the use of Point of Care Ultrasound (POCUS) for the evaluation of penetrating vascular injuries. Therefore, POCUS can only be recommended as an adjunct in the evaluation of these patients.

Box 17.4 Low Risk Injury

- Low to medium velocity weapon (<1,000 ft/sec)
- No hard or soft signs of injury
- Normal neurovascular examination
- Normal IEI
- No underlying fracture

Low Risk Penetrating Extremity Injury Management and Disposition

If after evaluation the patient has been found to be at low risk for penetrating extremity injury (Box 17.4), it is reasonable to observe the patent in the ED with serial examinations and IEI measurements. If the patient's symptoms and exam are reassuring, IEI remains >0.9, and the patient does not develop compartment syndrome, then wound irrigation, analgesia, and discharge with follow up with a surgeon is a reasonable option. This should be performed in accordance with predetermined policies at the institution or in consultation with a trauma surgeon.

Antibiotic therapy is not recommended for routine low velocity and uncomplicated gunshot wounds/penetrating wounds of the extremities.[40] There are some special situations which antibiotic therapy may be warranted; however, these fall out of the low risk category and include high velocity injuries, open fractures, heavy wound contamination, joint involvement, and hand injuries.[41] The most important aspect in the care of low risk injuries is to provide detailed discharge instructions and strict return precautions for complications of these injuries. In particular, compartment syndrome, sudden swelling, worsening bleeding or repeated soaking of dressings, fevers, and a cold distal extremity should be addressed with the patient.

Surgical Indications

Any patient not falling into the low risk category requires more definitive evaluation. Patients with hard signs of vascular injury stable for transport should be taken immediately to the OR. An unstable patient requires resuscitation until stable for transport and definitive repair.

Patients with soft or non-specific signs of vascular injury should undergo an IEI vs. CTA of the affected extremity based on availability. If there are signs of arterial disruption on CTA, or if the IEI is <0.9, then the patient should receive operative consultation and management for presumed vascular injury. An IEI <0.9 is often evaluated further with CTA. In patients who have a normal physical exam (no hard or soft signs) and a normal IEI, the likelihood of arterial injury is exceedingly low, and further testing does not need to be performed. Physical exam or IEI used in isolation does not have high enough sensitivity to exclude a vascular injury.[39]

Pitfalls in ED Evaluation and Management

- Not suspecting vascular injury with penetrating injury. Many of these may have no decrease in pulse, patients may be asymptomatic, or have subtle exam findings.
- Overzealous administration of fluids. Hemorrhage requires replacement of what is lost: RBCs, platelets, and clotting factors.

- Not aggressively controlling hemorrhage (failure to apply tourniquet).
- Not consulting the appropriate service when there is uncertainty about the injury.

Key Points
- Peripheral Vascular Injury is common and increasing. Emergency physicians should be well versed in their management.
- Hemorrhage control is the most important intervention. Direct pressure should work in most injuries, but there are other adjuncts for control of bleeding.
- Tourniquets are not bad. They save lives when used appropriately.
- Damage control resuscitation aims to eliminate the lethal triad of trauma.
- Hard signs of vascular injury warrant immediate operative intervention. Soft signs require further diagnostics.
- CTA is the diagnostic modality of choice when vascular injury is suspected.
- Not all penetrating extremity injuries need trauma surgery consultation. Select injuries may be managed conservatively, and outpatient follow up is reasonable.

References

1. CDC/National Center for Health Statistics. FastStats - Injuries. *CDC Fast Stats.* www.cdc.gov/nchs/fastats/injury.htm. 2016. Accessed October 11, 2017.

2. FBI Uniform Crime Reporting Program. FBI – Aggravated Assault. *FBI UCR.* https://ucr.fbi.gov/crime-in-the-u.s/2016/crime-in-the-u.s.-2016/topic-pages/aggravated-assault. 2016. Accessed January 15, 2018.

3. Nessen SC, Lounsbury DE, Hetz SP, eds. *War Surgery in Afghanistan and Iraq.* Washington: Borden Institute; 2008. https://ke.army.mil/bordeninstitute/published_volumes/war_surgery/Prologue_FINAL.pdf. Accessed October 11, 2017.

4. Lenhart M, Lounsbury DE Nessen SC, Hetz SP. Ch 7 Orthopedic trauma: open ulna fracture. In: Nessen SC, Lounsbury DE, Hetz SP, eds. *War Surgery in Afghanistan and Iraq.* Washington: Borden Institute; 2008, p. 273, fig 1.

5. Kotwal RS, Butler FK, Gross KR, et al. Management of junctional hemorrhage in tactical combat casualty care: TCCC guidelines? Proposed Change 13-03. *J Spec Oper Med.* 2013;13(4):85–93.

6. Lenhart M, Lounsbury DE, Nessen SC, Hetz SP. Ch 8 Vascular trauma. In: Nessen SC, Lounsbury DE, Hetz SP, eds. *War Surgery in Afghanistan and Iraq.* Washington: Borden Institute; 2008, p. 326, fig 1.

7. Cannon J, Morrison J, Lauer C, et al. Resuscitative endovascular balloon occlusion of the aorta (REBOA) for hemorrhagic shock. *Jt Theater Trauma Syst Clin Pract Guidel.* 2012;(March):1–18.

8. Lenhart M, Lounsbury DE, Nessen SC, Hetz SP. Ch 5 Abdominopelvic trauma: indirect effects of wounding. In: Nessen SC, Lounsbury DE, Hetz SP, eds. *War Surgery in Afghanistan and Iraq.* Washington: Borden Institute; 2008, p. 160, fig 1.

9. Van Waes O. Treatment of penetrating trauma of the extremities: ten years' experience at a Dutch level 1 trauma center. *Scand J Trauma Resusc Emerg Med.* 2013;21(2):1–6.

10. O'Brien PJCM. Stents in tents: Endovascular therapy on the battlefields of the global war on terror. *J Surg Radiol.* 2011;1(2):Photo found at: Wikimedia Commons contributors, "F.

11. Balogh Z, McKinley BA, Cocanour CS, et al. Supranormal trauma resuscitation

causes more cases of abdominal compartment syndrome. *Arch Surg.* 2003;138(6):633–37.

12. Cap AP, Pidcoke HF, Spinella P, et al. Joint Theater Trauma System Clinical Practice Guideline. Damage Control Resuscitation CPG. https://jts.amedd.army.mil/assets/docs/cpgs/JTS_Clinical_Practice_Guidelines_(CPGs)/Damage_Control_Resuscitation_03_Feb_2017_ID18.pdf. 2017;(June):1–34.

13. Duke MD, Guidry C, Guice J, et al. Restrictive fluid resuscitation in combination with damage control resuscitation: time for adaptation. *J Trauma Acute Care Surg.* 2012;73 (3):674–78.

14. Duchesne JC, Barbeau JM, Islam TM, et al. Damage control resuscitation: from emergency department to the operating room. *Am Surg.* 2011;77(2):201–6.

15. Holcomb JB, Tilley BC, Baraniuk S, et al. Transfusion of plasma, platelets, and red blood cells in a 1:1:1 vs a 1:1:2 ratio and mortality in patients with severe trauma: the PROPPR randomized clinical trial. *JAMA.* 2015;313(5):471–82.

16. Holcomb JB, del Junco DJ, Fox EE, et al. The prospective, observational, multicenter, major trauma transfusion (PROMMTT) study: comparative effectiveness of a time-varying treatment with competing risks. *JAMA Surg.* 2013;148 (2):127–36.

17. Jansen JO, Thomas R, Loudon MA, Brooks A. Damage control resuscitation for patients with major trauma. *BMJ.* 2009;338: b1778.

18. Williams-Johnson JA, McDonald AH, Strachan GG, Williams EW. Effects of tranexamic acid on death, vascular occlusive events, and blood transfusion in trauma patients with significant haemorrhage (CRASH-2) a randomised, placebo-controlled trial. *Lancet.* 2010;376 (6):23–32.

19. Afshari A, Wikkelsø A, Brok J, Møller AM, Wetterslev J. Thromboelastography (TEG) or thromboelastometry (ROTEM) to monitor haemotherapy versus usual care in patients with massive transfusion. *Cochrane database Syst Rev.* 2011;(3): CD007871.

20. da Luz LT, Nascimento B, Rizoli S. Thrombelastography (TEG®): practical considerations on its clinical use in trauma resuscitation. *Scand J Trauma Resusc Emerg Med.* 2013;21:29.

21. Wikkelsø A, Wetterslev J, Møller AM, Afshari A. Thromboelastography (TEG) or thromboelastometry (ROTEM) to monitor haemostatic treatment versus usual care in adults or children with bleeding. *Cochrane Database System Rev.* 2016;(8):CD007871.

22. Nickson C. Thromboelastogram. *LITFL.* https://lifeinthefastlane.com/ccc/thromboelastogram-teg/. 2014. Accessed January 1, 2017.

24. Geiderman JM, Katz D. General principles of orthopedic injuries. In: Walls R, Hockberger R, Gausche-Hill M, eds., *Rosen's Emergency Medicine – Concepts and Clinical Practice, 2-Volume Set.* Elsevier; 2014, pp. 511–33.e2.

25. Kragh JF, Littrel ML, Jones JA, et al. Battle casualty survival with emergency tourniquet use to stop limb bleeding. *J Emerg Med.* 2011;41(6):590–97.

26. Kragh JFJ, Dubick MA, Aden JK, et al. U.S. Military use of tourniquets from 2001 to 2010. *Prehospital Emerg Care.* 2015;19 (2):184–90.

27. Beekley AC, Sebesta JA, Blackbourne LH, et al. Prehospital tourniquet use in Operation Iraqi Freedom: effect on hemorrhage control and outcomes. *J Trauma.* 2008;64(2 Suppl):S28–37; discussion S37.

28. NAEMT. Tactical Combat Casualty Care Guidelines for Medical Personnel. 2015; (June).

29. Passos E, Dingley B, Smith A, et al. *Tourniquet Use for Peripheral Vascular Injuries in the Civilian Setting.* Vol 45. Elsevier Ltd; 2014.

30. Mayo Clinic. The return of tourniquets - For Medical Professionals - Mayo Clinic. www.mayoclinic.org/medical-professionals/clinical-updates/trauma/

combat-tested-tourniquets-save-lives-limbs. Accessed March 18, 2018.

31. Dayan L, Zinmann C, Stahl S, Norman D. Complications associated with prolonged tourniquet application on the battlefield. *Mil Med.* 2008;173(1):63–66.

32. Rasmussen T, Stockinger Z, Antevil J, et al. *Vascular Injury. Joint Trauma System Clinical Practice Guideline.* https://jts.amedd.army.mil/assets/docs/cpgs/JTS_Clinical_Practice_Guidelines_(CPGs)/Vascular_Injury_12_Aug_2016_ID46.pdf. 2016. Accessed March 18, 2018.

33. Clay JG, Grayson JK, Zierold D. Comparative testing of new hemostatic agents in a swine model of extremity arterial and venous hemorrhage. *Mil Med.* 2010;175(4):280–84.

34. Littlejohn LF, Devlin JJ, Kircher SS, et al. Comparison of Celox-A, Chitoflex, WoundStat, and combat gauze hemostatic agents versus standard gauze dressing in control of hemorrhage in a swine model of penetrating trauma. *Acad Emerg Med.* 2011;18(4):340–50.

35. Ivatury RR, Anand R, Ordonez C. Penetrating extremity trauma. *World J Surg.* 2015;39(6):1389–96.

36. Wallin D, Yaghoubian A, Rosing D, et al. Computed tomographic angiography as the primary diagnostic modality in penetrating lower extremity vascular injuries: a level I trauma experience. *Ann Vasc Surg.* 2011;25(5):620–23.

37. Patterson BO, Holt PJ, Cleanthis M, et al. Imaging vascular trauma. *Br J Surg.* 2012;99(4):494–505.

38. Mollberg NM, Wise SR, Banipal S, et al. Color-flow duplex screening for upper extremity proximity injuries: a low-yield strategy for therapeutic intervention. *Ann Vasc Surg.* 2013;27(5):594–98.

39. DeSouza IS, Benabbas R, McKee S, et al. Accuracy of physical exam, ankle-brachial index, and ultrasonography in the diagnosis of arterial injury in patients with penetrating extremity trauma: a systematic review and meta-analysis. *Acad Emerg Med.* 2017;8:994–1017.

40. Zalavras CG, Patzakis MJ, Holtom PD, Sherman R. Management of open fractures. *Infect Dis Clin North Am.* 2005;19(4):915–29.

41. Simpson BM, Wilson RH, Grant RE. Antibiotic therapy in gunshot wound injuries. *Clin Orthop Relat Res.* 2003;(408):82–85. www.ncbi.nlm.nih.gov/pubmed/12616042. Accessed October 24, 2017.

Chapter

18

Pelvic Trauma

Michael K. Abraham

Pelvic Fractures

Pelvic fractures are serious injuries, accounting for 20% of deaths due to trauma.[1] Most high energy pelvic fractures are due to motor vehicle accidents, including motorcycles, and falls from a significant height. Since these injuries can have major effects on hemodynamics, especially in the setting of multi-trauma, time is of the essence, with focus on early diagnosis and management.

Anatomy

- The pelvis is a complex structure that has a bony and ligamentous framework.
- Disruption of either ligaments, bones, or a combination of both can lead to pelvic instability and, subsequently, due to the rich vascular supply of the pelvis, hemodynamic instability.
- Hemorrhage may occur from surfaces of fractured bones, arterial injury, venous plexus injury, and extra pelvic sources (Figure 18.1). Pelvic hemorrhage is difficult to treat due to the myriad of potential sources of bleeding. The most common source of bleeding is the venous plexus (90%), which causes many treatment issues. The pelvis provides access to the retroperitoneal space, abdomen, and thighs, depending on the fracture. This access may result in significant blood loss before enough pressure forms to tamponade the vessels.[2]
- The hip joint is comprised of the acetabulum and the proximal femur (Figure 18.2). The dense bone, designed for weight bearing, takes a great deal of force to injure in younger people. In older patients, however, osteopenia contributes to greater risk of fracture.

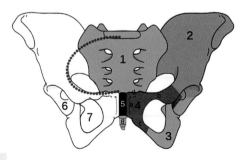

Figure 18.1 (1) Sacrum; (2) Ilium; (3) Ischium; (4) Pubis: (4a) Body of pubic bone, (4b) Superior pubic ramus, (4c) Inferior pubic ramus, (4d) Pubic tubercle; (5) Pubic symphysis; (6) Acetabulum; (7) Obturator foramen; (8) Coccyx, Red dotted line = Linea terminalis (from https://upload.wikimedia.org/wikipedia/commons/f/ff/Skeletal_pelvis-pubis.svg, reproduced here under CC BY-SA 4.0 license https://creativecommons.org/licenses/by-sa/4.0/)

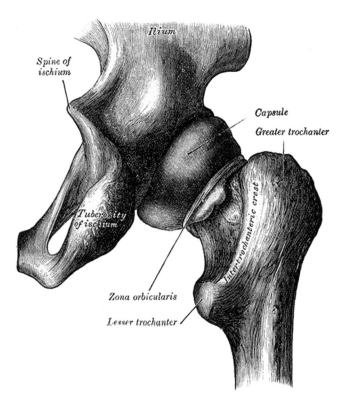

Figure 18.2 Drawing of the hip joint (from https:// en.wikipedia.org/wiki/ Intertrochanteric_crest#/media/File: Gray343.png)

- Acetabular fractures require a good deal of force and are usually associated with falls or motor vehicle injuries. A "dashboard injury" occurs when a flexed knee hits the dashboard of a car. This transmits forces into the posterior column of the acetabulum and often causes a posterior hip dislocation.
- Significant pelvic trauma and fractures are associated with multisystem injuries.

Diagnosis

- Due to the mechanism of injury and the forces needed to cause injury, pelvic and hip trauma are often apparent. The initial examination depends on the mechanism and patient age. An elderly female with a fall from standing may have the sole complaint of pain with bearing weight and a fracture. However, a young male is unlikely to sustain a fracture with the same mechanism. High energy mechanisms are associated with fractures in younger patients.
- Patients with pelvic injuries often have associated multi-system traumatic injuries. Isolated subtle pelvis and hip fractures may be more difficult to diagnose due to the lack of forceful mechanism, such as fall from a standing height.
- Examination includes inspection, palpation, mobility, and neurovascular assessment.
- Initial examination may be notable for differences in height or rotation of the iliac crests. Leg length discrepancy may be present if the acetabulum is involved. Pelvic stability should be assessed, with care to not excessively push down and out on the iliac crests. This mechanism may exacerbate unstable fractures and lead to greater

hemodynamic instability. Rather, the iliac crests should be gently compressed to evaluate instability. If instability is found, pelvic binding is recommended. Repeat examinations for instability are not recommended.

- Fracture communication with the vaginal or rectal areas should be evaluated, as these types of open fractures carry a much higher risk of complications.
- Patients with no debilitating injuries should be ambulated.
- The mainstay of diagnosis includes plain radiography, although the sensitivity is reported to be as low as 80% in some studies.[3,4] Several studies state that plain radiographs are unnecessary if the patient has a normal physical examination and is hemodynamically stable.[4] Depending on patient hemodynamic status, CT may be the highest yield. Alternatively, if the patient has significant hemodynamic instability, a prompt plain film can demonstrate significant pelvic fractures leading to hemorrhage (open book fracture) and indicate the necessity for operative repair without further diagnostic imaging.
- Pelvic x-ray is indicated for patients with hemodynamic instability, altered mental status, distracting injury, pediatrics, and if the CT abdomen/pelvis cannot be completed for another reason. Pelvic X-ray is not required if the patient is alert, able to ambulate, and has a normal examination.
  - . Normal findings on AP pelvis radiograph (Figure 18.3): Symphysis pubis = 0.5 cm; sacroiliac joint = 2 mm; small offset of pubic rami.[5]
- CT scan is the diagnostic test of choice due to increased sensitivity and specificity and the additional diagnostic information gained with the imaging of the abdominal and pelvic organs, as well as vasculature.
- Bedside ultrasonography is essential, with FAST. Bleeding from pelvic injury is typically confined to the retroperitoneal space and may be difficult to evaluate using US. FAST may be negative in this setting.[6,7]
- MRI for subtle hip and pelvic fracture is warranted if injury is strongly suspected with negative imaging and the patient is unable to bear weight.
- Pelvic fracture classifications include Tile and Young – Burgess (Tables 18.1 and 18.2). The classification of fractures is important to determine the need for operative management.[8–10]
- Laboratory assessment includes CBC, coagulation profile/thromboelastography, metabolic panel, and beta hCG in reproductive aged women.
- VBG for lactate and base deficit/excess can be helpful for evaluation of hemodynamic compromise.

Treatment

- Initial stabilization of the patient is paramount, as many patients with pelvic injuries will suffer from multiple injuries and can be hemodynamically unstable.
- If pelvic injury is suspected, obtaining a Type and Screen/Crossmatch is recommended, with the understanding that blood transfusions may be necessary either peri- or intraoperatively.
- Hemorrhage is one of the most worrisome sequelae of fractures. Studies have shown a correlation between type of fracture and volume of blood transfusions with unstable fractures.[11]

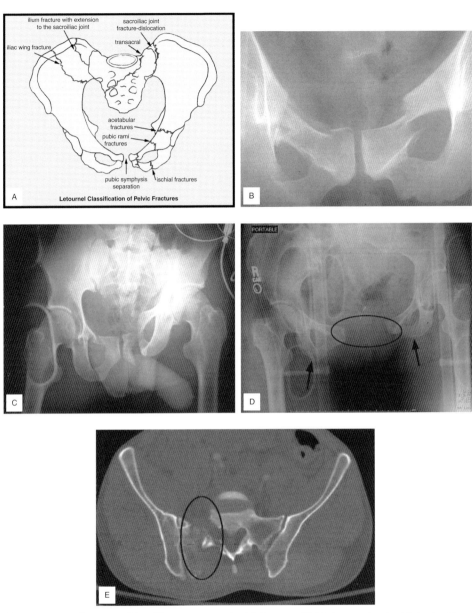

Figure 18.3 (A) Illustration of the different patterns of pelvic fractures. (B) Pelvic x-ray showing bilateral pubic and ischial rami fractures resulting in a "butterfly" fragment. This injury is often associated with significant bleeding. (C) Pelvic x-ray showing unstable Malgaigne fracture with widening of symphysis pubis, right acetabular fracture, left rami fracture, and left sacroiliac joint disruption. This type of fracture is always associated with severe bleeding. (D) Pelvic x-ray shows severe pubic symphysis diastasis. This is partially unstable and may be associated with significant bleeding. Arrows show bilateral inferior rami fractures. (E) CT scan shows fracture of the sacral bone with severe displacement. It is usually associated with severe bleeding from the presacral venous plexus or the iliac vessels (reproduced with permission from *Color Atlas of Emergency Trauma, Second Edition*, illustration at (A) by Robert Amaral)

Table 18.1 Tile[8] classification of pelvic fractures

Type	Description	Stability
A	All avulsion fractures, individual iliac wing fractures, isolated pubic rami fractures, minimally displaced ring fractures, and transverse fractures of the sacrum or coccyx	Yes
B	Posterior arch-incomplete disruption; AP (open book) and LC injuries; unilateral or bilateral	Partial
C	Posterior arch – complete disruption; includes iliac, sacroiliac, and vertical sacral injuries from vertical shearing forces; unilateral or bilateral.	No

Table 18.2 Young–Burgess classification of fractures[9]

	Stability
Anteroposterior Compression	
I. Symphysis diastasis <2.5 cm	Yes
II. Symphysis diastasis >2.5 cm, sacrospinous and anterior SI ligament disruption,	Partial
III. Symphysis diastasis >2.5 cm, with complete disruption of the anterior and posterior SI ligament	No
Lateral Compression	
I. Sacral crush injury on ipsilateral side	Yes
II. Sacral crush injury with disruption of posterior SI ligaments; iliac wing fracture may be present (crescent fracture); rotationally unstable	No
III. Severe internal rotation of ipsilateral hemipelvis with external rotation of contralateral side	No
Vertical Shear	
Vertical displacement of symphysis and sacroiliac	No
Combined Mechanisms	
Any combination of the above mechanisms	No

- Uncrossmatched blood should be available, as damage control resuscitation is paramount to initial resuscitation efforts.
- The pelvis should be stabilized (Figure 18.4). For "open book" fractures this requires a pelvic girdle or sheet forcefully tied around the pelvis at the level of the greater trochanters. For other unstable fractures the goal is to limit mobility of the pelvis, and splinting may be sufficient.
- The decision for surgical intervention is complex and not algorithmic. It will require discussion with consultant services and will vary depending on the resources available.
- The best course of treatment for a stable patient will be transfer to a trauma center if possible.

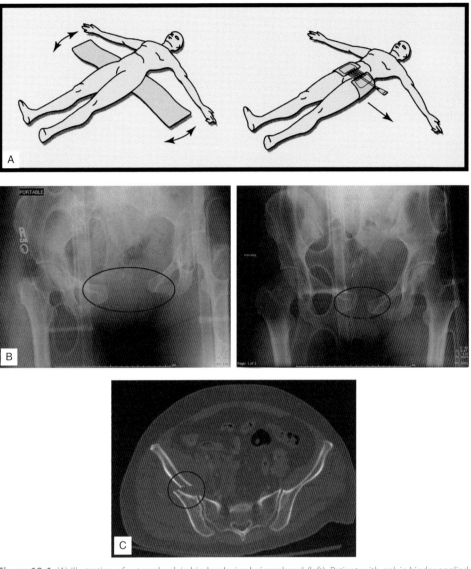

Figure 18.4 (A) Illustration of external pelvic binder device being placed (left). Patient with pelvic binder applied (right). (B) Radiographs of a patient with pubic symphysis diastasis before (left) and after (right) reduction and pelvic binder application. This type of immobilization is ideal for pubic symphysis diastasis, but not other types of pelvic fractures. (C) CT scan showing fracture of the right iliac wing (circle). Application of a pelvic binder in this type of fracture is contraindicated because it worsens the fracture displacement (reproduced with permission from *Color Atlas of Emergency Trauma, Second Edition*, illustration at (A) by Robert Amaral)

- Unstable patients with hemoperitoneum should go to the OR for laparotomy and possible packing of the pelvis – orthopedics can be consulted to perform external fixation of the pelvis at that time.
- Interventional Radiology, if available, may be able to perform angiography of the pelvic vessels with the goal of hemostasis (Figure 18.5).

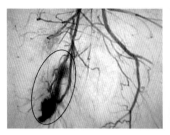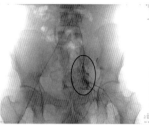

Figure 18.5 Angiograms of patients with complex pelvic fracture showing severe active bleeding (reproduced with permission from *Color Atlas of Emergency Trauma, Second Edition*)

- REBOA is a newer but promising treatment that may help temporize unstable patients with pelvic fractures and hemodynamic compromise.
- Fractures of the femur shaft should be brought to length using traction while awaiting orthopedic repair.
- Isolated acetabular fractures should be stabilized and prepared for orthopedic repair; reduction of any dislocations should be considered if operative repair is not imminent.

Pitfalls

- Delay in the stabilization of the pelvis can lead to exsanguination.
- Delay in consulting surgical consultants: trauma, orthopedics, vascular.
- Delay in obtaining blood for transfusion.
- Missing other injuries in the chest and abdomen, since one can be focused on issues from the pelvic injuries.

Key Points

- Pelvic fractures due to trauma are associated with significant morbidity and mortality.
- Stabilize the pelvis to limit hemodynamic instability and splint the pelvis.
- Select diagnostic imaging carefully, as patients may be too unstable for CT or MRI evaluations.
- Mobilize consultants in a timely fashion, including trauma surgery, orthopedics, and interventional radiology.
- Always complete a focused but complete secondary examination for other injuries, as pelvic trauma is usually present with multisystem injury.

Hip Fractures

The term "hip fracture" actually consists of proximal femur fractures. These injuries commonly affect the elderly, who experience greater rates of falls and bone disease. Hip fractures in younger patients are more commonly due to high-energy mechanisms. Unfortunately, 30 day all-cause mortality for isolated hip fracture approaches 22%, while mortality is 36% at one year.[12,13]

Anatomy

Fractures can be broken into intracapsular fractures (femoral head or neck fracture) and extracapsular fractures (intertrochanteric and trochanteric femur fracture) (Figure 18.6).

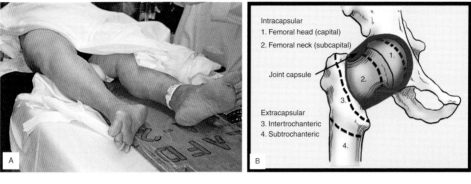

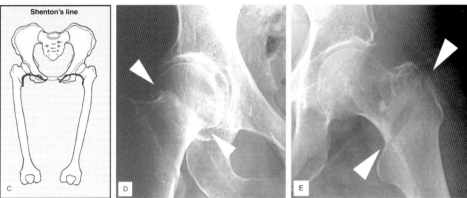

Figure 18.6 (A) Photograph of a shortened and externally rotated leg: the classic leg position after hip fracture. (B) Illustration of anatomic types of hip fracture. (C) Illustration of Shenton's line. (D) Hip radiograph of a femoral neck fracture. (E) Hip radiograph of an intertrochanteric hip fracture (reproduced with permission from *Color Atlas of Emergency Trauma, Second Edition*, illustrations at (B) and (C) by Robert Amaral)

- Intracapsular fractures have limited blood supply and may undergo avascular necrosis (AVN). However, extracapsular fractures are at low risk of AVN, due to excellent blood flow.

Diagnosis
- Patients will typically present with pain along the hip, medial thigh, or groin, as well as pain with internal or external rotation and logroll. Pain with axial loading of the leg is also suggestive of fracture.
- Examination includes inspection, palpation, mobility, and neurovascular assessment. The affected leg is often shortened and externally rotated. However, neurovascular function is usually intact.
- Standard radiographs for evaluation include AP pelvis and AP/lateral views of the proximal femur/hip. Close evaluation of the contralateral side may be required, as well as evaluation of the trabeculae and Shenton's line (Figure 18.6).
- Minor fractures may not be diagnosed on plain radiograph. CT or MRI may be required for patients with persistent pain and the inability to bear weight. Patients with adequate bony cortex (young patients) may be appropriate for CT; however, older patients or those with bone disease (osteoporosis) likely require MRI.[12]

Treatment

- Close evaluation and resuscitation of other injuries is required, along with orthopedic consultation.
- Analgesia is recommended, with nerve block a viable option for pain relief (fascia iliaca or 3-in-1 block). These blocks are associated with improved patient outcomes.[14]
- Most fractures are treated with open reduction internal fixation (ORIF), especially displaced fractures. However, isolated trochanteric fractures may not require surgical repair.
- Patients should receive type and cross/screen, as well as CBC, coagulation panel, and electrolytes.
- Disposition for those patients with diagnosed fracture is admission.

Pitfalls in ED Management

- Failure to consider intracapsular fractures as high risk for AVN.
- Failure to obtain further imaging in patients with hip pain and the inability to bear weight with negative radiographs.

Key Points

- Hip fractures come in two forms: intracapsular and extracapsular.
- Intracapsular are at high risk of AVN.
- Diagnosis is most commonly with radiographs, though further imaging may be required.
- Treatment includes analgesia, orthopedic consultation, and usually surgical repair.

Hip Dislocations

As seen in pelvic fractures, native hip dislocations also require a significant amount of force due to the ligamentous and structural design of the joint. The dislocation is classified using the femoral head in relation to the acetabulum. There are four types of dislocation: posterior, anterior, central, and inferior.[12,15]

- Posterior dislocations are far more common and account for 90% of dislocations.
- Anterior dislocations account for 10–15% and can be sub-classified into medial and lateral dislocations.
- Central dislocations are not true dislocations, as they are a result of a fracture of the acetabulum and the resultant movement medially of the femoral head.
- Inferior dislocations are extremely rare, with <5% of occurrences.

The anatomy of the joint is relevant, since the main nutrient artery of the femoral head is easily damaged in dislocations, and the risk of avascular necrosis increases with time. The femoral vessels and sciatic and femoral nerves can also be impacted depending on the direction of the dislocation.

- Posterior dislocations are associated with sciatic nerve damage, while anterior dislocations are associated with damage to the femoral nerve and vessels.

Diagnosis

- Due to the mechanism of injury and the forces needed to cause injury, hip trauma is often readily apparent. Unlike pelvic fractures, however, the inciting event may seem trivial, i.e. standing from a seated position or tripping and a ground level fall.
- Patients with pelvic or femur fractures will often have associated multi-system traumatic injuries.
- Examination includes inspection, palpation, mobility, and neurovascular assessment. Every patient presenting with hip or knee pain should have hip range of motion tested and documented.
- Initial physical examination may be notable for leg length discrepancy. Pelvic stability should be assessed, with care to not excessively push down and out on the iliac crests.
- Posterior dislocations will most commonly present with the affected leg in adduction, flexion, and internal rotation, while anterior dislocations present with extension and external rotation (Figure 18.7).
- The mainstay of diagnosis includes plain radiography, and almost all dislocations will be seen on AP and lateral views of the affected hip.

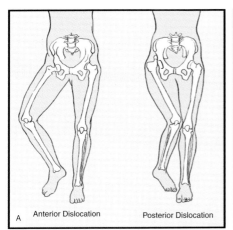
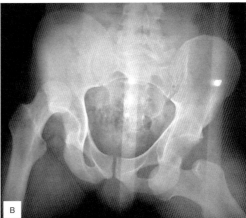
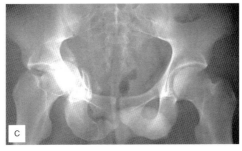

Figure 18.7 (A) Illustration of the classic position of adduction, flexion, and internal rotation seen in a posterior hip dislocation, and extension and external rotation seen in anterior hip dislocation. (B) Anteroposterior pelvis radiograph reveals both a posterior (right hip) and an anterior hip dislocation (left hip) occurring simultaneously in a patient involved in a motor vehicle crash. (C) Anteroposterior pelvis radiograph showing a right central hip dislocation with an acetabular fracture (reproduced with permission from *Color Atlas of Emergency Trauma, Second Edition*, illustration at (A) by Robert Amaral)

- If the patient presents after a significant trauma, a CT scan of the pelvis may aid in the diagnosis of acetabular and pelvic fractures.

Treatment

- The mainstay of treatment for dislocations is closed reduction and is a time sensitive procedure. Native hips should be reduced as soon as possible, as damage to surrounding structures increases with time.
- Reductions that occur greater than 12 hours or more from the time of injury are associated with a 50% rate of avascular necrosis.
- Patients with prosthetic hip joints do not have the same risk of avascular necrosis but can have damage to other neurovascular structures and should be reduced promptly as well.
- If the patient has an isolated dislocation, several possible techniques may be used to reduce the joint. This chapter discusses the Stimson, Allis, Captain Morgan, and Whistler techniques.
    - Choice of technique should take into account the patient's hemodynamic stability, patient size, practitioner size, presence of native or prosthetic joint, and other fractures of bones of the lower extremity.
- Procedural sedation will greatly assist all of the techniques; however, some patients will require general anesthesia for reduction.
- Contact consultants early in the process, as it may require time to arrange for anesthesia and operating room time if bedside reduction is unsuccessful.

Techniques

Allis Technique for Reduction of Posterior Hip Dislocation (Figure 18.8)[15]

1. Place the patient in the supine position, with the pelvis stabilized by an assistant.
2. The practitioner should be on the bed straddling the patients affected leg and hands placed in the popliteal fossa or on the calf.

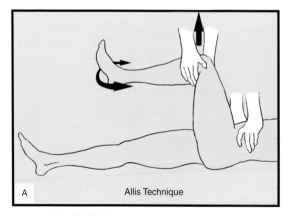
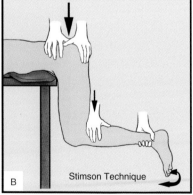

Figure 18.8 (A) Illustration of Allis closed reduction technique used for posterior dislocations. (B) Illustration of Stimson closed reduction technique used for posterior dislocation (illustrations by Robert Amaral, reproduced with permission from *Color Atlas of Emergency Trauma, Second Edition*)

3. Slowly bring the hip to 90° of flexion while applying steady upward traction and gentle rotation.
4. Ask the assistant to push the greater trochanter forward toward the acetabulum.
5. Bring the hip to the extended position while maintaining traction once you have achieved reduction.

Stimson's Technique for Reduction of Posterior Hip Dislocation (Figure 18.8)[15]

1. Place the patient in a prone position, with the leg hanging over the edge of the bed causing the hip and knee to be flexed at 90°.
2. Stabilize the pelvis.
3. Apply steady downward traction in line with the femur.
4. Gently rotate the femoral head while the assistant pushes the greater trochanter anteriorly toward the acetabulum.
5. Bring the hip to the extended position while maintaining traction once you have achieved reduction.

Captain Morgan Technique for Reduction of Posterior Hip Dislocation[16]

1. With the patient supine on the stretcher in its lowest position, secure the pelvis to the stretcher with a bed sheet or strap. Place the strap over the pelvis to prevent you from lifting the patient off the bed.
2. Stand at the side of the bed and place one foot up on the bed. Place the patient's ipsilateral leg over your leg so that your knee is resting in the patient's popliteal fossa.
3. While holding the ankle in position with slight downward pressure, lift up with both legs to apply traction on the femur and reduce the hip.
   a. DO NOT press the ankle or lower extremity down forcefully as this can damage or dislocate the knee as it levers against the providers knee.
4. If traction alone does not work, use your hands to internally and externally rotate the leg to achieve the reduction.

Whistler Technique for Reduction of Posterior Hip Dislocation[17]

1. Start with the patient lying and stabilized like the Captain Morgan technique.
2. Bend both legs so that the patient's knee is flexed 90° and the foot is on the bed.
3. Place your arm under the injured extremity knee and rest it on top of the uninjured knee and facing the patient's feet.
4. While holding the patient's ankle on the injured side with your other hand, slowly lift up with your legs, while keeping your arm straight and strong. This maneuver puts traction on the femur and should result in successful reduction.
5. If reduction is not achieved with traction alone, use your hand that is on the ankle to internally or externally rotate the leg to achieve the reduction.

Pitfalls

- Missing other injuries as you focus solely on the dislocation.
- Delaying the reduction as complications increase with time spent in a dislocated position.
- Forcing the lower leg down on your knee/shoulder when using the Captain Morgan or Whistler techniques, causing iatrogenic knee or ankle injury.

Key Points

- Time is of the essence, and reductions should be achieved as soon as reasonably possible.
- Do not overlook other injuries as a result of the inciting event, especially if significant trauma is suggested.
- Contact your consultant early in the process as it may take time to arrange for OR time.
- Become familiar with multiple techniques, as not every technique is suitable for every patient.

References

1. Schulman JE, O'Toole RV, Castillo RC, et al. Pelvic ring fractures are an independent risk factor for death after blunt trauma. *J Trauma*. 2010;68:903–34.

2. Hak DJ, Smith WR, Suzuki T. Management of hemorrhage in life-threatening pelvic fracture. *J Am Acad Orthop Surg*. 2009;17 (7):447–57.

3. Holmes JFWD. Indications and performance of pelvic radiography in patients with blunt trauma. *Am J Emerg Med*. 2012;30:1129–33.

4. Paydar S, Ghaffarpasand F, Foroughi M, et al. Role of routine pelvic radiography in initial evaluation of stable, high-energy, blunt trauma patients. *Emerg Med J*. 2013;30(9):724–27.

5. Rogers LFWO. *Imaging Skeletal Trauma*, 4th ed. Elsevier Ltd; 2015.

6. Verbeek DOF, Zijlstra IAJ. The utility of FAST for initial abdominal screening of major pelvic fracture patients. *World J Surg*. 2014;38:1719–25.

7. Uyeda J, Anderson SW, Kertesz J, Rhea JT, Soto JA. Pelvic CT angiography: application to blunt trauma using 64MDCT. *Abdom Imaging*. 2010;35 (3):280–86.

8. Tile M. Pelvic ring fractures: should they be fixed? *J Bone Jt Surgery, Br Vol*. 1988;70-B (1):1–12.

9. Burgess AR, Eastridge BJ, Young JW, et al. Pelvic ring disruptions: effective classification system and treatment protocols. *J Trauma*. 1990;30(7):848–56.

10. Aggarwal SBV. Classification of pelvis and acetabulum injuries. *Trauma Int*. 2016;2 (2):4–8.

11. Eastridge BJ, Starr A, Minei JP, O'Keefe GE, Scalea TM. The importance of fracture pattern in guiding therapeutic decision-making in patients with hemorrhagic shock and pelvic ring disruptions. *J Trauma*. 2002;53(3): 446–50.

12. Tornetta P, Court-Brown CM, Heckman JD, et al. *Rockwood, Green, and Wilkins Fractures in Adults and Children: Eighth Edition*, Vol 1–2. Philadelphia: Lippincott Williams & Wilkins; 2014.

13. Lawrence VA, Hilsenbeck SG, Noveck H, Poses RM, Carson JL. Medical complications and outcomes after hip fracture repair. *Arch Intern Med*. 2002;162 (18):2053–57.

14. Guay J, Parker MJ, Griffiths R, et al. Peripheral nerve blocks for hip fractures. *Cochrane Database Syst Rev*. 2017;5: CD001159.

15. Yang EC, Cornwall R. Initial treatment of traumatic hip dislocations in the adult. *Clin Orthop Relat Res*. 2000;(377):24–31.

16. Hendey GW, Avila A. The Captain Morgan technique for the reduction of the dislocated hip. *Ann Emerg Med*. 2011;58 (6):536–40.

17. Walden PD, Hamer JR. Whistler technique used to reduce traumatic dislocation of the hip in the emergency department setting. *J Emerg Med*. 1999;17 (3):441–44.

Chapter 19

Upper Extremity Trauma

Kristen Kann

Introduction

Upper extremity (UE) trauma is a common finding in patients presenting to the Emergency Department (ED), found in 31.6% of patients reported to the National Trauma Data Base,[1] and occurring with an estimated incidence of 1,130 upper extremity injuries per 100,000 persons per year.[2]

General rules of wound management should be followed, including cleaning of the wound, complete neurovascular examination, tetanus administration as indicated, and pain control as needed. In addition, any wound with neurovascular compromise requires immediate intervention and/or emergent orthopedic consultation (Table 19.1).

Hand and Finger Injuries

Bone

Distal Phalanges

- Tuft fracture: Distal, comminuted fracture. May be associated with nail bed injuries (Figure 19.1).[3]
- Shaft fractures: Reduce those with gross deformity or severe pain and immobilize with malleable splint.
- Dorsal intra-articular fractures: "Bony mallet finger," see section below on soft tissue injuries (Figure 19.2).

Table 19.1 Hand surgery consultation

Immediate Hand Surgery Consultation	Delayed Hand Surgery Consultation
Amputation	Tendon lacerations
Severe crush injury	Tendon ruptures (Jersey finger, mallet finger)
Open fracture	Closed fracture
Severe soft tissue loss	Ligamentous injuries/laxity or instability
Irreducible dislocations	Dislocations reduced in ER
Vascular injury	Nerve injury
Compartment syndrome	
High-pressure injection injury	

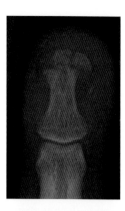

Figure 19.1 Tufts fracture

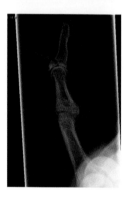

Figure 19.2 Mallet finger

- Volar intra-articular fracture: "Bony jersey finger," uncommon, presents with tenderness over the volar aspect of the distal phalanx – if patient also has palmar pain, assume rupture of the flexor digitorum profundus tendon. Treatment is volar splint and orthopedic follow up for likely surgical fixation.[3]

Proximal and Middle Phalanges

- Most fractures can be buddy taped or placed in a gutter splint (radial gutter for 2nd and 3rd phalanges, ulnar gutter for 4th and 5th) and followed up with primary care.[3]
- Intra-articular and unstable (displaced, spiral, oblique, comminuted) fractures should be reduced to anatomic position, placed in a gutter splint, and referred for orthopedic follow up.[4]

Metacarpal Head

Place in gutter splint with metacarpophalangeal (MCP) joint flexed >70° and follow up with a hand surgeon (many require fixation).[3,4]

Metacarpal Neck

- Boxer's fracture: Fracture of neck of the 4th or 5th metacarpal (MC) (Figure 19.3).[3]
- Acceptable angulation: <10° for 2nd and 3rd MCs, <30–40° in 4th and 5th MCs.[3,4]
- Reduce as needed, then place in gutter splint with wrist at 20° extension and MCP >70° flexion.[4]

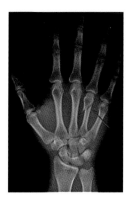

Figure 19.3 4th MC neck fracture

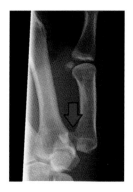

Figure 19.4 Bennett's fracture

Metacarpal Shaft

- Acceptable deformities:
  - Rotational: <10°.[5]
  - Dorsal angulation: <10° for 2nd and 3rd MCs, <10–20° for 4th and 5th MCs.[3]
  - Anything beyond these should be further reduced, and, if this is not possible, refer for likely operative fixation.

- Place in gutter splint with wrist extended about 30° and MCP joint in 90° flexion, IP joints in extension.[3]

Thumb Metacarpal

- Extra-articular:
  - Acceptable angulation <30°.[3]
  - Oblique and rotational fractures, often require pinning.[3,5]

- Intra-articular:
  - Bennett's: Fracture dislocation at the metacarpal joint, ulnar portion in anatomic position with displaced radial/distal portion (Figure 19.4). Place in thumb spica splint and refer to orthopedics.[5]
  - Rolando's: Comminuted intra-articular fracture. Place in thumb spica splint and refer to orthopedics.[5]

Table 19.2 Innervation of the hand

Nerve	Motor Exam	Sensory Exam
Radial nerve	Wrist and finger extension, thumb extension against resistance	Sensation at web space between thumb and index finger
Median nerve	Thumb–pinky opposition	Sensation at pad of index finger
Ulnar nerve	Resisted abduction of fingers	Sensation at pad of pinky finger

Joint Dislocations
- Distal interphalangeal (DIP) joint: Usually dorsal. Digital block and reduce with exaggeration/traction/re-approximation technique.
- Proximal interphalangeal (PIP) joint: Usually dorsal or lateral; reduce as with DIPs.
- MCP subluxations and dislocations: Usually dorsal. To reduce, flex the wrist and apply volar pressure over the proximal phalanx. Splint in MCP flexion, such as with a gutter splint.[5]
- Carpometacarpal joint dislocations: Usually dorsal. Reduce with traction, flexion, and pressure on the MC base. Volar dislocations should be referred.[5]

Nerve
Table 19.2 provides specific innervation of the hand.

Soft Tissue
- Up to 90% of a tendon can be lacerated with preserved ROM without resistance – always test with resistance and compare to uninjured side.[5]
- Tendon laceration – May be able to fix extensors in consultation with hand surgeon, but operative repair is becoming more common. For flexor tendon injury, consult hand surgeon, with loose closure and splint until follow up.[5]
- Specific injuries:
  - Mallet finger:[6]
    - Most common tendon injury in athletes.[5]
    - Complete laceration/rupture of extensor tendon resulting in inability to extend DIP joint.
    - Splint in extension, as no flexion is allowed for 6–10 weeks. Any flexion requires resplinting and restarting the immobilization period.[3-5]
    - Poor healing leads to Swan neck deformity, in which lateral bands slip dorsally and increase extension at the PIP.[5]
  - Jersey finger:[6]
    - Laceration/rupture of flexor tendon at insertion into distal phalanx.
    - Presents with pain/tenderness at volar DIP/distal phalanx, with digit held in relative extension.
    - Splint in flexion and refer to a hand surgeon, as operative repair is almost always necessary.

- Boutonniere deformity:

    - PIP flexion and DIP extension caused by laceration/rupture of central slip over the PIP and volar displacement of lateral bands.[7]
    - Splint with PIP in full extension and follow up with orthopedics/hand surgeon.

- Gamekeeper's/Skier's thumb:

    - Rupture or strain of ulnar collateral ligament (UCL).
        - Presents with pain and ecchymosis at thumb MCP, as well as pincer weakness.
    - >35° radial angulation, or >10° difference from uninjured thumb, indicates complete rupture and should be treated in consultation with a hand surgeon.
    - Place in thumb spica splint and obtain urgent orthopedics/hand surgery follow up for likely surgical repair.[8]

- High-pressure injection injury:

    - Orthopedic emergency: Benign early appearance progresses to edema, pallor, and exquisite tenderness to palpation.
      Treatment: Early orthopedic consult for surgical debridement.
    - While pending bedside consult, splint and elevate the extremity, update tetanus, and provide broad spectrum antibiotics and analgesia.[5]

Wrist and Distal Forearm Injuries

Bone
Distal Radius

- Colles' fracture:

    - Usually from a fall onto an outstretched hand (FOOSH) type injury, with distal fracture fragment of the radius dorsally angulated and displaced (Figure 19.5).[5]
    - Classic "dinner fork" deformity with gross dorsiflexion of the wrist.

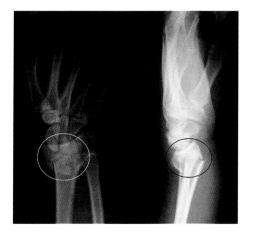

Figure 19.5 Colle's fracture

- > 20° angulation, intra-articular involvement, marked comminution, or >1 cm of shortening meets criteria for an unstable fracture.[5]
- Closed reduction with restoration of volar tilt (minimum of 0° angulation) and proper radial length and application of a sugar tong splint.[5]

- Smith's fracture is equivalent to reverse Colles' fracture:
  - Volar angulation of the distal radius after a fracture, known as "garden spade" deformity.[5]
  - Closed reduction and sugar tong splint application.

- Barton's fracture:
  - Rim fractures of the distal radius, frequently with carpal subluxation.
  - Sugar tong splint application and orthopedic follow up.[5]

- Radial styloid fracture:
  - Radial styloid is the insertion site of multiple major carpal ligaments.
  - Often accompanied by lunate dislocation.
  - Place in short arm splint with wrist in mild flexion and ulnar deviation and orthopedic referral.[5]

Distal Ulna

- Ulnar styloid fracture:
  - Rarely significant, unless extensive and involving the triangular fibrocartilage complex/distal radioulnar joint.
  - Treat with ulnar gutter splint with slight ulnar deviation and a neutral wrist.[5]

Carpal Fractures

- Scaphoid:
  - Most commonly fractured carpal bone (Figure 19.6).[5]
  - Clinical exam: pain along radial aspect of the wrist, specifically tenderness in the anatomic snuffbox. Exam may also reveal pain in the snuffbox with resisted supination or pronation, as well as pain on axial load of the thumb's MC joint.[5]

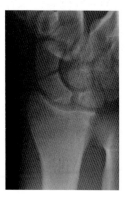

Figure 19.6 Scaphoid fracture

- If x-rays are negative but there is concern for scaphoid fracture, consider MRI or CT of the scaphoid.[9]
- Vascular supply to scaphoid enters distally, so fractures (especially proximal, oblique, or displaced fractures) can lead to proximal avascular necrosis.[5]
- For non-displaced fractures or those with negative x-rays but concern for scaphoid fracture, place in short arm thumb spica splint with dorsiflexion and radial deviation.[5]

- Triquetrum fractures:
    - Second most common carpal bone fracture:[5]
    - Tenderness dorsally, just distal to the ulnar styloid.
    - Dorsal avulsion fractures: "Flake" of bone over triquetrum on lateral x-rays, usually splinted for 1–2 weeks with excellent prognosis.[5]
    - Body fractures: Usually cast for 6 weeks. Displaced fractures may require fixation.[5]

- Lunate fractures: Rare in isolation. Distal blood supply, similar to the scaphoid, increases risk of avascular necrosis.[5]
    - Fractures require orthopedic consult and short arm thumb spica splint.

- Trapezium fracture: Painful thumb movement and weak pinch with tenderness at the snuffbox. Consult orthopedics and place in a short arm thumb spica splint.[5]
- Pisiform fracture: Localized tenderness over the pisiform, which can be palpated in the hypothenar eminence with the wrist flexed.
    - Consider carpal tunnel view or supination films.
    - Treat with compression dressing or splint in 30° flexion with ulnar deviation.[5]

- Hamate fracture: Usually involves the hook of the hamate, best visualized with carpal tunnel views, though consider a CT if negative x-rays and high index of suspicion.
    - Remember to examine for signs of injury to the ulnar nerve and artery, which pass through Guyon's canal.[5]
    - Splint and refer to orthopedics.

- Capitate fracture: Often occur in conjunction with a scaphoid fracture. Distal blood supply with danger of avascular necrosis, similar to the lunate and scaphoid.
    - Examination with tenderness and swelling just proximal to the 3rd MC.
    - Splint and consult orthopedics.[5]

- Trapezoid fracture: Rare, examination reveals tenderness on axial load of the index finger. Consider CT or MRI if negative x-rays and place thumb spica splint.[5]

Subluxations and Dislocations
- Distal radio-ulnar joint subluxation:
    - Rarely isolated, usually seen with intra-articular or distal radial shaft fractures (Galeazzi) or both-bone fractures of the forearm.[5]
    - True lateral X-ray will show displacement of the ulna (either volar or dorsal).
    - Examination with pain at radioulnar joint, prominent ulnar head, weak grip, and decreased ROM in pronation and supination.[5]

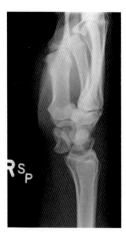

Figure 19.7 Lunate dislocation

- Peri-lunate and lunate dislocations:[10]
  - Parts of a continuous spectrum of high-energy injuries. Typically, there is little gross deformity on examination.
  - Lunate dislocation: "Spilled teacup" sign on lateral x-ray shows the lunate's concavity oriented towards the palm (Figure 19.7).
  - Both perilunate and lunate dislocations necessitate immediate orthopedic consultation.[5]

Soft Tissue

- Scapholunate ligament: Most commonly injured ligament of the wrist, most often from FOOSH.[5]
  - Scapholunate dissociation: "Terry Thomas sign" results from widening of the scapholunate joint space of >3 mm.[5]
  - If high suspicion, obtain a grip compression view or consider comparison views of uninjured hand.[10]
  - Treatment includes radial gutter splint or short arm volar posterior mold and orthopedic referral.
- Triquetrolunate ligament instability: The ulnar version of scapholunate injuries; usually a result of a FOOSH onto the hypothenar eminence. Treat with ulnar gutter splint and orthopedics referral.

Elbow and Forearm

Bone

Distal Humerus Fractures

- Fat pads:
  - Normal fat pads: Small anterior fat pad and no visible posterior fat pad.
  - Large anterior pad ("sail sign") or visible posterior pad: abnormal/hemarthrosis or joint effusion (Figure 19.8).

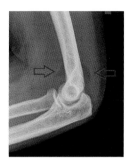

Figure 19.8 Abnormal anterior and posterior fat pads

- Supracondylar fractures:
  - Most common elbow fracture in children 5–10 years of age.[5]
  - 95% are extension type/posterior displacement.[5]
    - FOOSH with swelling and pain at elbow, prominent olecranon, and depression proximal to the elbow.[5]
    - If non-displaced, the only x-ray finding may be abnormal fat pads or disruption of anterior humeral line.[5]
    - Nondisplaced with <20° angulation: long arm posterior splint with elbow at 90° flexion and forearm neutral rotation, outpatient orthopedics follow up.
    - Displaced with >20° angulation should be reduced prior to splinting.
    - Consider admission for patients with severe edema (to monitor neurovascular status of arm) or severely displaced fractures.[5]
  - Complications:
    - Volkmann's ischemic contracture:
      - ○ Refusal to open the hand, pain with passive extension of the fingers, forearm tenderness, and/or lack of radial pulse accompanied by another of these signs.
      - ○ Loss of radial pulse is often not found until later in the course; do not use a present radial pulse to rule out compartment syndrome.
      - ○ Patient needs to go emergently to the OR for fasciotomy.[5]
    - Intercondylar fractures: Much more common in adults than supracondylar fractures.[5]
      - ○ Nondisplaced: Treat with long arm posterior splint with elbow at 90° and forearm neutral.[5]
      - ○ Displaced: Attempt reduction prior to splinting and arrange for orthopedic follow up.[5]
      - ○ Consider admission for patients with severe edema (to monitor neurovascular status of arm) or severely displaced fractures.[5]
    - Epicondyle fractures:
      - ○ Long arm posterior mold with elbow at 90° flexion and:
        - ▪ Medial epicondyle fracture: Forearm in PROnation.[5]
        - ▪ Lateral epicondyle fracture: Forearm in SUPination.[5]
    - Condyle fractures:
      - ○ Nondisplaced: Long arm posterior splint and orthopedic follow up.[5]
      - ○ Displaced or neurovascular compromise: Immediate orthopedic consultation.[5]

- Articular surface:
  - ○ Trochlea: Rare, x-rays can be subtle, consider CT or MRI if high suspicion. Long arm posterior splint and orthopedic consult for likely operative fixation.[5]
  - ○ Capitellum: Usually associated with radial head fractures. X-rays can be subtle, consider radial head/capitellum view and/or CT/MRI. Long arm posterior splint and orthopedic consult for likely operative fixation.

Ulnar Fractures[11]

- Coronoid: Usually associated with posterior elbow dislocations.[5]

  - Pain, swelling, and tenderness to palpation at AC fossa; can be subtle on x-ray, so consider CT/MRI.
  - Long arm posterior splint with elbow in flexion and forearm in supination; outpatient orthopedic consult.

- Olecranon: Up to 10% of UE fractures.[12] Insertion site of triceps, so active elbow extension is impaired. Pain/swelling/tenderness at posterior elbow. Long arm posterior splint with elbow in flexion and neutral forearm, orthopedic referral within 24 hours.[5]

- Ulnar shaft/Nightstick fracture:

  - Nondisplaced: Treat with short arm cast and orthopedic referral.
  - Fractures with >50% displacement, >10° angulation, or involving proximal 1/3 of ulna are unstable. Reduce and splint; orthopedic consult.[5]
  - Monteggia Fracture–Dislocation: Proximal ulnar fracture with radial head dislocation (Figure 19.9). Evaluate the radial head in all ulnar fractures, as the radial head injury can be subtle, but missed injuries lead to chronic pain and limited ROM.
  - Treatment: Orthopedics consult, as these usually require ORIF.[5]

Proximal Radius/Radial Head Fractures

- Essex-Lopresti lesion: Disruption of triangular fibrocartilage of the wrist and interosseous membrane between the radius and ulna, causing distal radioulnar join dissociation.

  - Clinically presents with radial head fracture and distal forearm/wrist pain.

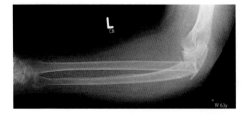

Figure 19.9 Monteggia fracture–dislocation

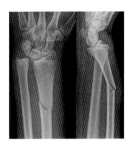

Figure 19.10 Galeazzi fracture–dislocation

- Radial head fractures can be subtle on x-ray, consider radial head-capitellum views.
  - Other signs: Abnormal displacement of the radiocapitellar line away from the center of the capitellum and/or abnormal fat pad (large anterior sail sign and/or visible posterior fat pad).[5]
- Treatment: Sling immobilization with elbow in flexion, orthopedic follow up within 1 week for nondisplaced fractures. Displaced fractures should be followed-up within 24 hours.[3]
- Radial Shaft Fractures: Proximal 2/3 and displaced fractures usually require internal fixation to prevent rotational deformity; consult orthopedics.[5]
- Galeazzi Fracture–dislocation: Fracture of the distal 1/3 of the radial shaft with dislocation of the distal radioulnar joint (Figure 19.10); consult orthopedics as this injury requires surgical repair.[5]

Elbow Dislocations

- This is the third most common major joint dislocation and frequently complicated/associated with fractures.[3,5]
- The "terrible triad" refers to an elbow dislocation with a radial head fracture and a coronoid fracture; unstable and requires reduction and surgical repair.[5]
- 90% of elbow dislocations are posterolateral.
- Examine for injuries to brachial artery and the ulnar, radial, and median nerves. Consider angiography if concerned about a vascular injury.[5]
- Reduction: Multiple techniques, all requiring adequate analgesia or sedation, stabilization of the humerus, distraction, and re-approximation of the olecranon into anatomical position.
  - Inability to maintain reduction through full ROM requires orthopedic consult for surgical repair.[5]
  - If stable through ROM, test for varus (rare) or valgus (more common) instability.
    - Mild instability that stabilizes with 90° flexion and pronation should be splinted in that position with orthopedic follow up.
    - Instability that cannot be stabilized requires orthopedic consult for possible surgical repair.[5]
  - Stable through ROM and stable with varus/valgus stress requires long arm posterior splint with elbow slightly <90° flexion and forearm in mild pronation with orthopedic follow up.[5]

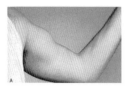

Figure 19.11 Popeye sign of biceps tendon rupture

Nerve Injury
For exam, see "Nerve Injury" in the preceding "Hand and Fingers" section.

Soft Tissue Injury
Biceps Tendon Rupture
- Snap or pop during contraction of biceps with pain at anterior shoulder. Firing the bicep (elbow flexion) will cause pain and may produce the "popeye sign" of a bulge in the midarm, showing the location of the distally retracted head of the biceps (Figure 19.11).
- Distal rupture less common, but similar story and pain at AC fossa.
- Distal biceps tendon ruptures occur more commonly in young males, while proximal tendon ruptures more typically occur in older patients.
- Treat with sling and orthopedic referral. Patients with distal biceps tendon rupture require immobilization and early orthopedics referral.

Triceps Tendon Rupture
- Rare, almost always distal.[13] Decreased or lost ability to extend the elbow. Obtain x-rays, as avulsion fractures of the olecranon are common.
- Treatment includes sling and obtain orthopedic follow up.[5]

Shoulder and Upper Arm
Bone
Proximal Humerus Fractures
- Complications:
  - Most commonly injured nerve is the axillary nerve (sensation over deltoid), then suprascapular nerve (abduction through supraspinatus and infraspinatus).[14]
  - Most commonly injured vessel is the axillary artery (weak distal pulses, paresthesias, pallor, or expanding hematoma).[5]
- Most common fractures involve surgical neck and greater tuberosity.[5]
- Nondisplaced requires sling and swathe with orthopedic referral. Displaced/angulated or fracture dislocations require orthopedic consult, closed reduction vs. operative management.[5]

Humeral Shaft Fractures
- Complications include injury to brachial artery/vein or radial/ulnar/median nerves.
  - Most common is the radial nerve, which courses along the spiral groove in the posterior humerus.[5]

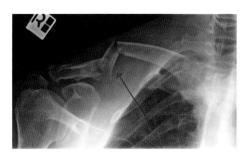

Figure 19.12 Comminuted clavicular fracture

- Most closed fractures of the humeral shaft are managed non-operatively, and a 2012 Cochrane review found no difference in outcomes between operative and non-operative management.[15]
  - . Treat with sugar tong splint vs. simple sling and swathe with orthopedic follow up for casting.

Distal Humerus Fractures

Complex due to surrounding neurovascular structures. See section on supracondylar fractures.

Clavicular Fractures

- Proximal 1/3: More concerning due to proximity to mediastinal and intrathoracic structures as well as forces involved. Emergent consultation for mediastinal disruption, otherwise orthopedic referral in 1–2 weeks and sling.
- Middle 1/3: Typically managed non-operatively, but consider orthopedic referral in cases with comminution, severe tenting of the skin, athletes, or patients with cosmetic concerns (Figure 19.12). Treat with sling and primary care follow up for minimally displaced, orthopedic follow up for others.[3,5]
- Distal 1/3 Clavicle:
  - . Type I: Distal to coracoclavicular ligaments, and ligaments remain intact. Treatment includes sling and primary care follow up.[16]
  - . Type II: Distal to coracoclavicular ligaments, but ligaments are disrupted. Orthopedic consult for possible operative repair.[17]
  - . Type III: Intra-articular through AC joint. Managed with sling and primary care follow up.[16]

Scapular Fractures

- Often a high-energy mechanism, so maintain a high level of suspicion for associated injuries to the upper extremity, spine, and thorax.
- While fractures can be identified on x-rays, consider CT given association with other significant injuries.
- Treatment includes sling and orthopedic referral.

Dislocation

- Anterior glenohumeral (GH) x-rays to confirm diagnosis and absence of fractures, unless neurovascular compromise necessitates immediate reduction (Figure 19.13).

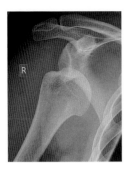

Figure 19.13 Anterior shoulder dislocation

- Nerve injury occurs in 10–25% of acute dislocations, usually axillary nerve traction neuropraxia resulting in decreased sensation over the deltoid, weakness in shoulder abduction/external rotation.[5]
- Vascular injuries: Rare but usually axillary artery leading to hematoma, bruising, axillary bruit, and decreased/absent radial pulse.[5]
- Reduction: Pain control (systemic or intraarticular) or sedation. There are numerous reduction methods, which all involve some aspect of at least one of the following: traction, leverage, scapular manipulation.
- Post-reduction: Sling and swath/shoulder immobilizer, orthopedic follow up (1–2 days for any bony or soft tissue associated injury, and 1 week otherwise).[5]

- Anterior GH dislocation with fractures:
  - Hill-Sachs: Humeral head bony defect; treat with orthopedic follow up.
  - Bankart: Glenoid labrum (soft Bankart) defect or glenoid defect (bony Bankart); treat with orthopedic follow up.

- AC subluxation and dislocation:
  - Usually due to direct trauma. Diagnosis is clinical, but x-rays can help to determine grade of injury.
    - Rockwood types I (pain at AC joint but no ligament rupture) and II (ligament rupture but <100% displacement of clavicle) should be managed with sling.
    - >100% displacement of the clavicle, ±A/P displacement, requires orthopedic referral for likely surgical management.[18]

- Posterior GH dislocation:
  - Clinically, prominence of posterior shoulder with flattened anterior shoulder. Patient will be unable to externally rotate or abduct the arm.
  - Reduction: After proper analgesia ± sedation, apply traction to adducted humerus and gently push humeral head anteriorly. Place in sling/shoulder immobilizer and follow up with orthopedics.[5]

- Luxatio erecta:
  - Hyperabduction mechanism: Patient presents with arm fully abducted and forearm dropped onto or behind the head.[5]
  - Reduction: Traction upward and outward with assistant providing countertraction.[5]

.   After reduction, place in sling/shoulder immobilizer and follow up with orthopedics. These injuries frequently result in severe rotator cuff injuries that may require operative repair.[5]
.   May require operative reduction if humeral head buttonholes through the rotator cuff.[5]

- Sternoclavicular rupture/strain/dislocation:[3,5]
    .   Direct blow or transmitted force from shoulder injury.
    .   Dislocations: Pain at sternoclavicular joint with either prominent (anterior dislocation) or sunken (posterior dislocation) medial clavicle. In posterior dislocations, patient may have airway symptoms due to displacement of the superior mediastinum, as well as high risk of vascular injury.[5]
    .   More minor trauma: Sprain/strain, which will present with pain/swelling at the sternoclavicular joint without deformity.
    .   CT is imaging of choice, due to low sensitivity of x-rays.[5]

Vessel Injury

- Mechanism usually traction injury, though also can occur with blunt or penetrating injury to the shoulder/neck.
- Often delayed diagnosis due to other injuries – significant forces involved, and motor and sensory deficits are often overshadowed/complicated by severe fractures and soft tissue injuries.
- Perform a detailed neurologic examination of the upper extremity in patients with concerning history, such as traction injuries to the neck/shoulder.

Pitfalls

- Subtle ligamentous injuries can be missed without a focused exam and comparison to the uninjured extremity/digits.
- Do not underestimate a high-pressure injection injury to the hand.
- Many carpal bone fractures can be easily missed on x-ray. When in doubt, obtain a CT.
- Pay attention to the fat pads of the elbow – they can reveal injuries that would otherwise be easily missed.

Key Points

- Upper extremity injuries are commonly encountered in the ED, and targeted examination of the upper extremity, including vessels, ligaments, and bony landmarks, is critical for an efficient and effective assessment.
- Be aware of the immediate hand surgery consultation guidelines. Most other injuries can be reduced as needed, splinted, and provided with routine orthopedic follow up.
- Close evaluation of imaging is necessary, with consideration of commonly missed injuries.
- Consult Orthopedics for any irreducible fractures or dislocations, concerns for compartment syndrome, and/or neurovascular compromise.

References

1. The National Trauma Data Bank Annual Report. In: Vincent JL, Hall JB, eds. *Encyclopedia of Intensive Care Medicine.* Berlin: Springer; 2016.

2. Oortes D, Lambers KT, Ring DC. The epidemiology of upper extremity injuries presenting to the emergency department in the United States. *Hand.* 2012;7(1):18–22.

3. Manthey DE, Askew K. Hand. In: Sherman SC, ed. *Simon's Emergency Orthopedics,* 7th ed. New York, NY: McGraw-Hill; 2014.

4. Egol KA, Koval KJ, Suckerman JD. *Handbook of Fractures,* 4th ed. New York, NY: Lippincott Williams & Wilkins; 2010.

5. Davenport M, Tang P. Injuries to the hand and digits. In: Tintinalli JE, Stapczynski J, Ma O, et al., eds. *Tintinalli's Emergency Medicine: A Comprehensive Study Guide,* 8th ed. New York, NY: McGraw-Hill; 2016.

6. Bachoura A, Ferikes AJ, Lubahn JD. A review of mallet finger and jersey finger injuries in the athlete. *Curr Rev Musculoskel Med.* 2017;10(1):1–9.

7. Grandizio LC, Klena JC. Sagittal band, boutonniere, and pulley injuries in the athlete. *Curr Rev Musculoskel Med.* 2017;10(1):17–22.

8. Samora JB, Harris JD, Griesser MJ, Ruff ME, Awan HM. Outcomes after injury to the thumb ulnar collateral ligament – a systematic review. *Clin J Sport Med.* 2013;23(4):247–54.

9. Carpenter CR, Pines JM, Schuur JD, et al. Adult scaphoid fracture. *Acad Emerg Med.* 2014;21(2):101–21.

10. Morrell NT, Moyer A, Quinlan N, Shafritz AB. Scapholunate and perilunate injuries in the athlete. *Curr Rev Musculoskel Med.* 2017;10(1):45–52.

11. Logan AJ, Lindau TR. The management of distal ulnar fractures in adults: a review of the literature and recommendations for treatment. *Strategies Trauma Limb Reconstr.* 2008;3(2):49–56.

12. Anderson ML, Larson AN, Merten SM, Steinmann SP. Congruent elbow plate fixation of olecranon fractures. *J Orthop Trauma.* 2007;21:6.

13. Yeh PC, Dodds SD, Smart LR, Mazzocca AD, Sethi PM. Distal triceps rupture. *J Am Acad Orthop Surg.* 2010;18:31.

14. Khmelnitskaya E, Lamont LE, Taylor SA, et al. Evaluation and management of proximal humerus fractures. *Adv Orthop.* 2012;2012:861598.

15. Gosler MW, Testroote M, Morrenhof JW, Janzing HM. Surgical versus non-surgical interventions for treating humeral shaft fractures in adults. *Cochrane Database Syst Rev.* 2012;(1):Cd008832.

16. Anderson K. Evaluation and treatment of distal clavicle fractures. *Clin Sports Med.* 2003;22:319.

17. van der Meijden OA, Gaskill TR, Millett PJ. Treatment of clavicle fractures: current concepts review. *J Shoulder Elbow Surg.* 2012;21:423.

18. Bradley JP, Elkousy H. Decision making: operative versus nonoperative treatment of acromioclavicular joint injuries. *Clin Sports Med.* 2003;22(2):277–90.

Chapter 20

Lower Extremity Trauma

Ryan LaFollette and Jeffery Hill

Femur

Mechanism of Injury

Usually results from high-energy mechanisms (i.e. high speed MVC), but low-energy mechanisms (falls) are possible in elderly patients as well.[1]

Physical Examination

- Obvious external deformity of the thigh is common with femur fractures.[1,2]
- Palpate the compartments of the thigh to assess the degree of hematoma formation and screen for possible compartment syndrome (Figure 20.1).
- Neurovascular exam:
  - Popliteal, dorsalis pedis, and posterior tibial pulses distal to the site of fracture pre- and post-reduction, splinting, or application of traction.
  - Calculate Ankle Brachial Indices (ABIs) if diminished pulses are found on initial examination.
  - Assess for sensory and motor deficits in sciatic and peroneal nerve distributions pre- and post-reduction and traction/splinting.[2]

Femoral Shaft Fractures

- Anatomic considerations: The femoral shaft extends from 5 cm distal from the lesser trochanter to 6 cm proximal to the adductor tubercle.
  - Three soft tissue compartments (see Figure 20.1): anterior, medial, posterior
- Types of fractures:
  - Spiral, transverse, or oblique fractures
  - Comminuted
  - Open
- Imaging: AP and lateral plain x-rays of the femur, as well as imaging of the ipsilateral hip and knee.
- Associated injuries/complications:
  - Ipsilateral femoral neck fracture: 1–9% incidence with 20–50% missed on initial evaluation.[1,3]

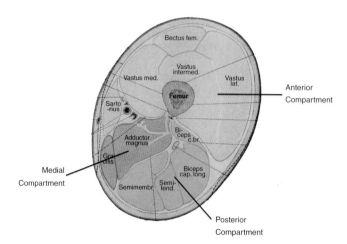

Figure 20.1 Compartments of the thigh (adapted from the 1921 German edition of *Anatomie des Menschen* by Hermann Braus)

- Bleeding – closed fractures can result in significant bleeding (1–1.5 L) into the soft tissue compartments of the thigh. However, this bleeding is usually not sufficient in and of itself to result in hypotension.[1,2]
  - Thigh Compartment Syndrome is relatively uncommon due to the large size of the compartment.[2] Suspect this condition when physical examination reveals a tense compartment with palpation, pain out of proportion to exam, and associated neurovascular compromise.
  - Anterior compartment is most commonly affected.
  - Urgent consultation with an orthopedic surgeon is needed as definitive management is surgical with fasciotomy.[2]

- Neurovascular:
  - Sciatic nerve injuries are uncommon in blunt mechanisms of injury. Higher incidence of injuries noted with penetrating trauma.[2]
  - Peroneal nerve injuries are uncommon as a result of the fracture itself but can result from traction/splinting.

- Management:
  - Non-operative management is by placement of a long leg cast. Preferred when multiple medical comorbidities preclude operative management.[1]
  - Surgical management within 24 hours is preferred with intramedullary (IM) nailing vs. open reduction and internal fixation (ORIF) with plate fixation.[1]

Distal Femur Fractures

- Represent <1% of all fractures and 3–6% of all femur fractures (though frequency increases with periprosthetic fractures).[1]
  - Bimodal distribution with increased incidence in young, healthy males (usually as a result of high-energy mechanism of injury) and elderly osteopenic females (usually as a result of low-energy mechanism of injury).[4]

- AO/Orthopedic Trauma Association Classification:[1]
  - Type A – Extra-articular (supracondylar)
  - Type B – Partial articular with extension into the medial or lateral condyle (partial condylar)
  - Type C – Intra-articular with extension into the intercondylar region (intercondylar)
- Imaging: AP and lateral x-ray are adequate for visualization, though CT may be needed to evaluate for intra-articular extension and can help with operative planning.
  - Consider angiography if diminished distal pulses on exam.
- Associated injuries:
  - Ligamentous injuries to the knee in 20% of patients.[2]
  - Vascular injury – thrombosis, pseudoaneurysm, and dissection of femoral artery/popliteal artery.
  - Nerve injury – overall uncommon, but peroneal nerve injury is possible.
- Management:
  - Operative therapy is common, but non-operative management is considered for non-displaced fractures, non-ambulatory patients, non-reconstructable injuries, or patients with comorbidities precluding operative management.[5]
  - Non-operative management includes a hinged knee brace with immediate range of motion and non-weight bearing for 6 weeks.[4]

Traction vs Splinting

Stabilization of midshaft femur fractures through traction or splinting may improve analgesia.[6] It may also improve bony/soft tissue alignment and could benefit resuscitation if there is a large femoral compartment bleed as a result of the fracture (Table 20.1).[2,7]

Pediatric Femur Fractures

- Thorough history and physical examination are mandated to evaluate for the potential for non-accidental trauma as a cause of the fracture.
- There is typically no difference in the type of fracture observed in non-accidental trauma vs. accidental trauma.[11]
- Non-accidental trauma is more likely in patients 0–18 months of age.[11,12]
- If the child is old enough to run, they are old enough to fall and sustain a femur fracture (a fall with twisting rotational force can lead to spiral midshaft femur fracture).[11]

Knee

Physical Examination: Evaluate for fracture/deformity of the distal femur, patella, and proximal tibia, dislocation, or subluxation of the knee joint, as well as significant ligamentous injury.

- Inspect for deformity, wounds, skin changes, or any other abnormality.
- Careful evaluation for joint effusion as lipohemarthrosis is the most sensitive indicator of knee fracture.[13]

Table 20.1 Types of traction

	Traction Splints	Cutaneous Traction	Skeletal Traction
Description/ Example	KTD Splint/Hare Traction	Foam padded boot with weighted distraction	Temporary traction pin placed into distal femur/ proximal tibia with weighted distraction[9]
Complications	Peroneal nerve injury, skin breakdown, pain[8]	Skin breakdown	Skin infection, osteomyelitis, septic arthritis (0.7% w/proper technique), fracture, regional neuromuscular injury, ligamentous injury[6,10]
Indications	Pre-hospital temporary stabilization of isolated midshaft femur fractures	In-hospital stabilization of midshaft or distal femur fractures	In-hospital stabilization of diaphyseal femur fractures
Contraindications	Ipsilateral hip dislocation, multiple ipsilateral leg fractures	Ligamentous knee injury, multiple ipsilateral leg fractures[6]	Existing fractures at pin placement sites

- Neurovascular examination distal to the site of the injury – evaluate dorsalis pedis and posterior tibial pulses with ABIs if diminished pulses are present.
- Active range of motion (normal is 10° of extension with 130° of flexion).[13]
- Palpation along medial and lateral joint lines, varus and valgus testing, assessment of patellar tendon/quadriceps tendon function.

Tibial Plateau Fractures

Anatomic Considerations: The tibial plateau is comprised of the medial and lateral condyle of the proximal articular surface of the tibia. The plateau slopes 10° from anterior to posterior.[14]

Fracture classification is with the Schatzker Classification (Table 20.2, Figure 20.2).[2,13]

Mechanism of Injury

- Axial and rotational forces (falls from height).
- Direct blows to the proximal tibia (pedestrian struck):
  - Forceful abduction causing lateral tibial plateau fractures.
  - Forceful adduction causing medial tibial plateau fractures.

Segond Fracture

- Avulsion fracture of the lateral tibial plateau that is frequently associated with ACL disruption.[13,15]
- Mechanism of injury: Flexion of the knee with excessive internal rotation and varus stress.

Table 20.2 Schatzker classification of tibial plateau fractures

Schatzker Classification	Morphologic Description	Condyle Involved	Mechanism of Injury Energy
I	Lateral Split Fracture	Lateral Condyle	Lower
II	Lateral Split Fracture with Medial Depression (Split-Depression Fracture)	Lateral Condyle	Lower
III	Lateral Depression Fracture	Lateral Condyle	Lower
IV	Medial Condyle Fracture	Medial Condyle	High
V	Bicondylar	Medial and Lateral Condyle	High
VI	IV or V Fracture with Disruption of Metaphysis and Diaphysis	Either	High

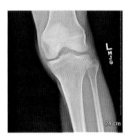

Figure 20.2 Non-displaced bicondylar tibial plateau fracture (Schatzker Class V) (image: Jeffery Hill, MD Med)

Reverse Segond Fracture

- Elliptical avulsion fracture of the medial proximal tibia associated with tears of medial meniscus and PCL.[16]
- Uncommon (0.64% of fractures seen in acute knee trauma presentations).[15] Usually found in association with other fractures in the bones of the knee.

Imaging Considerations

- Lateral tibial plateau fractures are commonly missed in the Emergency Department.[17]
- AP and lateral x-rays are the initial imaging of choice (79% sensitive for the detection of lateral tibial plateau fractures).[16]
  - Oblique views increase sensitivity to 85%.[16]
  - Plateau view: AP view with a 10° tilt to account for anterior to posterior slope of the tibial plateau.[17]
  - Layering of lipohemarthrosis on lateral x-ray is highly suggestive of fracture.[13,17]
- CT can identify fractures not seen on x-ray and assists in operative planning of severely comminuted fractures.[2,14]

Complications and Associated Injuries

- Tibial plateau fractures are often associated with ligamentous injuries and joint instability.[2]

- Peroneal nerve injuries are possible.
- Popliteal artery injuries – typically from the high energy mechanism of injury, usually associated with Schatzker type IV fractures.[2,17]
- Compartment syndrome is an uncommon complication from isolated tibial plateau fracture.[2]

Management

- Initial stabilization of fracture site with knee immobilizer and non-weight bearing status until evaluated by orthopedist.
- Non-operative management: Hinged knee brace and partial weight bearing.[17]
  - Considered for patients with minimally displaced fractures, nonambulatory patients, or low energy mechanism of injury with stable varus/valgus alignment.
- Operative management for displaced fractures or joint instability.

Tibial Spine Fracture

- Uncommon fractures of the intercondylar eminence that are more commonly seen in adolescents (8–14 years) and is roughly the equivalent of an ACL tear in an adult.[2,14]
- Examination: May have a block to full knee extension due to fracture fragment or tense hemarthrosis.[14]
- Imaging: Standard AP and lateral views are typically sufficient, but may need plateau or tunnel view to fully identify fractures.[14,18]
- Management:
  - Reduction: Extend knee to within 20° of full extension and observe for fracture reduction.[18]
  - Aspiration of hemarthrosis can improve reduction and decrease patient pain.[18]
  - Immobilization in 0–20° of flexion with knee immobilizer.

Knee Dislocation

Classification (Kennedy Classification) based on direction of tibia in relation to the femur – Anterior (most common), Posterior, Lateral, Medial, Rotatory (rare).[2]

Mechanism of Injury

- High-energy: MVC with dashboard causing axial load on flexed knee (2/3 of cases), falls from height.[2]
- Low-energy: Rotational component, patients with morbid obesity are at increased risk.

Examination

- May see obvious deformity, severe ecchymosis, and swelling, but should consider any grossly unstable knee following a trauma to be a dislocation until proven otherwise.[2]
  - 50% of injuries spontaneously reduce prior to presentation.
- Distal vascular exam is crucial, but may be insufficient for detecting arterial injuries.
  - Sensitivity of pulse exam for popliteal injury is 80%.[19]

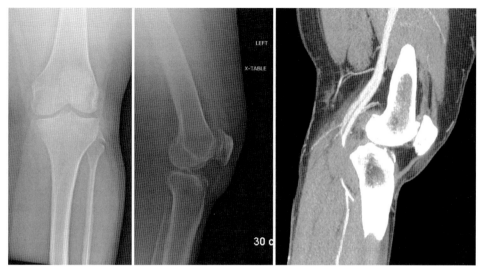

Figure 20.3 Obese patient with low mechanism of injury and diminished lower extremity pulses on exam. AP and Lateral Knee films with tibial spine and proximal fibula fracture. CTA of lower extremity with complete occlusion of popliteal artery (images courtesy of Peter Toth, MD)

Associated Injuries (Figure 20.3)

- Popliteal artery injuries (dissection, thrombosis):
  - Popliteal artery injuries are common (up to 50% incidence) with anterior/posterior dislocations.[20]
  - Have a high index of suspicion and a low threshold for ordering CT angiography.
  - 86% of patients with a delay in repair >8 hours undergo amputation.[2]
- Nerve injuries: Tibial and common peroneal nerve injuries in 16–40% of cases.[2]
- Severe ligamentous and soft tissue disruption are likely with any knee dislocation.

Imaging

- AP and lateral x-rays may be normal in appearance if dislocation reduced prior to presentation.
- CT angiography:
  - Should be performed for all patients with signs of ischemia prior to reduction, even if pulse returns to normal after reduction.[2,21]
  - Consider for all patients with suspected dislocation, even if pulse examination is normal.[2]
- Intraoperative angiography: For patients with persistent signs of ischemia after reduction.[2,21]

Initial Management

- Reduction by exerting longitudinal traction on the lower leg and directing the tibia anteriorly or posteriorly (depending on the initial direction of the dislocation).[2]
- Post-reduction, splint with a long leg posterior splint in 15–20° of flexion.[2,20]

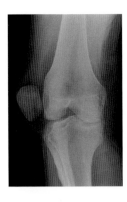

Figure 20.4 Patella dislocation (image courtesy of Hellerhoff, reproduced here under CC BY-SA 3.0 license http://creativecommons.org/licenses/by-sa/3.0)

Definitive Management

Surgical repair emergently for irreducible dislocations, open fracture/dislocations, or persistent vascular compromise.[14,20]

Patella Dislocations

- Lateral dislocation is most common (Figure 20.4).
- Mechanism of injury: Direct blow (less common) or twisting motion of lower extremity with foot planted and knee flexed.[2,22]
- Imaging:
  - Diagnosis is typically apparent based on clinical examination alone if patella is still displaced.
  - Post-reduction x-ray is recommended to identify associated fractures.
- Initial management:
  - Lateral dislocations reduced by flexing the ipsilateral hip while extending the knee and pushing the dislocated patella medially.[2]
  - Horizontal or intra-articular dislocations require operative reduction.[2]
  - Post-reduction, place patient in a knee immobilizer with full weight bearing and follow up with orthopedic surgery.[2]

Patella Fractures

Mechanism of injury is most commonly from a direct blow to the patella. It can also be indirect from contraction of the quadriceps.[2,23]

Examination – Superior Displacement of the Patella ("High Riding")

Test extensor function of the quadriceps to ensure it is intact.

Imaging – AP, Lateral, and "Sunrise" Views (Figure 20.5)

Displacement seen best on lateral view and correlates with disruption of extensor function.[23]

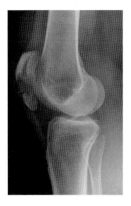

Figure 20.5 Horizontal patella fracture (image courtesy of Hellerhoff, reproduced here under CC BY-SA 3.0 license http://creativecommons.org/licenses/by-sa/3.0)

Initial Management

- Consider aspiration of tense hemarthrosis.
- Splint in full extension with knee immobilizer or posterior long leg splint.[2] Weight bear as tolerated in full extension.[2]

Definitive Management

Nonoperative management for those patients with intact extensor function, intact articular surface, and <2 mm of displacement.[2,23]

Evaluation for an Open Knee Joint

Any disruption of the skin surface near the knee joint should raise suspicion for the possibility of an open knee joint. These can occur as a result of simple lacerations, open fractures, or projectiles.

- Patients with open joints should receive antibiotics and undergo urgent irrigation and debridement to decrease the possibility of septic arthritis.[24,25]

Saline Load Test

- Injection of sterile saline into the knee joint (either superomedial or inferomedial approach) until saline comes through the open wound or unable to continue to inject due to high pressure.[24]
- The mean volume needed to detect an open knee joint is 64 mL in the inferomedial approach and 95 mL in the superomedial approach, but up to 175 mL of saline may be needed in order to detect 99% of open knee joints.
- With advent of CT, saline load test is not as commonly used.

CT

- Intraarticular air on CT is diagnostic of open knee joint. CT has a higher sensitivity and specificity than the saline load test and is recommended as the diagnostic modality of choice for open joints.[25]
- One study found that patients with an absence of intra-articular air and no other signs of open joint did not experience septic arthritis.[25]

Proximal Third Tibial Fractures

Subcondylar tibial fractures are typically transversely or obliquely oriented and most importantly can extend intra-articularly and can be associated with tibial plateau fractures.[2]

Initial Management

- Long leg posterior splint and orthopedic consultation.
- Non-operative management for patients with non-displaced and non-angulated transverse fractures.[2,26]

Tibial Shaft Fractures

Tibial shaft fractures are the most common leg fracture, and they can be associated with vascular injury, although this is rare.[2]

Anatomy

- The interosseous membrane is a fibrous structure connecting most of the tibia and fibula, stabilizing their relative positions. Either the fibula or tibia may be fractured independently; however, the most common injury pattern is a both bone spiral fracture.[27]
- Concurrent fractures of the distal tibia or deltoid ligament in combination with a proximal fibula fracture is concerning for interosseous membrane injury (Maisonneuve fracture) which requires surgical repair to stabilize the ankle mortise.[28]

Imaging

AP x-rays are adequate for diagnosis of mid-shaft injuries.

Vascular Injuries – Compartment Syndrome

- Risk of compartment syndrome is 4.3% after closed tibia fractures (highest risk fracture).
  - This occurs most commonly in the anterior compartment, with deep peroneal nerve compression and neuropraxia.
- If the compartment pressure is greater than the venous pressure, there is a risk of neurovascular compromise and high morbidity.
- Compartment pressures >30 mmHg or delta pressure (calculated by subtracting the compartment pressure from the diastolic blood pressure) <30 mm Hg is suggestive of compartment syndrome.[29,30]
- In an awake patient, increasing pain is concerning. If comatose, use clinical suspicion with compartment pressure assessment and specialist consultation.
- Open fractures are still at risk for compartment syndrome.
- Patients at risk for compartment syndrome include younger patients, and missed compartment syndrome occurs more often in comatose and intoxicated patients.[31]
- Penetration injury: ABI >0.9 and absence of soft or hard signs of vascular injury can reliably exclude vascular injury.[32]

- Indications for admission include open fractures, concerns for compartment syndrome, or neurovascular compromise. Immobilization in a long posterior splint is warranted.

Proximal Fibula Fractures

- Rarely isolated fracture; consider concomitant ankle fracture or knee ligamentous injury.
- Management depends on other injuries, and isolated proximal fibula fractures rarely need operative repair.
- Patients are usually appropriate for early mobilization.[2]

Ankle

The articular surface (mortise) consists of the medial malleolus (tibia), lateral malleolus (fibula), and posterior malleolus (tibia), making the trimalleolar structure which articulates inferiorly with the talus.

- Most common injury is an inversion injury with progressive ligamentous to bony injury.
- Treatment based on radiographic and clinical stability and amount of dislocation (Table 20.3).
- Bimalleolar fractures (medial + lateral) typically require operative therapy and non-weight bearing status.
- Axial load intra-articular fractures (pilon/plafond) require orthopedic evaluation and surgical intervention. Highly variable fracture patterns may require ORIF or ex-fix depending on soft tissue swelling and extent of displacement.
- Non-displaced medial malleolar fracture

  - Management includes weight bearing as tolerated if the joint is stable. If the joint is unstable or significant pain is present, place in a splint and discuss need for non-weight bearing to prevent further articular damage.

- Displaced fractures

  - If widened or unstable, reduce, place in short leg splint, and consult orthopedics.

Table 20.3 Ankle dislocation types

Dislocation Type	Associated Injuries	Reduction Method	Caveats
Lateral	Medial malleolar fracture or Deltoid ligament rupture > Lateral malleolar fracture	Traction and Medial Manipulation	Evaluate vascular integrity, posterior splint
Posterior	Posterior malleolar fracture, capsular tears	Plantar flexion, anterior traction	Posterior splint
Anterior	Distal tibia ± malleolar fracture	Dorsiflexion and downward traction	
Superior	Capsular Disruption	Traction	Rare
Tibiotalar Dislocations	Capsular Disruption	Traction, as above	

Table 20.4 Splints of the lower leg

Splint Type	Splint Anatomy	Injury Indications
Posterior Short Leg	90° ankle flexion, toes to proximal calf posteriorly	Distal leg fractures (medial/lateral malleolar), Talus/Calcaneus fractures
Equinus Splint	Forced plantar flexion by anterior splint	Achilles tendon rupture

Imaging

- AP, Lateral, and Oblique views are required to visualize the mortise.
- >7 mm of space of the medial malleolus indicates instability.
- Weight-bearing views can help establish ligamentous instability if the mortise widens.[33]

Isolated Distal Fibular Fractures

- Treatment based upon stability of the deltoid ligament medially (Table 20.4).
- Weight-bearing with less than 7 mm mortise widening can be treated conservatively.[33]

Foot

Anatomically divided into hindfoot (calcaneus, talus), midfoot (cuboid, navicular, cuneiforms), and forefoot (metatarsals, phalanges) (Figure 20.6).

Imaging

- AP, lateral, and 45° oblique x-rays.
- On AP, the medial 2nd metatarsal should align with the medial 2nd cuneiform.
- On the oblique view, the medial 3rd cuneiform should be aligned to the medial 3rd metatarsal.

Hindfoot

Talus Fractures

- Fractures often occur from translational load or with high energy mechanism and are associated with other injuries including ankle dislocation.
- Head, neck, and body fractures common (see Table 20.5 for Hawkins classifications).
- High risk of concurrent foot fractures, and CT is recommended for diagnosis and delineation.
- Subtalar dislocations:
  - High energy mechanism injury.
  - Medial (72%) > Lateral (22%).
  - 15% open fractures.
  - 75% have successful closed reduction under anesthesia.[35]
  - Short leg splint should be used for immobilization.

Table 20.5 Hawkins classifications of talar neck fractures[36]

Talar Neck Fracture	Description	Risk of AVN	ED Management
Hawkins I	Nondisplaced	0–13%	Posterior splint, CT, non-weight-bearing
Hawkins II	Subtalar Dislocation	20–50%	Reduction, consult
Hawkins III	Subtalar and Tibiotalar Dislocation	20–100%	Reduction, consult
Hawkins IV	Subtalar, Tibiotalar, and Talonavicular Dislocation	70–100%	Reduction, consult

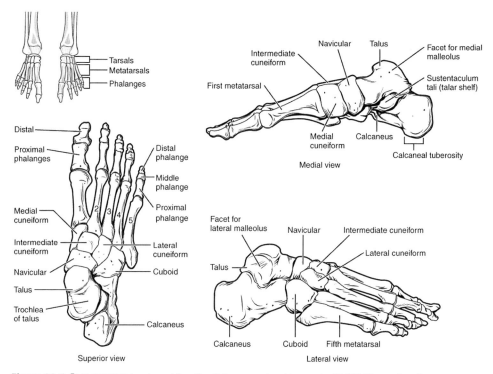

Figure 20.6 Foot anatomy (courtesy of OpenStax College, reproduced here under CC BY 3.0 license (http://creativecommons.org/licenses/by/3.0)[34]

Calcaneal Fractures

- Primarily an axial load injury associated with high morbidity.
- These are often intra-articular (75%) and depressed (75%).[37]
- Consider other axial load injuries and polytrauma. May be associated with spinal compression fracture (7.5%).[38]
- Pain out of proportion to exam is hallmark symptom and may require admission for pain control. Also consider compartment syndrome of the foot (associated with 10% of fractures).
- AP and lateral x-rays are adequate for most cases; if the provider has concern for intra-articular (primarily subtalar) extension, CT should be obtained.

- Bohler's angle for fracture is measured on lateral foot x-ray with angle made between lines connecting the posterior and superior calcaneus with the superior and anterior aspects of the calcaneus. Normal angle should be 20–40°. Less than 20° is concerning for fracture.[39]
- Treatment includes immobilization with posterior ankle splint, non-weight bearing, and orthopedics referral.

Midfoot

Cuboid, Navicular, Cuneiform Fractures
- Diagnosed with typical AP, lateral, oblique imaging.
- Navicular dorsal avulsion fracture most common.[2]

  . Nondisplaced, nonarticular fractures with weight bearing as tolerated.

- Cuboid and cuneiform fractures often occur concurrently.

  . Often due to direct crush injuries.
  . Nondisplaced fractures should be non-weight bearing.
  . Displaced fractures will require operative fixation.

Lisfranc Fracture
- The Lisfranc joint includes the articulation of the first, second, and 3rd–5th tarsometatarsal joints.
- Primarily an axial load injury but can be low impact mechanism with forced dorsiflexion and abduction/external rotation.
- Instability of the mid foot after disruption of the joint.
- These are fractures that often go undiagnosed on an initial visit (20–50%).[40]
- Plain film radiography is 84% sensitive for diagnosis. CT increases sensitivity and is the diagnostic gold standard.[41]
- High miss rate can lead to rapid osteoarthritis and chronic pain.
- Operative management can prevent early osteoarthritis.[42]

Forefoot Fractures
- Imaging: AP, lateral and oblique views as above.
- Metatarsal fractures:

  . Mechanisms

    – Direct trauma, dorsiflexion, rotation, stress fractures.
    – First metatarsal takes ~50% of weight and is a higher consequence fracture.

  . Closed fractures

    – Single non-displaced distal or shaft metatarsal fracture or displaced <3–4mm or angulated >10 degrees.[43]
      ○ Treatment with hard shoe and outpatient follow up.

- Displaced >3–4 mm
  - Closed reduction with application of a posterior splint.
  - Non-weight bearing until outpatient follow up.

. Proximal 5th metatarsal fractures

- Jones fractures
  - Meta-diaphyseal 5th phalanx fracture, thought to be due to adduction and plantar flexion injury.[44]
  - High chance of nonunion (15–30%) due to watershed vascular supply.
  - Treatment is non-weight bearing, referral for likely operative screw, short leg splint.[45]

. Pseudo Jones fractures

- Fracture of the proximal tuberosity of the 5th metatarsal (proximal to articulation with 4th metatarsal).
- Treatment is a hard-soled shoe, early return to activity. If displaced, has >30% articular surface involvement with step off, or pain precludes weight bearing, treat with splint, crutches, and referral.

. Diaphyseal stress fractures

- 1.5 cm from ligamentous attachment. Typically with a less acute presentation.

Phalanx Fractures

- Most common forefoot fracture.
- Phalanx fractures can be buddy taped (gauze between toes, tape to adjacent toe) with excellent results with conservative management.[46]
- 1st phalanx fractures are associated with greater morbidity. Treatment includes buddy taping and hard sole shoe. A posterior splint may be applied if significant pain is present, and the patient should be referred to orthopedics if more than 25% of the articular surface is involved.
- If displaced, digital block and traction reduction followed by taping as above.

Pitfalls

- Knee dislocations spontaneously reduce 50% of the time and can have normal plain film radiographs.
- Failing to look for lipohemarthrosis on plain film x-rays (may miss occult fractures).
- Failing to evaluate for syndesmotic disruption (by compressing the proximal lower leg) in patients with ankle fractures or sprains.

Key Points
- Have a high clinical suspicion for knee dislocation and pursue CT imaging in patients with a concerning story, completely unstable knees, or vascular exam abnormalities.

- Tibial plateau fractures are frequently missed by plain film radiographs; consider CT imaging in patients with effusion/lipohemarthrosis.
- Midfoot pain after axial load injury is concerning for Lisfranc disruption; use CT, weight bearing images, and splint if concerned.
- Proximal 5th metatarsal fractures should be carefully evaluated for extension through the metatarsal to distinguish between Jones' fractures (high morbidity) and Pseudo Jones' fracture (weight bearing, good recovery).

References

1. Karadsheh M, Taylor B. Femoral shaft fractures. orthobullets.com Web site. www.orthobullets.com/trauma/1040/femoral-shaft-fractures. 2019. Accessed March 29, 2019.

2. Simon R, Sherman S, Koenigsknecht S. *Emergency Orthopedics: The Extremities*, 5th ed. New York, NY: McGraw-Hill Publishing; 2007.

3. Tornetta PI, Kain MSH, Creevy WR. Diagnosis of femoral neck fractures in patients with a femoral shaft fracture: improvement with a standard protocol. *J Bone Joint Surg Am.* 2007;89(1):39–43.

4. Day M. Distal femur fractures. orthobullets.com Web site. www.orthobullets.com/trauma/1041/distal-femur-fractures?expandLeftMenu=true. 2019. Accessed March 29, 2019.

5. Gangavalli AK, Nwachuku, CO. Management of distal femur fractures in adults. *Orthop Clin North Am.* 2016;47(1):85–96.

6. Even J, Richards J, Crosby CG, et al. Preoperative skeletal versus cutaneous traction for femoral shaft fractures treated within 24 hours. *J Orthop Trauma.* 2012;26(10):177–82.

7. Bumpass DB, Ricci WM, McAndrew CM, Gardner MJ. A prospective study of pain reduction and knee dysfunction comparing femoral skeletal traction and splinting in adult trauma patients. *J Orthop Trauma.* 2015;29(2):112–18.

8. Wood SP, Vrahas M, Wedel SK. Femur fracture immobilization with traction splints in multisystem trauma

patients. *Prehosp Emerg Care.* 2009;7(2):241–43.

9. Althausen PL, Hak DJ. Lower extremity traction pins: indications, technique, and complications. *Am J Orthop.* 2002;31(1):43–47.

10. Austin DC, Donegan D, Mehta S. Low complication rates associated with the application of lower extremity traction pins. *J Orthop Trauma.* 2015;29(8):e259–65.

11. Hoytema van Konijnenburg EM, Vrolijk-Bosschaart TF, Bakx R, Van Rijn RR. Paediatric femur fractures at the emergency department: accidental or not? *BJR.* 2016;89(1061):20150822–27.

12. Thomas S, Rosenfield N, Leventhal J, Markowitz R. Long-bone fractures in young children: distinguishing accidental injuries from child abuse. *Pediatrics.* 1991;88(3):471–76.

13. Allen D. History and physical examination of the knee. orthobullets.com Web site. www.orthobullets.com/sports/3003/history-and-physical-exam-of-the-knee. 2016. Accessed September 11, 2017.

14. Lyn E, Pallin D, Antosia R. Knee and lower leg. In: Rosen P, Marx JA, Hockberger RS, Walls RM, Adams J, eds., *Rosen's Emergency Medicine Concepts and Clinical Practice*, 6th ed. Philadelpha, PA: Mosby Elsevier; 2006, pp. 770–807.

15. Peltola EK, Lindahl J, Koskinen SK. The reverse Segond fracture: not associated with knee dislocation and rarely with posterior cruciate ligament tear. *Emerg Radiol.* 2014;21(3):245–49.

16. Pulfrey S, Lahiffe B. Two fractures of the lower extremity not to miss in the emergency department. *Can Fam Physician*. 2013;59(10):1069–72.

17. Karadsheh M. Tibial plateau Fractures. orthobullets.com Web site. www.orthobullets.com/trauma/1044/tibial-plateau-fractures. 2019. Accessed March 29, 2019.

18. Karadsheh M. Tibial eminence fracture. orthobullets.com Web site. www.orthobullets.com/pediatrics/4022/tibial-eminence-fracture. Accessed September 12, 2017.

19. Green NE, Allen BL. Vascular injuries associated with dislocation of the knee. *J Bone Joint Surg Am*. 1977;59(2):236–39.

20. Patel A. Knee dislocation. orthobullets.com Web site. www.orthobullets.com/trauma/1043/knee-dislocation. 2019. Accessed March 29, 2019.

21. Barnes CJ, Pietrobon, R, Higgins, LD. Does the pulse examination in patients with traumatic knee dislocation predict a surgical arterial injury? *A meta-analysis*. J Trauma. 2002;53(6):1109–14.

22. Krause E, Lin C-W, Ortega H, Reid S. Pediatric lateral patellar dislocation: is there a role for plain radiography in the emergency department? *JEM*. 2013;44(6):1126–31.

23. Abbasi D. Patella fracture. orthobullets.com Web site. www.orthobullets.com/trauma/1042/patella-fracture. 2018. Accessed March 29, 2019.

24. Nord RM, Quach T, Walsh M, Pereira D, Tejwani NC. Detection of traumatic arthrotomy of the knee using the saline solution load test. *J Bone Joint Surg Am*. 2009;91(1):66–70.

25. Sanjit R, Konda MD, Roy I, et al. Open knee joint injuries: an evidence-based approach to management. *Bull Hosp Joint Dis*. 2014;72(1):61–69.

26. Sheth U. Proximal third tibia fracture. orthobullets.com Web site. www.orthobullets.com/trauma/1062/proximal-third-tibia-fracture?

27. expandLeftMenu=true. 2019. Accessed March 29, 2019.

27. Larsen P, Elsoe R, Hansen S, et al. Incidence and epidemiology of tibial shaft fractures. *Injury*. 2015;46(4):746–50.

28. Stufkens SA, van den Bekerom MPJ, Doornberg JN, Niek van Dijk C, Kloen P. Evidence-based treatment of Maisonneuve fractures. *J Foot Ankle Surg*. 2011;50(1):62–67.

29. Nelson JA. Compartment pressure measurements have poor specificity for compartment syndrome in the traumatized limb. *J Emerg Med*. 2013;44(5):1039–44.

30. von Keudell AG, Weaver MJ, Appleton PT, et al. Diagnosis and treatment of acute extremity compartment syndrome. *Lancet*. 2015;386(10000):1299–310.

31. McQueen MM, Duckworth AD, Aitken SA, et al. Predictors of compartment syndrome after tibial fracture. *J Orthop Trauma*. 2015;29(10):451–55.

32. deSouza IS, Benabbas R, McKee S, et al. Accuracy of physical examination, ankle-brachial index, and ultrasonography in the diagnosis of arterial injury in patients with penetrating extremity trauma: a systematic review and meta-analysis. *Acad Emerg Med*. 2017;24(8):994–1017.

33. Seidel A, Krause F, Weber M. Weightbearing vs gravity stress radiographs for stability evaluation of supination-external rotation fractures of the ankle. *Foot Ankle Int*. 2017;38(7):736–44.

34. Bones of the Foot. Anatomy & Physiology, Connexions Web site. http://cnx.org/content/col11496/1.6/. June 19, 2013. Accessed March 18, 2018.

35. Byrd Z, Ebraheim M, Weston J, Liu J, Ebraheim N. Isolated subtalar dislocation. *Orthopedics*. 2013;36:714–20.

36. Hawkins L. Fractures of the neck of the talus. *J Bone Joint Surg Am*. 1970;52(5):991–1002.

37. Perron A, Brady W. Evaluation and management of the high-risk orthopedic emergency. *Emer Med Clin North Am*. 2003;21(1):159–204.

38. Walters JL, Gangopadhyay P, Malay DS. Association of calcaneal and spinal fractures. *J Foot Ankle Surg.* 2014;53 (3):279–81.

39. Kang O, Amini B. Böhler angle. radiopaedia.org Web site. https://radiopaedia.org/articles/bohler-angle-2. Accessed October 29, 2017.

40. Rammelt S, Schneiders W, Schikore H, et al. Primary open reduction and fixation compared with delayed corrective arthrodesis in the treatment of tarsometatarsal (Lisfranc) fracture dislocation. *J Bone Joint Surg Br.* 2008;90 (11):1499–506.

41. Haapamaki VV, Kiuru MJ, Koskinen SK. Ankle and foot injuries: analysis of MDCT findings. *AJR Am J Roentgenol.* 2004;183 (3):615–22.

42. Myerson MS, Fisher RT, Burgess AR, Kenzora JE. Fracture dislocations of the tarsometatarsal joints: end results correlated with pathology and treatment. *Foot Ankle.* 1986;6(5):225–42.

43. Hatch R, Alsobrook J, Clugston J. Diagnosis and management of metatarsal fractures. *Am Fam Phys.* 2007;76 (6):817–26.

44. Theodorou DJ, Theodorou SJ, Kakitsubata Y, Botte MJ, and Resnick D. Fractures of proximal portion of fifth metatarsal bone: anatomic and imaging evidence of a pathogenesis of avulsion of the plantar aponeurosis and the short peroneal muscle tendon. *Radiology.* 2003;226(3):857–65.

45. Metzl J, Olson K, Davis WH, et al. Clinical and radiographic comparison of two hardware systems used to treat Jones fracture of the fifth metatarsal. *Foot Ankle Int.* 2013;34(7):956–61.

46. Van Vliet-Koppert S, Cakir H, Van Lieshout E, et al. Demographics and functional outcome of toe fractures. *J Foot Ankle Surg.* 2011;50:307–10.

Chapter 21

Burns and Electrical Injuries

Ashley Brady

Burns

In the United States alone, burns are responsible for 450,000 emergency department visits, 45,000 hospitalizations, and 3,500 deaths every year.[1] Roughly half of those hospital admissions are to specialized regional burn centers.[2] In 2009, there were 128 regional burn centers in 43 states, and 40% of admissions were due to fire or flame burns, while another 30% were due to scald injuries. The majority of scald injuries occur in children under the age of 5 years.[3,4] Therefore, understanding the management of the burn patient is essential to all emergency physicians. Not only do burns cause local damage to the affected site, but large burns can also result in fluid and electrolyte abnormalities, metabolic acidosis, inflammatory response, and even myocardial dysfunction in severe cases.[5]

Pathophysiology[6]

- Local tissue damage is classified into three zones from the center out, termed the zone of coagulation, zone of stasis, and zone of hyperemia (Figure 21.1).

    . *Zone of coagulation* is the area of maximal injury containing irreversible tissue coagulation and necrosis.

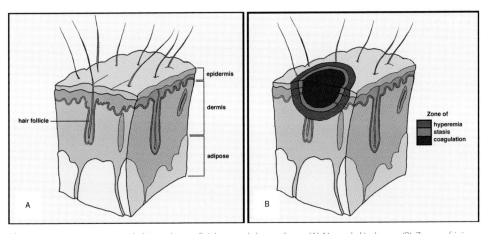

Figure 21.1 Layers in normal skin and superficial second-degree burn. (A) Normal skin layers. (B) Zones of injury with a superficial second-degree burn. The central coagulation zone is irreversibly damaged tissue. The zone of stasis may progress to necrosis or may recover, depending on good resuscitation and prevention of infection (illustrations by Robert Amaral, reproduced with permission from *Color Atlas of Emergency Trauma, Second Edition*)

- *Zone of stasis* has decreased tissue perfusion but is potentially reversible. The tissue is at high risk for irreversible damage if any additional insults occur and is the area most targeted by therapies.
- *Zone of hyperemia* is the outermost zone and has increased perfusion initially. Tissue in this zone should recover.

- Burn injuries cause the release of cytokines and other inflammatory mediators to the site of the injury. However, in large burns, typically >20–30%, this inflammatory response can have systemic effects. Capillaries become more permeable, and fluids are lost to the interstitial space. Vasoconstriction occurs peripherally and in the splanchnic circulation, in addition to decreased overall myocardial contractility causing diffuse hypoperfusion. Bronchoconstriction and acute respiratory distress syndrome may also occur.

ED Evaluation and Management

- As with all trauma evaluations, airway, breathing, circulation, disability, and exposure must be quickly evaluated in a primary survey.
- Once the primary survey is completed and the patient has been stabilized, a complete secondary survey should be performed.
- Remember to assess for all traumatic injuries, in addition to the burn, as many of these patients have been thrown, fallen, or were even in a motor vehicle accident.
- Hypotension is rare in a burn patient. Any patient with hemodynamic instability and burn requires evaluation and resuscitation for the associated type of shock.

Airway Management

- Always consider an inhalational injury, as airway swelling can occur very quickly.
- Indicators for a possible inhalation injury include: burns to the face or neck, singed nasal or facial hairs, hoarse voice, soot in the airway, dyspnea, wheezing, or stridor.[1,2,5]
- If any of the above indicators are present and there is concern for inhalational injury, early intubation is recommended.
- Other therapies that may be helpful are humidified supplemental oxygen and bronchodilators. However, do not delay intubation to attempt these therapies if there is concern for significant inhalational injury.[5]
- Always consider carbon monoxide and cyanide poisoning in patients presenting with burns from fires, especially house fires or any other enclosed space.[5]

Estimating Burn Size and Depth

- It is important to estimate burn size and depth as it will help guide management in the emergency department (Table 21.1 and Figures 21.2–21.4).
- When estimating total body surface area (TBSA) burned, only partial thickness and full thickness burns are included.[7,8]
- The "rule of nines" provides a quick estimation of TBSA burned in adults (Figure 21.5).
- For children, the Lund-Browder diagram is available to help estimate TBSA (Figure 21.6).
- Another quick estimation is to use the palm of the patient's hand as approximately 1% TBSA.[1,5]

Table 21.1 Burn classification

Depth of Burn	Structures Involved	Clinical Features
Superficial	Epidermis	Pain, erythema (similar to a sunburn), dry
Superficial partial thickness	Epidermis + superficial dermis	Intense pain, clear blisters, weeping
Deep partial thickness	Epidermis + deep dermis	Intense pain, red, clear, and hemorrhagic blisters, weeping, mottled skin, nonblanching
Full thickness	Epidermis + dermis + fat/muscle/nerve	No pain in the primary burn area (surrounding areas painful), white, charring, leathery

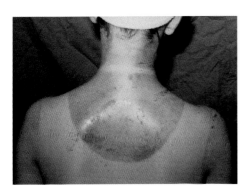

Figure 21.2 Sunburn is a typical first-degree burn. The skin is erythematous and painful, but without blistering (reproduced with permission from *Color Atlas of Emergency Trauma, Second Edition*)

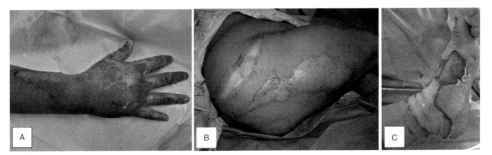

Figure 21.3 Deep second-degree burns. (A) Superficial and deep second-degree burn from hot-water scald to the hand. (B) Deep second-degree burn with central third-degree burn. Notice the classic color differentiation. (C) Foot scald injury consisting of largely nonblanching pale appearing third-degree burn and erythematous deep second-degree burn over the medial forefoot (reproduced with permission from *Color Atlas of Emergency Trauma, Second Edition*)

Fluid Resuscitation

- Patients with TBSA >20% will need fluid resuscitation.[9] The area affected no longer has the normal skin layer which acts as a semipermeable barrier to help avoid fluid loss through evaporation.[5,10] Fluid resuscitation is also beneficial to prevent burn shock from the systemic inflammatory reaction and prevent hypoperfusion to end organs and salvageable burn tissue.[11] However, burn patients should not be hypotensive. If so, other etiologies of shock need to be investigated, such as cyanide poisoning, sepsis, trauma, hemorrhage, or myocardial infarction.[9]

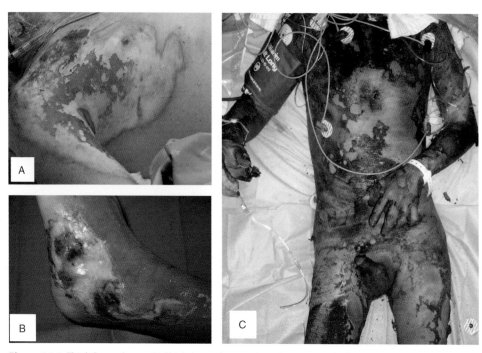

Figure 21.4 Third-degree burns. (A) Third-degree burn with its characteristic leathery appearance and lack of tissue edema. (B) Third-degree burn of the foot from hot cooking-oil splash. (C) Fatal 95% TBSA fourth-degree burn from a household fire (reproduced with permission from *Color Atlas of Emergency Trauma, Second Edition*)

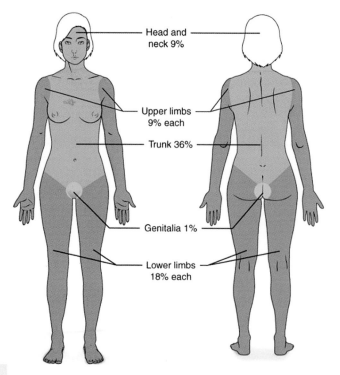

Head and neck 9%

Upper limbs 9% each

Trunk 36%

Genitalia 1%

Lower limbs 18% each

Figure 21.5 "Rule of Nines" to estimate adult TBSA burned (from https://cnx.org/contents/ FPtK1zmh@6.27:CHzzQ6Vf@4/ Diseases-Disorders-and-Injuries-of-the-Integumentary-System; reproduced here under CC BY 4.0 license https:// creativecommons.org/licenses/by/ 4.0/)

Estimating Percent Total Body Surface Area in Children Affected by Burns

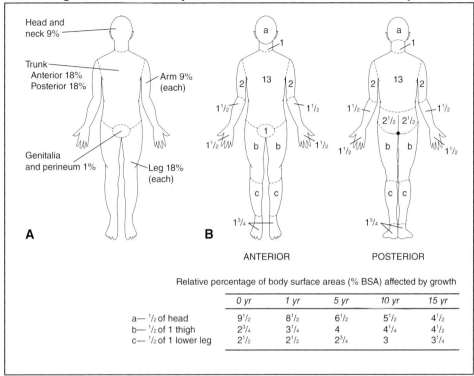

(A) Rule of "nines"
(B) Lund-Browder diagram for estimating extent of burns

Figure 21.6 Lund-Browder diagram (image courtesy of the US Department of Health & Human Services, at www.remm.nlm.gov/burns.htm)

Parkland Formula[1]
24 hr replacement fluids (L) = 4 mL × kg × % TBSA burned 1st half given over 8 hours, then the remaining over the next 16 hours

Brooke Formula[1]
24 hr replacement fluids (L) = 2 mL × kg × TBSA burned 1st half given over 8 hours, then the remaining over the next 16 hours

ISR "Rule of 10"[12]
Hourly fluid rate (mL/hr) = TBSA to the nearest 10 × 10 (for patients between 40–80 kg) For every 10 kg >80 kg, add 100 mL/hr

Figure 21.7 Burn resuscitation formulas

- Intravenous access is ideally placed in an unaffected area but may be placed through burned skin if necessary. Once obtained, the access must be sufficiently secured, which may require suturing if in a burned area.[10]
- Several different formulas exist to calculate the rate of the fluid resuscitation (Figure 21.7).[11–13]
- Lactated ringers (LR) is generally preferred over normal saline. LR is more similar to human plasma, while normal saline is less physiologic, with greater risk of metabolic

Box 21.1 Escharotomy Considerations[14]

Keys to Performing an Escharotomy:

- Full thickness burns require no anesthesia, but deep partial thickness burns may require analgesia.
- Incise just through the skin until the subcutaneous fat is exposed and the eschar is released. This should result in only minimal bleeding that can be controlled by local pressure.
- Always reassess perfusion after the procedure to ensure adequate release.
- Wound care over the escharotomy incisions is the same as to the adjacent burned tissue.

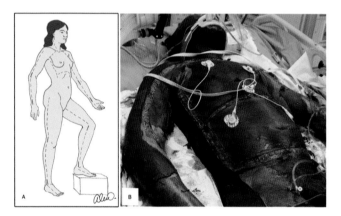

Figure 21.8 Escharotomy for circumferential burn. (A) Illustration of the recommended escharotomy incisions. (B) Truncal and extremity escharotomies in a household fire victim (reproduced with permission from *Color Atlas of Emergency Trauma, Second Edition*, illustration at (A) by Alexis Demetriades)

and renal disturbance. Therefore, in large volumes normal saline can induce a hyperchloremic acidosis.[11-13]

- Patients receiving fluid resuscitation should be monitored for signs of volume overload, especially concerning the development of pulmonary edema or acute respiratory distress syndrome, or in the chronically volume overloaded patient.
- A urinary catheter should be placed for adequate input and output monitoring. The goal urine output is 1 mL/kg/hr.[5]

Escharotomies

- Circumferential burns may require an escharotomy in the emergency department (Box 21.1 and Figure 21.8). This can be assessed for by delayed capillary refill, decreased pulse oximetry distal to the burned area (<95% in a non-hypoxic patient), decreased Doppler signals, and absence of a palpable pulse in the affected extremity. If the patient is awake and alert, he/she may also complain of increasing pain, numbness, or tingling. Loss of motor activity and loss of pulses are late signs, but, if present, should prompt immediate escharotomy.[14]
- Trunk escharotomies may also be required if the patient cannot be adequately ventilated due to chest constriction or if abdominal compartment syndrome develops. It is

important to routinely monitor a patient's ventilation status, including airway pressures, as well as oxygenation, and measure bladder pressures in patients that are at risk.[2,5,14–16]

- To perform an escharotomy, standard sterile precautions should be used. For extremities, use a scalpel to create an incision on both the lateral and medial aspects from 1 cm proximal to 1 cm distal of the constricted tissue. These incisions may need to cross joints. Be very careful in these areas to avoid damaging underlying blood vessels and nerves. For the trunk, create an incision in the anterior axillary line bilaterally from the clavicle to below the costal margin or to the entire abdomen as needed. Then create a transverse incision to connect the two incisions at the superior chest and subcostal margin.[14]

Carbon Monoxide Poisoning

- Carbon monoxide poisoning should always be considered in burn patients, especially those with inhalational injuries and any patient from a house fire or enclosed space.
- There are no specific symptoms or signs for carbon monoxide poisoning, and patients presenting with trauma and burn injuries may be even more difficult to assess. The clinician must maintain a high degree of clinical suspicion in these patients. Patients may present with mild headache, confusion, chest pain, ataxia, seizures, hypotension, tachypnea, tachycardia, and even coma.[5]
- For diagnosis, a carboxyhemoglobin level should be obtained. A co-oximeter can also be used. VBG or ABG can be used. Pulse oximetry cannot be relied upon because it does not differentiate between the wavelengths for carboxyhemoglobin and oxyhemoglobin and may give a falsely normal oxygen saturation. In severe poisoning, the patient may also have an elevated lactate, troponin, and anion gap metabolic acidosis.[5]
- Treatment is supplemental oxygen. Hyperbaric oxygen can be considered in patients with neurologic symptoms, levels >25%, and pregnant women with levels >15%; however, this may be difficult given the patient's need for trauma evaluation and burn care management.[5]

Cyanide Poisoning

- Cyanide can be found in plastics, wool, nylon, silk, polyurethane, and several other chemicals. Therefore, when any of these products burn, they can release cyanide into the air, causing inhalational exposure.[5]
- Cyanide poisoning should be considered in all burn patients presenting from a house fire or other enclosed space.
- Clinical features are nonspecific but include mild headache, dyspnea, seizures, coma, apnea, tachycardia, hypotension, and even cardiac arrest.[5]
- Diagnosis is often clinical. A cyanide level can be obtained; however, treatment should be initiated immediately if the patient is believed to have significant cyanide toxicity. Laboratory abnormalities include elevated lactate (>10 demonstrates sensitivity over 85%) and anion gap metabolic acidosis. Patients with significant carbon monoxide poisoning are more likely to have cyanide toxicity as well.[5]
- Treatment includes supplemental oxygen and the use of a cyanide treatment kit. Patients are given 10 mL of intravenous 3% sodium nitrite followed by 50 mL of intravenous

> **Box 21.2   Burn Center Considerations**
>
> Indications for Transfer to a Regional Burn Center:
>
> - Any inhalational injury
> - >20% TBSA burned in adults
> - >10% TBSA burned in children or elderly
> - >5% TBSA full thickness burn
> - Any burns involving the face, genitalia, hands, feet, or over major joints
> - Circumferential burns
> - Additional traumatic injuries or patients with other significant comorbidities

25% sodium thiosulfate solution. Sodium thiosulfate can then be repeated. Caution must be taken as nitrites can cause severe hypotension and methemoglobinemia. Sodium nitrite is contraindicated if carbon monoxide toxicity is present or suspected. Given this side-effect, 5 g intravenous hydroxocobalamin given over 30 minutes is first line if available. It is presumed to have less side-effects than nitrites but can also cause transient hypotension and anaphylaxis. However, it is more expensive and has a short shelf life so may not be stocked by many hospitals.[5]

Other Considerations

- All patients with moderate to large burns should have laboratory testing, including a CBC, electrolytes, BUN/creatinine, CK, and urinalysis. Hyperkalemia and rhabdomyolysis can be fatal complications of burns.[2]
- Be sure to avoid hypothermia, as patients with large burns are at high risk.[15] Provide warm blankets, warm intravenous fluids, or devices such as the Bair Hugger.[2]
- Prophylactic antibiotics or steroids are not beneficial and may increase the incidence of systemic fungal infections.[10]

Transfer to a Burn Center

Small burns can be managed in any emergency department; however, there are several situations when a patient should be transferred to a regional burn center (Box 21.2).[5,15]

Wound Care

- Superficial and partial thickness burns can be very painful, especially during wound care. Ensure adequate analgesia for the patient which may require intravenous narcotics or anxiolytics.
- Wounds should be cleaned and debrided if necessary. Most blisters can be left intact, but any large blisters that may restrict movement, such as over a joint, should be debrided.[5]
- Tetanus vaccination status should be obtained and updated if last vaccination was >5 years ago.
- Either silver sulfadiazine or Bacitracin may be used to cover the affected area. Avoid using silver sulfadiazine on the face or neck and in any patients with a sulfa allergy.[1,5]
- After applying the ointment, a sterile dressing should be placed.

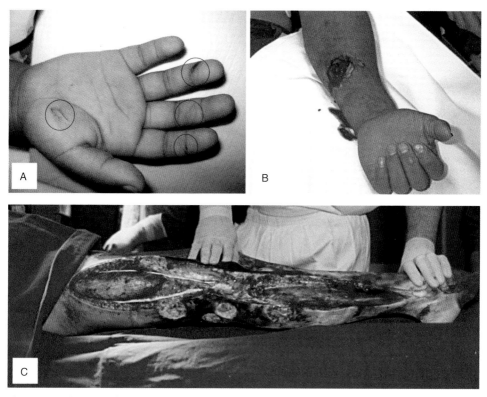

Figure 21.9 Electrical burns. (A) Low-voltage electrical burns to the hand from holding a defective electrical cord. (B) High-voltage electrical injury to the forearm of an electrician. (C) High-voltage electrical burn requiring lower extremity fasciotomies (reproduced with permission from *Color Atlas of Emergency Trauma, Second Edition*)

- Minor burns can follow up with a primary care physician, but all others should follow up with a burn specialist.
- Patients should be instructed on how to change their dressings daily and to return to the emergency department for any symptoms or signs of infection.[5]

Electrical Injuries

Electrical injuries are less common than thermal burns, accounting for approximately 500 deaths every year in the United States. However, the nonfatal injuries can also carry a high morbidity. Injuries in children generally occur at home from electrical cords or sockets, while most injuries to adults occur at their workplace.[17] Electrical injuries are the sixth leading cause of injury-related occupational deaths.[18] Lightning strikes kill >50 people a year in the United States, with the majority being males between the ages of 20–44 years old (Figure 21.9).[19,20]

Mechanism of Injury

The severity of the injury depends on the current, voltage, and duration of contact. For example, lightning strikes only last for a brief millisecond, but the immense amount of current can cause immediate cardiac arrest, while a lower current household appliance can cause just as devastating of an injury if sustained contact occurs.

Table 21.2 Current effects

Current	Effect
1 mA	Tingling sensation
3–5 mA	Max current an average child can "let go"
16 mA	Max current an average adult can "let go"
50–100 mA	Ventricular fibrillation
>2 A	Asystole
240 A	Max intensity allowed for household current in the United States

Table 21.3 Voltage characteristics

Lightning Strike	High Voltage	Low Voltage
>200,000 A	>1,000 A	<240 A
DC current	DC or AC current	AC current

Current

- Current is either alternating current (AC) or direct current (DC).
- AC is the most commonly used type in homes and offices and consists of electrons flowing back and forth through a conductor. AC is much more efficient but also more dangerous. It creates tetanic muscle contractions which can prolong the contact with the victim because he/she cannot move or "let go" (Table 21.2).[5,17]
- DC is when the electrons only flow in one direction and is more commonly found in batteries or pacemakers/defibrillators. Lightning is DC and generally only lasts for 1–2 milliseconds, but the voltage exceeds 1 million volts and generates currents over 200,000 amperes (A). This current can generate temperatures up to 50,000°F (Table 21.2).[17]

Voltage

Electrical injuries are divided into high or low voltage. Most household injuries are low voltage, while power lines injuries can be high voltage (Table 21.3).

Contact

- Direct contact will create a burn to the area that was directly touched (entry point).
- Indirect contact causing an electrical injury is when a current spark occurs between two objects, creating an arc. This is usually in high voltage injuries.[17] This can cause very high temperatures and even lead to the ignition of clothing in addition to the electrical burn injury.[1]
- Regardless of how the electrical injury occurs, the electricity can then travel through the body from the entry point to an exit point and create injury along the way.

Box 21.3   Goals of ED Management

ED Goals:

- Stabilize the patient
- Evaluate for any other trauma
- ECG to evaluate for dysrhythmia
- Laboratory studies: CBC, CMP, CK, UA
- Troponin and other tests may be indicated in certain situations
- Evaluate for compartment syndrome

- The electricity is most likely to travel along nerves, blood, and muscles because they have the least resistance, causing thermal damage to any structures it passes.[5]

ED Evaluation and Management

- Initial management includes a primary survey and intervention as needed, followed by a complete secondary survey (Box 21.3).

Clinical Features

Cardiopulmonary Injury

Immediate death is usually from electrical current induced ventricular fibrillation, asystole, and paralysis of respiration control center or muscles.[17,21] The most common dysrhythmias after lightning strike are asystole and ventricular fibrillation. In contrast to other causes of asystole, lightning strike patients in asystole with no signs of life have a high rate of return of spontaneous circulation with good neurologic outcome given prompt resuscitation.[22] Supraventricular tachycardias, bradycardias, or conduction delays including QT prolongation are rare but have occurred.[23] An elevated troponin is concerning for significant cardiac muscle injury. Elevated troponin may be secondary to vasospasm or direct muscle injury such as myocardial contusion. It may also be elevated from cardiac ischemia, especially with ST elevation on the electrocardiogram. It is unclear if these patients benefit from immediate percutaneous coronary intervention.[22] This should be discussed with cardiology on a case by case basis.

Nervous System Injury

Approximately half of all patients presenting with high voltage electrical injury will have a neurological issue. This ranges from transient loss of consciousness to seizures, paralysis, and coma. Always consider a CT head and C-spine to rule out other traumatic causes of these symptoms.[5]

Vascular and Muscle Injury

These are more common in high voltage injuries. Peripheral arteries may spasm leading to diminished pulses and later thrombosis formation.[5] Muscle inflammation and associated edema in the nerve sheath may lead to rhabdomyolysis or compartment syndrome.[1] A creatinine kinase (CK) should be checked in these patients to evaluate for rhabdomyolysis. If elevated, the patient will need aggressive intravenous fluids and close observation of their fluid status and urinary output to evaluate for developing renal failure. It is estimated that up to one third of patients with rhabdomyolysis will develop renal failure.[24]

GI Injury

Severe intra-abdominal and GI injuries have been reported after high voltage electrical injuries. Consider abdominal imaging or surgical consultation if concerned.

Cutaneous Injury

Cutaneous burns may be evident at both the entry and exit points as well as diffusely from associated flash burns. Lightning strikes can create a Lichtenberg burn which produces a fern pattern. The cutaneous injuries may be much worse than they initially appear.[21]

ENT Injury

The rupture of tympanic membranes is common after high voltage injuries (Figure 21.10). Additionally, cataracts can occur in high voltage injury but do not occur acutely (Figure 21.11).[5,17] An estimated 6% of lightning strike victims will go on to develop cataracts at some point.[25]

Lip Burns in Children

Children often present with full thickness burns to their lips from putting an electrical cord in their mouth. Make sure to warn the parents about delayed labial artery bleeding after the

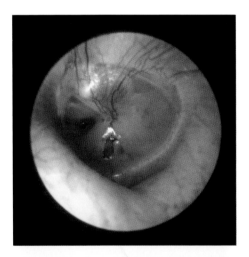

Figure 21.10 Tympanic membrane rupture (image courtesy of Michael Hawke, MD, reproduced under CC BY 4.0 license; https://creativecommons.org/licenses/by/4.0/)

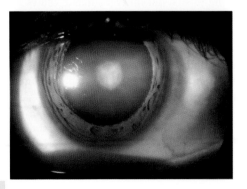

Figure 21.11 Ocular cataract (image courtesy of Rakesh Ahuja, MD, reproduced under CC BY-SA 3.0; https://creativecommons.org/licenses/by-sa/3.0)

eschar falls off, which may be several days to even weeks after the initial injury.[5,17] If this occurs, direct pressure should be immediately placed on the bleed, and they should return to the nearest emergency department. Patients generally have minimal pain that can be controlled with over the counter pain medications if needed. Ensure pediatric immunizations have been completed and, if not, provide tetanus immunization. The patient should follow up with ENT or burn plastics to ensure adequate healing and because lip contractures and scarring may require subsequent intervention.[26]

Lightning Strikes

A lightning strike causes a rapid but intense thermal burn from current flow through the body. In addition to the previously mentioned injuries, this can also cause internal organ contusions, paralysis – usually worse in the lower extremities – termed keraunoparalysis, and autonomic dysfunction including dilated or pinpoint pupils not related to a brain injury.[5]

Disposition

Most patients with a low voltage injury with an unremarkable evaluation in the emergency department can be safely discharged home. Any patient with abnormal cardiac or neurologic findings or severe burns should be admitted to the ICU or transferred to a regional burn center. Admission should also be considered for anyone with a history of heart disease, high voltage injury, any abnormal ECG, or loss of consciousness for observation and telemetry.[17]

- Patients who are asymptomatic on arrival with normal ECG have no increased risk for later dysrhythmias.[5,21,27]
- Pregnant women over 20 weeks gestation should have fetal monitoring for 4–6 hours after the injury.

Pitfalls in ED Evaluation and Management

- Do not forget to evaluate for all traumatic injuries as the burn or electrical injury may have resulted in the patient being thrown, falling, tetanic muscle contractions, or carbon monoxide/cyanide poisoning.
- Intubation should not be delayed in an inhalation injury. Once the airway swelling is present, an airway will be extremely difficult to obtain.
- Avoid hypothermia in the burn patient.
- Remember to consider injuries to internal structures when evaluating an electrical injury, including the development of compartment syndrome over the first 24 hours.

Key Points

- Burns and electrical injuries cause significant morbidity and mortality every year.
- Emergency department escharotomies may be required in the limbs, chest, or abdomen to combat compartment syndrome or improve ventilation of the patient.
- Early transfer to a regional burn center in a moderate to large burn patient or high voltage electrical injury is beneficial.
- Obtain an ECG on all electrical injury patients and consider observation if any abnormalities are discovered.

References

1. Schofer JM, Mattu A. Cutaneous injuries. *Emerg Med: A Focused Review of the Core Curriculum*. 2015;2:20–22.

2. White CE, Renz EM. Advances in surgical care: management of severe burn injury. *Crit Care Med*. 2008;36(7):318–24.

3. Al-Mousawi AM, Mecott-Rivera GA, Jeschke MG, Herndon DN. Burn teams and burn centers: the importance of a comprehensive team approach to burn care. *Clin Plast Surg*. 2009;36 (4):547–54.

4. Brusselaers N, Monstrey S, Vogelars D, Hoste E, Blot S. Severe burn injury in Europe: a systematic review of the incidence, etiology, morbidity, and mortality. *Crit Care*. 2010;14:R188.

5. Tintinalli JE, Schwartz LR, Balakrishnan C. Thermal burns, electrical injuries, lightning injuries, carbon monoxide, metabolic toxins. In: Tintinalli JE, ed., *Tintinalli's Emergency Medicine: A Comprehensive Study Guide*, 7th ed. New York: NY: McGraw-Hill Medical; 2011, pp. 1317–20, 1410–13, 1374–80, 1386–94.

6. Hettiaratchy S, Dziewulski P. Pathophysiology and types of burns. *BMJ*. 2004;328:1427–29.

7. Toussaint J, Singer A. The evaluation and management of thermal injuries: 2014 update. *Clin Exp Emerg Med*. 2014;1 (1):8–18.

8. Hettiaratchy S, Papini R. Initial management of a major burn: II – assessment and resuscitation. *BMJ*. 2004;329:101–3.

9. Hettiaratchy s, Papini R. Initial management of a major burn: I – overview. *BMJ*. 2004;328:1555–57.

10. Friedstat J, Endorf FW, Gibran NS. Burns. In: Brunicardi FC, Andersen DK, Billiar TR, et al., eds. *Schwartz's Principles of Surgery*. New York, NY: McGraw Hill; 2014, p. 10.

11. Haberal M, Abali AES, Karakayali H. Fluid management in major burn injuries. *Indian J Plast Surg*. 2010;43:S29–36.

12. Chung KK, Salinas J, Renz EM, et al. Simple derivation of the initial fluid rate for the resuscitation of severely burned adult combat casualties: in silico validation of the rule of 10. *J Trauma*. 2010;69:S49–54.

13. Todd SR, Malinoski D, Muller PJ, Schreiber MA. Lactated Ringer's is superior to normal saline in resuscitation of uncontrolled hemorrhagic shock. *J Trauma*. 2007;62(3):636–39.

14. Roberts JR, ed. Emergency escharotomy. *Roberts and Hedges' Clinical Procedures in Emergency Medicine*, 6th ed. Philadelphia, PA: Saunders; 2014, pp. 786–87.

15. Latenser BA. Critical care of the burn patient: the first 48 hours. *Crit Care Med*. 2009;37(10):2819–26.

16. Kupas DF, Miller DD. Out-of-hospital chest escharotomy: a case series and procedure review. *Prehosp Emerg Care*. 2010;14(3):349–54.

17. Koumbourlis AC. Electrical injuries. *Crit Care Med*. 2002;30(11):424–30.

18. Cawley JC, Homce GT. Trends in electrical injury in the US 1992–2002. Petroleum and Chemical Industry Conference; 2006.

19. Krider E, Uman M. Cloud-to-ground lightning: mechanisms of damage and methods of protection. *Semin Neurol*. 1995;15:227–32.

20. Adekoya N, Nolte KB. Struck-by-lightning deaths in the United States. *J Envir Health*. 2005;67(9):45–50.

21. Blackwell N, Hayllar J. A three year prospective audit of 212 presentations to the emergency department after electrical injury with a management protocol. *Postgrad Med J*. 2002;78:283–85.

22. Christophides T, Khan S, Ahmad M, Fayed H, Bogle R. Cardiac effects of lightning strikes. *Arrhythm Electrophysiol Rev*. 2017;6(3):114–17.

23. Varol E, Ozaydin M, Altinbas A, Dogan A. Low-tension electrical injury as a cause of atrial fibrillation. *Tex Heart Inst J*. 2004;31 (2):186–87.

24. Coban YK. Rhabdomyolysis, compartment syndrome and thermal injury. *World J Crit Care Med*. 2014;3(1):1–7.

25. Colwell C. *Lightning injuries.* Emerg Med Clini Essentials. 2013;132:1148–52.

26. LeCompte EJ, Goldman BM. Oral electrical burns in children – early treatment and appliance fabrication. *Ped Dentistry*. 1982;4 (4):333–37.

27. Arrowsmith J, Usgaocar RP, Dickson WA. Electrical injury and the frequency of cardiac complications. *Burns*. 1997;23 (1–8):576–78.

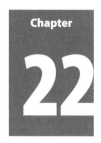

Procedural Sedation and Analgesia in Trauma

Steven G. Schauer and Jason F. Naylor

Background

Procedural sedation and analgesia (PSA) is a core competency for emergency physicians (EP) that is commonly practiced.[1-4] PSA entails suppressing a patient's level of consciousness with sedative or dissociative agents to alleviate pain, anxiety, and suffering to enhance medical procedure performance and patient experience (Table 22.1).[1,5]

Indications

- Traumatic injuries account for the greatest number of sedations in the emergency department (ED).[6-12]
- ED PSA for the severely injured trauma patient may be limited to life-saving interventions (LSI). Tube thoracostomy and cricothyrotomy may require PSA in addition to injection of local anesthetic agents.[13]
- LSI and emergent procedures necessitate procedural performance in the ED. For urgent and non-urgent procedures, however, lengthy procedures and higher risk patients may benefit from PSA in the operating room or with anesthesiology staff support in the ED.
- Agitated trauma patients may require sedation for diagnostic procedures, such as neuroimaging (Box 22.1).[14]

Preparation

- The American Society of Anesthesiology (ASA) physical status classification is a useful tool for risk stratifying patients by their medical history.[14-16] ASA Class I and II are associated with significant adverse event rates <5%, while risk increases with greater ASA Classes (Table 22.2).[16,17]
- Evaluate for difficult bag valve mask ventilation, difficult intubation, allergies, and PSA agent contraindications.
- Be prepared to respond to airway obstruction, apnea/hypoventilation, hypotension, dysrhythmia, and emesis.[14-16]
- Fasting state is often considered, but aspiration of emesis during ED PSA is rare, and preprocedural fasting does not decrease risk.[1,19]
- End tidal carbon dioxide monitoring is not required, but it may detect apnea/hypoventilation before pulse oximetry, especially in patients on supplemental oxygen.[20-22]
- Important equipment recommended for procedural sedation is listed in Box 22.2.

Table 22.1 American College of Emergency Physicians (ACEP) Clinical Policy for PSA[1]

Depths of Sedation	Definition
Minimal Sedation	Near-baseline level of alertness. A pharmacologically induced state during which patients respond normally to verbal commands. Although cognitive function and coordination might be impaired, ventilatory and cardiovascular functions are unaffected.
Moderate Sedation	Depression of consciousness during which patients respond purposefully to verbal commands, either alone or accompanied by light tactile stimulation. No interventions are required to maintain a patent airway, and spontaneous ventilation is adequate. Cardiovascular function is usually maintained.
Dissociative Sedation	Trance-like cataleptic state characterized by profound analgesia and amnesia, with retention of protective airway reflexes, spontaneous respirations, and cardiopulmonary stability.
Deep Sedation	Depression of consciousness during which patients cannot be easily aroused, but respond purposefully after repeated or painful stimulation. The ability to independently maintain ventilatory function may be impaired. Patients may require assistance in maintaining a patent airway, and spontaneous ventilation may be inadequate. Cardiovascular function is usually maintained.
General Anesthesia	Unresponsiveness to all stimuli and the absence of airway protective reflexes. The ability to independently maintain ventilatory function is often impaired. Patients often require assistance in maintaining a patent airway, and positive-pressure ventilation may be required because of depressed spontaneous ventilation or drug-induced depression of neuromuscular function. Cardiovascular function may be impaired.

Box 22.1 Indications For PSA in Trauma Patients
- Tube thoracostomy
- Surgical airway
- Fracture reduction
- Joint dislocation reduction
- Laceration repair
- Wound and burn debridement
- Foreign body removal
- Central venous catheterization
- Diagnostic imaging in agitated or uncooperative patients

Medication Choices
- Consider airway status, ventilatory function, hemodynamic state, and previous opioid analgesic administrations when selecting the appropriate agent and dose.
- Reduced doses titrated to sedation goals are appropriate in hypovolemic, elderly, and obese patients.[15,16]

Table 22.2 American Society of Anesthesiologists physical status classification[18]

Class	Definition	Example
I	A normal healthy patient	Healthy, non-smoking, no or minimal alcohol use.
II	A patient with mild systemic disease	Mild diseases only without substantive functional limitations. Examples include (but not limited to): current smoker, social alcohol drinker, pregnancy, obesity (30< BMI <40), well-controlled DM/HTN, mild lung disease.
III	A patient with severe systemic disease	Substantive functional limitations; one or more moderate to severe diseases. Examples include (but not limited to): poorly controlled DM or HTN, COPD, morbid obesity (BMI ≥40), active hepatitis, alcohol dependence or abuse, implanted pacemaker, moderate reduction of ejection fraction, ESRD undergoing regularly scheduled dialysis, premature infant, PCA <60 weeks, or history (>3 months) of MI, CVA, TIA, or CAD/stents.
IV	A patient with severe systemic disease that is a constant threat to life	Examples include (but not limited to): recent (<3 months) MI, CVA, TIA, or CAD/stents, ongoing cardiac ischemia or severe valve dysfunction, severe reduction of ejection fraction, sepsis, DIC, ARDS, or ESRD not undergoing regularly scheduled dialysis.
V	A moribund patient who is not expected to survive without the operation	Examples include (but not limited to): ruptured abdominal/thoracic aneurysm, massive trauma, intracranial bleed with mass effect, ischemic bowel in the face of significant cardiac pathology, or multiple organ/system dysfunction.
VI	A declared brain-dead patient whose organs are being removed for donor purposes.	

Box 22.2   Equipment for PSA[1,14–16]

- Oxygen
- NRB
- BVM
- LMA
- Intubation
- Suction
- Monitor
- (Required) Blood pressure, pulse oximetry
- (Recommended) Cardiac, capnography
- IV access
- Defibrillator
- Reversal and resuscitation medications

Ketamine

- Favorable adverse effects (AE) profile with respect to ventilation and hemodynamics.[14,15] However, transient apnea/hypoventilation and hypotension may occur, especially if given rapidly.[5,16]
- Recent research counters previous concerns for ketamine-induced elevations in intracranial and intraocular pressures with resultant adverse outcomes.[5,23-28] Recent guidelines for ketamine as an ED PSA agent removed head injury as a relative contraindication.[5]
- Prophylactic antisialagogue for hypersalivation and prophylactic benzodiazepines for emergence reaction are not recommended.[5]
- Prophylactic antiemetics may be given, as post-PSA emesis is common.[5]

Propofol

- Fewer contraindications and a shorter recovery period than ketamine, but it is associated with decreased blood pressure and hypoventilation.[14-16]
- Caution with hypovolemic trauma patients and significant traumatic brain injury, as hypotension should be avoided in these situations.[15,16,29]
- Adjunctive analgesic recommended, as it has no analgesic properties.[14-16]

Ketofol (Ketamine and Propofol)

- Theoretical advantage of limiting AE of each agent by reducing the total dosage of each agent given and intrinsic properties of each agent counteracting some AE of the other. Additionally, analgesic properties of ketamine may obviate opiate co-administration.[9,11,30,31]
- 1:1 mixture of 10 mg/mL ketamine and 10 mg/mL propofol in a single syringe given in 0.1–0.5 mL/kg aliquots (5 mg of each agent in each mL) produces reliable sedation effects.[8,9,11,30]

Etomidate, Midazolam, and Fentanyl

- Etomidate has the most favorable hemodynamic profile.[14-16]
- Although not common, all agents may produce hypoventilation, especially if given rapidly or after other agents for analgesia (i.e. opiates) and anxiolysis (i.e. benzodiazepines).[14-16]
- Etomidate may produce transient myoclonus (up to 20% of patients) that may interfere with procedural completion.[15,16]
- Midazolam is associated with paradoxical agitation (up to 15% of patients) that may be reversed with flumazenil.
- Fentanyl administered rapidly in large doses (>5–15 μg/kg) may result in the rare AE of rigid chest syndrome that is irreversible with naloxone and may require intubation and mechanical ventilation.[15,16]
- Tables 22.3–22.5 discuss medication options.

Discharge Considerations

- The ability to urinate or tolerate PO prior to discharge is not universally required; the need for this may be case-by-case specific.[34]

Table 22.3 PSA agents[5,9,14–16,30,32]

Agent	Dosing	Contraindications	Adverse Effects
Ketamine	IV: Adult: 1.0 mg/kg Peds: 1.5–2.0 mg/kg Redose: 0.5 mg/kg q3min IM: Adult: 4.0–5.0 mg/kg Peds: same dose Redose: half or full IN: 6.0 mg/kg	Absolute: <3 months old Schizophrenia Relative: Active asthma Active URI (peds) Airway instability (e.g. tracheal stenosis, laryngomalacia) CAD/CHF/HTN	Laryngospasm Emergence phenomenon Nausea, vomiting Hypersalivation Random movements
Propofol	IV: Adult: 0.5–1.0 mg/kg Peds: 0.5 mg/kg Redose: 0.5 mg/kg q1–3min	Absolute: Allergy egg protein Allergy soy protein Relative: Hypovolemia	↓BP ↓RR Injection pain
Ketofol 1:1 mix 10 mg/mL Ketamine 10 mg/mL Propofol 1 mL = 5 mg each	IV: Adult: 0.1–0.5 mL/kg aliquots Peds: same dose Redose: half or full q30–60sec	Same as above, but lower rates of AE	
Etomidate	IV: Adult: 0.1–0.2 mg/kg Peds: 0.1 mg/kg Redose: 0.1 mg/kg q2min		↓RR Myoclonus Nausea, vomiting Adrenal suppression
Midazolam	IV: Adult: 0.05–0.2 mg/kg Peds: 0.1 mg/kg Redose: 0.05 mg/kg q2min IM: Adult: 0.1 mg/kg Peds: same dose Redose: half or full IN (Peds): 0.2 mg/kg PO (Peds): 0.5 mg/kg	Relative: Hypovolemia	↓RR Paradoxical agitation Nausea, vomiting Hiccups, cough
Fentanyl	IV: Adult: 1.0–3.0 µg/kg q1–3min Peds: same dose Redose: half or full TM (Peds): 10.0 µg/kg		↓RR Rigid chest syndrome Nausea, vomiting Pruritis

Table 22.4 PSA agent characteristics[9,14–16,30]

Agent	Route	Onset (minutes)	Duration (minutes)
Ketamine	IV	1–3	10–20
	IM	5–20	30–60
	IN	5–10	30–120
Propofol	IV	1–2	5–10
Etomidate	IV	0.5–1	5–10
Midazolam	IV	1–3	30–60
	IM	10–30	60–120
	IN	10–15	45–60
	PO	15–30	60–90
Fentanyl	IV	0.5–2	30–60
	TM	10–30	60–120

Table 22.5 Potential adjunctive treatments[5,14-16,32,33]

Medication	Dosing	Indication
Naloxone	IV: Adult: 0.4–2.0 mg Peds (<20 kg): 0.1 mg/kg Peds (≥20 kg): 2.0 mg	Opiate reversal
Flumazenil	IV: Adult: 0.1–1.0 mg Peds (>1-year-old): 0.02 mg/kg	Benzodiazepine reversal
Crystalloids	IV: Adult: 250–500 mL Peds: 10–20 mL/kg	Hypotension
Phenylephrine	IV: Adult: 20–200 µg q2–5min Peds: 0.1–0.5 µg/kg/min	Hypotension
Midazolam	IV: Adult: 0.01 mg/kg Peds: 0.05–0.01 mg/kg	Emergence phenomenon
Ondansetron	IV: Adult: 4.0–8.0 mg Peds (8–30 kg): 0.15 mg/kg Peds (≥31 kg): 4.0 mg	Nausea, vomiting
Glycopyrrolate	IV: Adult: 0.2 mg Peds: 0.01 mg/kg	Hypersalivation

---

Box 22.3 Discharge Criteria Following ED PSA[34]

- Patient is alert and oriented to baseline
- Hemodynamic status is at acceptable level specific to the patient
- Protective reflexes, specifically airway, are intact
- Pain is adequately controlled
- Patient ambulation status at or near baseline (may not always be applicable)
- Responsible adult will be present with patient after discharge
- Patient is able to verbalize understanding of discharge instructions

---

- All patients should be required to have another responsible party with them prior to discharge.
- No data has demonstrated a required amount of time post-sedation before discharge.[34]
- ED should have sedation-specific discharge instructions to provide the patient.
- Discharge time needs to be adjusted if a reversal agent was given based on drug-specific pharmacokinetics.
- Box 22.3 depict discharge criteria after PSA.

Special Populations – Pediatrics

- Pediatric patients frequently require sedation for additional reasons beyond adults (e.g. psychological challenges, developmental delays).
- Ketamine is frequently used with a large safety margin[35]; ketamine-associated emesis and agitation are more frequent with older children.[36]
- Barbiturates are not recommended; they have no intrinsic analgesic properties.[37]
- Sedation in children is often more difficult to titrate, with greater variability in the level of sedation achieved.[38,39]
- Consider alternative routes of administration in order to obviate challenges associated with IV placement (e.g. oral midazolam, oral ketamine, intranasal ketamine, intramuscular ketamine); consider IV placement after sedation is achieved.[40]
- Advanced airway equipment specific to patient size should be readily available.[41]
- Use of an independent observer of patient hemodynamic/respiratory status reduces the risks of adverse events (does not have to be physician, consider having a dedicated nurse or qualified technician, if available).[41]
- Pediatric-specific protocols may reduce adverse events, especially in very young children.[42]
- NPO status is a consideration; but ED-based procedures are often not "elective" and, thus, clinicians must evaluate each patient encounter risk/benefit.[1,43]
- ACEP Clinical Policy states: "Do not delay procedural sedation in adults or pediatrics in the ED based on fasting time. Preprocedural fasting for any duration has not demonstrated a reduction in the risk of emesis or aspiration when administering procedural sedation and analgesia." (Level B recommendation)[1]
- Table 22.6 discusses key considerations in oral intake before sedation from the AAP and ASA, though ACEP recommends that no fasting is required before sedation.

Table 22.6 AAP and ASA recommendations for duration of NPO before elective sedation[43,44]

Age Group	Solid and Non-Clear Liquids (Infant Formula, Breast Milk, Non-Human Milk) (hours)	Clear Liquids (hours)
<6 months	4–6	2
6–36 months	6	2
>36 months	6–8	2

Note: May be adjusted depending on the urgency of the procedure, as not all ED-based procedural sedation is elective.

Table 22.7 University of Michigan Sedation Scale (UMSS)[45]

Score	Depth of Sedation
0	Awake and alert
1	Minimally sedated: tired/sleepy, appropriate response to verbal conversation and/or sound
2	Moderately sedated: somnolent/sleeping, easily aroused with light tactile stimulation or a simple verbal command
3	Deeply sedated: deep sleep, arousable only with significant physical stimulation
4	Unarousable

Box 22.4   AAP Guidelines For Discharge of Children After Sedation[46]

1. Cardiovascular function and airway patency are satisfactory and stable.
2. The patient is easily arousable, and protective reflexes are intact.
3. The patient can talk (if age appropriate).
4. The patient can sit up unaided (if age appropriate).
5. For a very young or handicapped child incapable of the usually expected responses, the presedation level of responsiveness or a level as close as possible to the normal level for that child should be achieved.
6. The state of hydration is adequate.

- Consider using the University of Michigan Sedation Scale (UMSS) to guide sedation goals, which is simple and reproducible (Table 22.7).[45]
- Box 22.4 depicts discharge criteria for pediatric patients after PSA.

Special Populations – Pregnancy

- There is very little data to guide PSA in the pregnant patient. ACEP does not have a specific clinical policy on this population.[4]
- Significant physiologic changes occur in pregnancy: plasma volume and cardiac output increase along with a commensurate increase in respiratory volume and rate to compensate for metabolic demands → decreased ability to compensate during hemodynamic stress and more rapid deoxygenation.[47]

- Regional anesthesia may be used as an alternative (lidocaine is pregnancy class B).
- Meperidine (pregnancy class B) may be preferred over morphine (pregnancy class C).[48]
    - May be reversed with naloxone (pregnancy class B).
- Propofol is the preferred agent (pregnancy class B).[48]
- Avoid benzodiazepines (pregnancy class D; known teratogenic effects).
    - Flumazenil risk unclear (pregnancy class C).

Special Populations – Elderly

- Age, in and of itself, is not a contradiction to sedation.[49]
- Very little ED-specific data on sedation in the elderly; most data are extrapolated from anesthesia and dental literature.
- Generally, elderly patients often require lower dosing and have higher risk of adverse events compared to other patient populations.[50,51]
- For propofol, consider administering an "age based" test dose. A rough estimate may be 100 mg minus the patient's age (e.g. for a 75 year old patient, start with 25 mg).[52]
- In elderly >70 years, half-dose titration of propofol and benzodiazepines is preferred to avoid adverse events.[49,50,53–55]
- While ketamine has some theoretical risks in the elderly, that has not been borne out in the data. Ketamine use appears safe in the elderly.[56–58]
- While we do not recommend etomidate for procedural sedation due to the high-risk of myoclonic reactions, it appears safe for use in the elderly.[59]

Pitfalls

- Pushing additional boluses of PSA agents (especially propofol) too quickly and inducing hypotension or hypopnea – wait an appropriate length of time for the drug to take effect before repeat dosing to reduce adverse event risk, which may have dose-dependent effects.[52]
- Drugs can have stacking-effects when given together. Drugs given before the sedation may potentiate the likelihood of an adverse event.[60]
- Airway related complications are not always predictable; have appropriate airway equipment available and ready before starting sedation.
- Consider adjusting dosing for patient characteristics that may affect medication metabolism (e.g. age, body mass, liver function, kidney function).

Key Points

- Tube thoracostomy and cricothyrotomy may require PSA in addition to injection of local anesthetic agents.
- Lengthy procedures and higher risk patients may benefit from PSA in the operating room or with anesthesiology staff support in the ED.
- Reduced doses of PSA agents titrated to sedation goals are appropriate in hypovolemic, elderly, and obese patients.

References

1. Godwin SA, Caro DA, Wolf SJ, et al. Clinical policy: procedural sedation and analgesia in the emergency department. *Ann Emerg Med.* 2005;45(2):177–96.

2. Miner JR, Krauss B. Procedural sedation and analgesia research: state of the art. *Acad Emerg Med.* 2007;14(2):170–78.

3. Bellolio MF, Gilani WI, Barrionuevo P, et al. Incidence of adverse events in adults undergoing procedural sedation in the emergency department: a systematic review and meta-analysis. *Acad Emerg Med.* 2016;23(2):119–34.

4. Godwin SA, Burton JH, Gerardo CJ, et al. Clinical policy: procedural sedation and analgesia in the emergency department. *Ann Emerg Med.* 2014;63(2):247–58, e218.

5. Green SM, Roback MG, Kennedy RM, Krauss B. Clinical practice guideline for emergency department ketamine dissociative sedation: 2011 update. *Ann Emerg Med.* 2011;57(5):449–61.

6. Burton JH, Miner JR, Shipley ER, et al. Propofol for emergency department procedural sedation and analgesia: a tale of three centers. *Acad Emerg Med.* 2006;13(1):24–30.

7. Newstead B, Bradburn S, Appelboam A, et al. Propofol for adult procedural sedation in a UK emergency department: safety profile in 1008 cases. *Br J Anaesth.* 2013;111(4):651–55.

8. Andolfatto G, Abu-Laban RB, Zed PJ, et al. Ketamine-propofol combination (ketofol) versus propofol alone for emergency department procedural sedation and analgesia: a randomized double-blind trial. *Ann Emerg Med.* 2012;59(6):504–12, e501–2.

9. Willman EV, Andolfatto G. A prospective evaluation of "ketofol" (ketamine/propofol combination) for procedural sedation and analgesia in the emergency department. *Ann Emerg Med.* 2007;49(1):23–30.

10. Ruth WJ, Burton JH, Bock AJ. Intravenous etomidate for procedural sedation in emergency department patients. *Acad Emerg Med.* 2001;8(1):13–18.

11. Miner JR, Moore JC, Austad EJ, et al. Randomized, double-blinded, clinical trial of propofol, 1:1 propofol/ketamine, and 4:1 propofol/ketamine for deep procedural sedation in the emergency department. *Ann Emerg Med.* 2015;65(5):479–88, e472.

12. Uri O, Behrbalk E, Haim A, Kaufman E, Halpern P. Procedural sedation with propofol for painful orthopaedic manipulation in the emergency department expedites patient management compared with a midazolam/ketamine regimen: a randomized prospective study. *J Bone Joint Surg Am.* 2011;93(24):2255–62.

13. Vassallo J, Smith JE, Bruijns SR, Wallis LA. Major incident triage: a consensus based definition of the essential life-saving interventions during the definitive care phase of a major incident. *Injury.* 2016;47(9):1898–902.

14. Adams JG, Barton ED, Collings J, et al. *Emergency Medicine: Expert Consult – Online.* Amsterdam, The Netherlands: Elsevier Health Sciences; 2008.

15. Walls R, Hockberger R, Gausche-Hill M. *Rosen's Emergency Medicine: Concepts and Clinical Practice: 2-Volume Set.* Amsterdam, The Netherlands: Elsevier; 2017.

16. Tintinalli J, Stapczynski J, Ma OJ, et al. *Tintinalli's Emergency Medicine: A Comprehensive Study Guide,* 8th ed. New York, NY: *McGraw-Hill Education*; 2015.

17. Miner JR, Martel ML, Meyer M, Reardon R, Biros MH. Procedural sedation of critically ill patients in the emergency department. *Acad Emerg Med.* 2005;12(2):124–28.

18. Daabiss M. American Society of Anaesthesiologists physical status classification. *Indian J Anaesth.* 2011;55(2):111–15.

19. Green SM, Krauss B. Pulmonary aspiration risk during emergency department procedural sedation – an examination of the role of fasting and sedation depth. *Acad Emerg Med.* 2002;9(1):35–42.

20. Burton JH, Harrah JD, Germann CA, Dillon DC. Does end-tidal carbon dioxide

monitoring detect respiratory events prior
to current sedation monitoring practices?
Acad Emerg Med. 2006;13(5):500–4.

21. Campbell SG, Magee KD, Zed PJ, et al.
End-tidal capnometry during emergency
department procedural sedation and
analgesia: A randomized, controlled study.
World J Emerg Med. 2016;7(1):13–18.

22. Dewdney C, MacDougall M, Blackburn R,
Lloyd G, Gray A. Capnography for
procedural sedation in the ED: a systematic
review. *Emerg Med J.* 2017;34(7):476–84.

23. Zeiler FA, Teitelbaum J, West M, Gillman
LM. The ketamine effect on ICP in
traumatic brain injury. *Neurocrit Care.*
2014;21(1):163–73.

24. Zeiler FA, Teitelbaum J, West M, Gillman
LM. The ketamine effect on intracranial
pressure in nontraumatic neurological
illness. *J Crit Care.* 2014;29(6):1096–106.

25. Zeiler FA, Sader N, Gillman LM, et al. The
cerebrovascular response to ketamine: a
systematic review of the animal and human
literature. *J Neurosurg Anesthesiol.* 2016;28
(2):123–40.

26. Oddo M, Crippa IA, Mehta S, et al.
Optimizing sedation in patients with acute
brain injury. *Crit Care.* 2016;20(1):128.

27. Drayna PC, Estrada C, Wang W, Saville
BR, Arnold DH. Ketamine sedation is not
associated with clinically meaningful
elevation of intraocular pressure. *Am
J Emerg Med.* 2012;30(7):1215–18.

28. Halstead SM, Deakyne SJ, Bajaj L,
Enzenauer R, Roosevelt GE. The effect of
ketamine on intraocular pressure in
pediatric patients during procedural
sedation. *Acad Emerg Med.* 2012;19
(10):1145–50.

29. Carney N, Totten AM, O'Reilly C, et al.
Guidelines for the management of severe
traumatic brain injury, *fourth edition.*
Neurosurgery. 2017;80(1):6–15.

30. Andolfatto G, Willman E. A prospective
case series of single-syringe ketamine-
propofol (Ketofol) for emergency
department procedural sedation and
analgesia in adults. *Acad Emerg Med.*
2011;18(3):237–45.

31. Miner J. Ketamine or ketofol: Do we have
enough evidence to know which one to use?
Acad Emerg Med. 2017:24(12):1511–13.

32. Green SM, Krauss B. Clinical practice
guideline for emergency department
ketamine dissociative sedation in children.
Ann Emerg Med. 2004;44(5):460–71.

33. Meredith JR, O'Keefe KP, Galwankar S.
Pediatric procedural sedation and
analgesia. *J Emerg Trauma Shock.* 2008;1
(2):88–96.

34. Apfelbaum JL, Silverstein JH, Chung FF,
et al. Practice guidelines for postanesthetic
care: an updated report by the American
Society of Anesthesiologists Task Force on
Postanesthetic Care. *Anesthesiology.*
2013;118(2):291–307.

35. Green SM, Clark R, Hostetler MA, et al.
Inadvertent ketamine overdose in children:
clinical manifestations and outcome. *Ann
Emerg Med.* 1999;34(4 Pt 1):492–97.

36. Green SM, Kuppermann N, Rothrock SG,
Hummel CB, Ho M. Predictors of adverse
events with intramuscular ketamine
sedation in children. *Ann Emerg Med.*
2000;35(1):35–42.

37. Rodriguez E, Jordan R. Contemporary
trends in pediatric sedation and analgesia.
Emerg Med Clin North Am. 2002;20
(1):199–222.

38. Motas D, McDermott NB, VanSickle T,
Friesen RH. Depth of consciousness and
deep sedation attained in children as
administered by nonanaesthesiologists in a
children's hospital. *Paediatr Anaesth.*
2004;14(3):256–60.

39. Dial S, Silver P, Bock K, Sagy M. Pediatric
sedation for procedures titrated to a desired
degree of immobility results in
unpredictable depth of sedation. *Pediatr
Emerg Care.* 2001;17(6):414–20.

40. Maxwell LG, Yaster M. The myth of
conscious sedation. *Arch Pediatr Adolesc
Med.* 1996;150(7):665–67.

41. Cote CJ, Notterman DA, Karl HW,
Weinberg JA, McCloskey C. Adverse
sedation events in pediatrics: a critical
incident analysis of contributing factors.
Pediatrics. 2000;105(4 Pt 1):805–14.

42. Morton NS, Oomen GJ. Development of a selection and monitoring protocol for safe sedation of children. *Paediatr Anaesth.* 1998;8(1):65–68.

43. Green SM. Fasting is a consideration – not a necessity – for emergency department procedural sedation and analgesia. *Ann Emerg Med.* 2003;42(5):647–50.

44. Agrawal D, Manzi SF, Gupta R, Krauss B. Preprocedural fasting state and adverse events in children undergoing procedural sedation and analgesia in a pediatric emergency department. *Ann Emerg Med.* 2003;42(5):636–46.

45. Malviya S, Voepel-Lewis T, Tait AR, et al. Depth of sedation in children undergoing computed tomography: validity and reliability of the University of Michigan Sedation Scale (UMSS). *Br J Anaesth.* 2002;88(2):241–45.

46. American Academy of Pediatrics, American Academy of Pediatric Dentistry, Cote CJ, Wilson S, Work Group on Sedation. Guidelines for monitoring and management of pediatric patients during and after sedation for diagnostic and therapeutic procedures: An update. *Paediatr Anaesth.* 2008;18(1):9–10.

47. Soma-Pillay P, Nelson-Piercy C, Tolppanen H, Mebazaa A. Physiological changes in pregnancy. *Cardiovasc J Afr.* 2016;27(2):89–94.

48. Qureshi WA, Rajan E, Adler DG, et al. ASGE guideline: guidelines for endoscopy in pregnant and lactating women. *Gastrointest Endosc.* 2005;61(3):357–62.

49. Weaver CS, Terrell KM, Bassett R, et al. ED procedural sedation of elderly patients: is it safe? *Am J Emerg Med.* 2011;29(5):541–44.

50. Yano H, Iishi H, Tatsuta M, et al. Oxygen desaturation during sedation for colonoscopy in elderly patients. *Hepatogastroenterology.* 1998;45(24):2138–41.

51. Taylor DM, Bell A, Holdgate A, et al. Risk factors for sedation-related events during procedural sedation in the emergency department. *Emerg Med Australas.* 2011;23(4):466–73.

52. Green SM, Andolfatto G. Managing propofol-induced hypoventilation. *Ann Emerg Med.* 2015;65(1):57–60.

53. Kitagawa E, Iida A, Kimura Y, et al. Responses to intravenous sedation by elderly patients at the Hokkaido University Dental Hospital. *Anesth Prog.* 1992;39(3):73–78.

54. Campbell RL, Smith PB. Intravenous sedation in 200 geriatric patients undergoing office oral surgery. *Anesth Prog.* 1997;44(2):64–67.

55. Patanwala AE, Christich AC, Jasiak KD, et al. Age-related differences in propofol dosing for procedural sedation in the Emergency Department. *J Emerg Med.* 2013;44(4):823–28.

56. Stefansson T, Wickstrom I, Haljamae H. Hemodynamic and metabolic effects of ketamine anesthesia in the geriatric patient. *Acta Anaesthesiol Scand.* 1982;26(4):371–77.

57. Jabre P, Combes X, Lapostolle F, et al. Etomidate versus ketamine for rapid sequence intubation in acutely ill patients: a multicentre randomised controlled trial. *Lancet.* 2009;374(9686):293–300.

58. Wickstrom I, Holmberg I, Stefansson T. Survival of female geriatric patients after hip fracture surgery. A comparison of 5 anesthetic methods. *Acta Anaesthesiol Scand.* 1982;26(6):607–14.

59. Cicero M, Graneto J. Etomidate for procedural sedation in the elderly: a retrospective comparison between age groups. *Am J Emerg Med.* 2011;29(9):1111–16.

60. Hughes CG, McGrane S, Pandharipande PP. Sedation in the intensive care setting. *Clin Pharmacol.* 2012;4:53–63.

Chapter 23

Commonly Missed Traumatic Injuries

Matthew Greer and Brian T. Wessman

Introduction

The terms "missed injury" and "delayed diagnosis" have undergone evolution in their academic meaning over the last several decades of trauma care. Missed injury is typically reserved for an unidentified injury for which the opportune moment for intervention has passed. A delayed diagnosis is the term given to injuries not identified on the primary or secondary survey of the initial trauma evaluation. There is obvious overlap in the ways these terms are employed throughout trauma care, and specific institutions may possess their own interpretations. Many emergency medicine texts list a missed injury as one that is discovered after the patient has left the Emergency Department (ED), whether discharged home or admitted. This version of the "missed injury definition" would include possible injuries which were suspected in the ED (not truly "missed"), though not officially found due to appropriate delays in imaging while more acute issues are being resolved in the operating room (OR) or Intensive Care Unit (ICU). The national trauma database of the American College of Surgeons defines missed injury as an "injury-related diagnosis discovered after initial workup is completed and admission diagnosis is determined."[1] Delayed diagnosis was proposed to describe diagnoses that were not found on primary and secondary survey. The tertiary survey was intended to identify many of these injuries,[2] though some literature still defines injuries found during the tertiary survey as "delayed."[3,4] In any case, the use of a tertiary survey should be employed in all trauma evaluations, as it leads to a reduction in clinically significant initially unidentified injuries.[5] Trauma surgery has also created leveling algorithms based on the mechanism of injury to help activate appropriate resources for trauma patients. Finally, multiple evidence-based decision tools (i.e. Ottawa knee rules, Canadian head computed tomography rules, etc.) exist to help delineate imaging decisions.

Scope of the Problem

The reported rate of missed injury varies widely (from 0.4% to 65%) depending on multiple factors: how the study defines the "miss," the specialty (i.e. orthopedics vs. vascular) the study focuses on, and whether the study is prospective or retrospective.[6,7] In 1990, Enderson et al.[2] introduced the tertiary survey as a means of capturing unidentified diagnoses before they became "missed." Yet, some studies still list all injuries found during the tertiary survey as "missed," claiming they occur after the initial trauma survey.[4,8] The percentage of unrecognized injuries discovered in a literature review by Pfeifer and Pape[8] found a range of 1.3–39%, with mean around 9%. Few studies break down the number of clinically significant missed injuries (a problem additionally confounded by publication bias), however, clinically significant missed injuries are noted to be a minority of overall missed injuries, found to range between 12% and 15% in studies reviewed by Lee and Bleetman[6] and 15% and 22.3% in a series by Pfeifer and Pape.[8] Another proposed way to evaluate the scope of this problem is to identify "rate of change in treatment," with some studies showing this rate to be as high as 55.1%.[4]

Predominant missed injuries by location:[9]

- Limbs (33.3%)
- Head (30.2%)
- Thorax (19.1%)

Patients at greatest risk for missed injuries:[3,8,10]

- Increased injury severity
- Intubated/noncommunicative
- Low GCS
- Receiving blood transfusions within 24 hours
- Undergoing emergency surgery
- Intoxication/drugs of abuse
- Pediatric
- Geriatric
- Pregnant

Missed Injuries by Location

Head

- Systems at risk:
  - . Nervous: brain, cranial nerves, eyes.
  - . Skull: cranium (including sinuses) as well as skull base.
- Common blunt injuries: motor vehicle collisions (MVC), assaults, falls.
- Common penetrating injuries: gunshot wounds (GSW), stab wounds, shrapnel.
- Tables 23.1 and 23.2 depict findings.

Neck

- Systems at risk:
  - . Nerves: recurrent laryngeal, vagus.
  - . Vasculature: carotid arteries, internal/external jugular veins.
  - . Respiratory: trachea.
  - . Gastrointestinal (GI): esophagus.
- Blunt neck injuries are most often from MVCs. However, assault, strangulation, and hanging may also be precipitating factors. Blunt trauma of the neck leads to a much higher incidence of missed injury (compared to penetrating trauma) due to the fact that external physical exam signs may be subtle.[12]
- Penetrating neck trauma makes up approximately 0.55–5% of all traumatic injuries. Mechanisms include GSW, stab wounds, and shrapnel. Cervical-collars are believed to

Table 23.1 Physical exam findings to consider

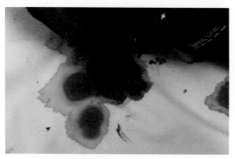

Halo sign (image: Matthew Greer, MD)

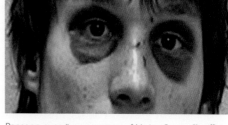

Raccoon eyes (image courtesy of Marion County Sheriff's Office)

CSF Halo Sign:
- Seen best on white sheet
- Indicates fracture of ethmoid sinus/cribriform plate from nose
- Indicates mastoid/temporal bone fracture from ear

Raccoon Eyes:
- Indicative of basilar skull fracture

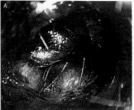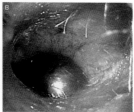

Hemotympanum with tympanic membrane perforation (reproduced with permission of Wolters Kluwer Health Inc.)[11]

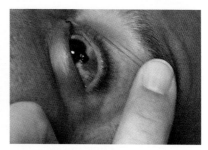

By Bobjgalindo (own work) (reproduced here under CC BY-SA 4.0 license, https://creativecommons.org/licenses/by-sa/4.0/)

Hemotympanum:
- Often indicates temporal bone fracture

Eye-lid laceration:
- Make sure to pull back lid to ensure eye does not have globe injury which can be occult/hidden under lid

be of extremely low yield in penetrating neck trauma, and early removal allows for easier management of airway and vascular injuries.[12]

- Table 23.3 and Box 23.1 depict exam and imaging findings requiring attention.

Spine

- Systems at risk:
  - Nervous: spinal cord.

Table 23.2 Imaging findings to consider

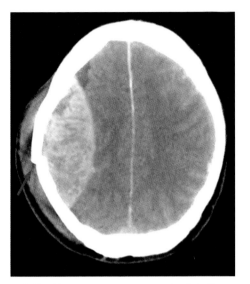

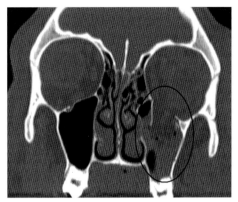

Blow out fracture (images courtesy of James Heilman, MD, reproduced here under CC BY-SA 3.0 license; https://creativecommons.org/licenses/by-sa/3.0)

Epidural hematoma (image courtesy of Hellerhoff, reproduced here under CC BY-SA 3.0 license; https://creativecommons.org/licenses/by-sa/3.0/)

Epidural Hematoma:
- Look for underlying skull fracture

Maxillary sinus fracture/orbital wall blowout:
- Look for ocular muscle entrapment
- Patient will be unable to look up or have limited intraocular muscle movements

- Vasculature: runs the entire thorax and lays next to aorta and IVC.
- Respiratory: lungs.
- GI: lumbar spine can be anvil against which bowels and abdominal organs are crushed.
- GU: none.

- Common blunt injuries: MVCs account for approximately 40% of all spinal injuries; falls make up a lower proportion and predominantly effect the lumbar spine.[13]
- Common penetrating injuries: GSWs, less often stab wounds.
- Box 23.2 depicts important exam findings.
- Imaging findings to consider:
  - One spine fracture should prompt the clinician to look for a second.
  - Consider vertebral artery injury with cervical spine fracture.
  - Consider descending aortic injury with a thoracic spine injury.
  - Consider abdominal aortic injury with a lumbar spine injury.

Table 23.3 Physical exam findings to consider[12]

Hard Signs (Need Urgent Surgical Intervention)	Soft Signs (Need Close Observation/Reevaluation)
• Expanding hematoma • Severe active bleeding • Shock not responding to fluids • Decreased or absent radial pulses • Vascular bruit or thrills • Cerebral ischemia • Airway obstruction	• Hemoptysis/hematemesis • Oropharyngeal blood • Dyspnea • Dysphonia/dysphagia • Subcutaneous air/mediastinal air • Chest tube air leak • Non-expanding hematoma • Nausea and vomiting • Focal neurologic deficits

---

Box 23.1 Imaging Findings to Consider

Air outside trachea:

• Concern for trachea or esophageal injury/perforation

Box 23.2 Physical Exam Fndings to Consider

Abnormal abdominal breathing:

• Consider phrenic nerve injury from possible C3/4 injury

Severe head and facial trauma:

• 5–10% chance of cervical spine injuries
• Consider spine immobilization until definitive imaging

Thoracic

• Systems at risk:
  · Nervous: vagus nerve, phrenic nerve.
  · Cardiovascular: cardiac (right ventricle anteriorly, left atria posteriorly), major cardiac vessels (aorta and pulmonary arteries, superior vena cava), subclavian arteries and veins.
  · Respiratory: lungs, diaphragm.
  · GI: esophagus.
  · GU: none.

• Common blunt injuries: MVCs are the most common cause of injuries leading to death in the United States, with immediate deaths often due to rupture of a myocardial wall or the thoracic aorta.

Table 23.4 Physical exam findings to consider

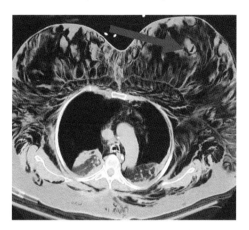

Subcutaneous emphysema

Crepitus/subcutaneous emphysema ("Rice-crispy sign"):
- Usually indicates more serious thoracic injury
- Consider pneumothorax
  Friction rub/Hamman's crunch (crackling sound with each heart beat):
- Look for pneumomediastinum
- Could be from esophageal or tracheal injury

- Common penetrating injuries: GSW, stab wounds, debris.
- Tables 23.4 and 23.5 depicts important exam findings.

Abdomen

- Systems at risk:
  - Nervous: vagus nerve.
  - Vasculature: abdominal aorta, celiac and superior mesenteric arteries, inferior vena cava, renal arteries/veins, splenic artery/vein.
  - Respiratory: diaghragmatic injury may result in herniation of abdominal contents into the thorax, and abdominal compartment syndrome may also worsen respiratory function.
  - GI: liver/gallbladder, spleen, pancreas, stomach, small intestine, colon.
  - GU: kidneys, ureters.

- Blunt injuries: There is greater risk of mortality and missed injuries (compared to penetrating trauma) due to unreliable symptoms/signs and more severe injuries occurring in these patients. Further caution should be exercised when co-existing severe extra-abdominal injuries are present (i.e. head trauma) which may limit the historical exam or ability for the patient to cooperate.[14]

Table 23.5 Imaging findings to consider

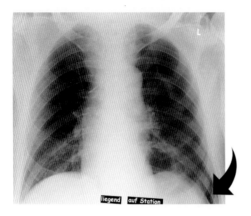

Deep sulcus (image courtesy of Braegel, reproduced here under CC BY-SA 3.0 license; https://creativecommons.org/licenses/by-sa/3.0/)

Deep sulcus sign:

- Anterior pneumothorax may only be demonstrated as a deep sulcus sign on supine CXR
  Fracture of 1st or 2nd rib or scapula:
- Consider aortic injury (dissection)
  Fracture of ribs 9–11:
- Associated with intra-abdominal injury
- Right sided = liver injury
- Left sided = splenic injuries
  Two or more rib fractures at any level:
- Higher incidence of internal injuries

- The most commonly injured abdominal organ in blunt trauma is the spleen, followed by the liver and intestines.
- Presence of blunt splenic and/or hepatic injuries predicts a higher risk of hollow viscus injury, and there is a correlation between severity of splenic injury and incidence of hollow viscous injury.[15,16]

- Penetrating injuries: stabbing injuries occur with 3-times more frequency than injuries from firearms, though the mortality rate is much higher from firearms.

  - The most commonly injured organ in penetrating trauma is the small intestines, followed by the liver and colon.
  - Stab wounds have a higher likelihood to injure the liver (more surface area).
  - Box 23.3 and Box 23.4 depict important exam findings.

Pelvis

- Systems at risk:

  - Nervous: sacral plexus, obturator.
  - Vasculature: iliac and femoral arteries/veins.
  - Respiratory: none.

Box 23.3   Physical Exam Findings to Consider

"Seat belt sign":

- Consider pancreatic or small bowel injury
- If only lap belt (no shoulder belt), consider chance fracture of L1

Abdominal compartment syndrome (ACS):

- Intraabdominal pressure >20 mm Hg
- Undifferentiated shock state
- Decreased urine output
- Undifferentiated abdominal organ dysfunction
- Compromised respiratory tidal volumes; increased peak airway pressures
- Metabolic acidosis

Chest injury:

- Risk factor for coincident intraperitoneal pathology (especially important with concommittant head injury which limits a patient's ability to communicate effectively)

Head injury with shock:

- Head injury unlikely to explain shock response, keep vigilant for potential occult abdominal injury

Box 23.4   Imaging Findings to Consider

Traumatic lumbar hernia >4 cm

- 100% chance of bowel injury[17]

Intraperitonial fluid without spleen or liver laceration

- Be wary of mesenteric injury

A negative Focused Assessment with Sonography for Trauma (FAST) does NOT rule out intra-abdominal injuries

Box 23.5   Physical Exam Findings to Consider

Examine all folds, creases, scrotum, rectum

- Look for additional penetrating wounds, bruising, or deformities which would alert to additional injury

Blood at urethral meatus

- Concern for urethral injury (do not pass Foley catheter until definitive imaging)

Imaging findings to consider:
Pelvic fractures

- Increased risk of rectal/vaginal laceration
- Urethral injury at highest risk with straddle fractures (all 4 rami involved)
- 80% of blunt bladder injuries are associated with fractures of bony pelvis

Table 23.6 Physical exam findings to consider

Posterior knee dislocation
- Popliteal artery rupture
  No plantar flexion w/calf squeeze (Thompson test):
- Achilles tendon rupture
- 2nd most frequently ruptured tendon
- Missed 25% of the time
  Unable to bear weight → get imaging
- Knee: tibial plateau fractures can happen with something as simple as axial load bearing in osteoporotic patient
- Hip: femoral neck fractures are most commonly missed fracture in adult; may be able to walk but trouble with rotation; may be occult in 2–9% of patients (usually because of osteoporosis)
  Pain over dorsal tarsal-metatarsal joint with plantar ecchymosis, or broadened foot:
- Lisfranc fracture–dislocation
- <1% of all orthopedic trauma, but missed on initial presentation 20% of time
- Passive pronation
- Consider comparison views of contralateral foot
- Fracture at base of metatarsal bone heightens suspicion of Lisfranc injury

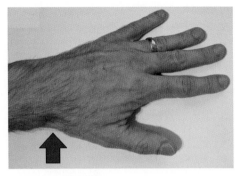

Anatomic snuffbox (images courtesy of James Heilman, MD, reproduced here under CC BY-SA 4.0 license; https://creativecommons.org/licenses/by-sa/4.0/)

Pain at anatomic snuffbox
- Scaphoid fracture
- 2% of "sprained wrist" diagnoses are actually scaphoid fractures
- Also pain with telescoping of thumb
- Treat with splint (thumb spica) and follow up in 7–10 days

Closed tendon injuries of the hand:
- Examine the hand and fingers carefully for function; it is easy to miss tendon injuries that are not associated with a laceration or fracture
- If a tendon injury is left untreated, it can lead to long lasting deformities such as Mallet finger or Boutonniere deformity

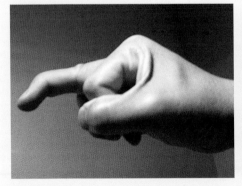

Mallet finger (image courtesy of Howcheng, reproduced here under CC BY-SA 3.0 license; https://creativecommons.org/licenses/by-sa/3.0/)

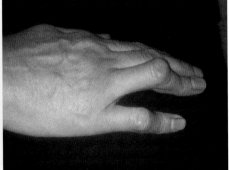

Boutonniere deformity (image courtesy of Alborz Fallah, reproduced here under CC BY-SA 3.0 license; https://creativecommons.org/licenses/by-sa/3.0/)

Table 23.7 Imaging findings to consider

First fracture → look for second
Pediatric growth plate injuries
- These are radiolucent, so must have high index of suspicion
- Consider contralateral films as "self control image" to evaluate spacing of growth plates
Knee:
- Hemarthrosis is almost always associated with another injury
- 75% are anterior cruciate ligament (ACL) tears
- Majority of remainder are patellar subluxation or patellar fracture

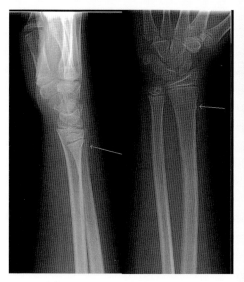

Greenstick fracture (Image courtesy of Lucien Monfils, reproduced here under CC BY-SA 3.0 license; https://creativecommons.org/licenses/by-sa/3.0/)

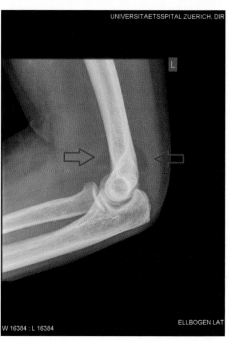

Anterior/posterior fat pad sign (Image courtesy of RSatUSZ (Own work), reproduced here under CC BY-SA 3.0 license; https://creativecommons.org/licenses/by-sa/3.0/)

Greenstick fracture of distal radius:
- Often missed in wrist images as provider is looking at carpal bones and does not examine the distal radius

Posterior fat pad/Anterior sail sign on lateral elbow x-ray
- Indicates hemarthrosis
- Radial head fracture in adults
- Supracondylar fracture in children
- Posterior fat pad is always abnormal

- GI: colon (sigmoid) and rectum.
- GU: uterus/ovaries, urethra, testicles, bladder.

- Blunt injuries: 2/3 of bladder injuries are from blunt trauma, with MVC accounting for 90% of these injuries (from vehicle ejection or seat belt against a distended bladder).

Table 23.8 Common sites where fractures lead to vascular or nerve compromise[18]

Fracture/Dislocation	Vascular/Nerve at Risk
Clavicle/first rib	Subclavian vessel, brachial plexus
Humerus neck	Axillary artery/nerve
Mid-shaft humerus/supracondylar area	Brachial artery/radial nerve
Acetabulum	External iliac, superior gluteal and femoral vessels, sciatic nerve
Femoral shaft	Superficial femoral artery
Supracondylar femur	Popliteal vessels
Proximal tibia	Popliteal artery, tibioperoneal trunk, tibial artery, peroneal artery/peroneal nerve
Distal tibia	Tibial, peroneal artery
Cervical spine	Vertebral artery
Thoracic spine	Descending aorta
Lumbar spine	Abdominal aorta
Shoulder dislocation	Axillary artery/nerve
Elbow dislocation	Brachial artery, radial, ulnar, median nerves
Hip dislocation	Femoral artery/sciatic nerve
Knee dislocation	Popliteal artery; peroneal/tibial nerves
Ankle dislocation	Posterior tibial artery/posterior tibial nerve

- Penetrating injuries: GSW, stab wounds, or impalement.
- Box 23.5 demonstrates important exam findings.

Extremities
- Systems at risk:
  - Nervous: brachial plexus, femoral nerves, all peripheral nerves.
  - Vasculature:
    - Major arteries of the upper extremity (axillary, brachial, radial, ulnar).
    - Major arteries of the lower extremity (iliac, femoral, popliteal).
  - Respiratory: none.
  - GI: none.
  - GU: none.
- Tables 23.6–23.8 depict important exam findings.

Key Points

- This chapter presents a small representation of the missed injuries that can occur with trauma patients.
- Most undiagnosed injuries occur because the physical exam was not thorough enough, or the performer/physician was too junior or inexperienced.[19]
  - Ensure systematic review of all diagnostics by competent Attending-level provider within 24 hours (tertiary survey).
  - Perform serial patient physical exams when available.
  - Ensure follow up clinic availability.
- Having a systematic way of handling trauma patients will ensure that a formalized approach to patient evaluation is followed every time. Protocolized methods have proven to improve this catchment of "missed" diagnosis.
- Remember to perform a tertiary survey on every trauma patient, a recent addition to the Advanced Trauma & Life Support (ATLS) course.
- Always attempt to understand the mechanism of the injury (i.e. height of fall, speed of MVC, etc.) to help delineate the extent and modality of imaging, regardless of initial physical exam findings.
- Open lines of communication between medical providers, radiology, consultants, and other ED and surgical team members help minimize unrecognized injuries and keeps care patient-centered.

References

1. Lawson CM, Daley BJ, Ormsby CB, Enderson B. Missed injuries in the era of the trauma scan. *J Trauma*. 2011;70:452–56.

2. Enderson BL, Reath DB, Meadors J, et al. The tertiary trauma survey: a prospective study of missed injury. *J Trauma*. 1990;30:666–69.

3. Giannakopoulos GF, Saltzherr TP, Beenen LFM, et al. Missed injuries during the initial assessment in a cohort of 1125 level-1 trauma patients. *Injury*. 2012;43:1517–21.

4. Vles WI, Veen EJ, Roukeme JA, Meeuwis JD, Leenen LPH. Consequences of delayed diagnosis in trauma patients. *J Am Coll Surg*. 2003;197:596–602.

5. Hajibandeh S, Hajibandeh S, Idehen N. Meta-analysis of the effect of the tertiary survey on missed injury trauma patients. *Injury*. 2015;46:2474–82.

6. Lee C, Bleetman A. Commonly missed injuries in the accident and emergency department. *Trauma*. 2004;6:41–51.

7. Tammelin E, Handolin L, Soderlund T. Missed injuries in polytrauma patients after trauma tertiary survey in trauma intensive care unit. *Scan J Surg*. 2016;105:241–47.

8. Pfeifer R, Pape HC. Missed injuries in trauma patients: a literature review. *Patient Saf Surg*. 2008;2:20.

9. Budduhan G, McRitchie DI. Missed injuries in patients with multiple trauma. *J Trauma*. 2000;49:600–5.

10. Sharma OP, Scala-Barnett DM, Oswanski MF, Aton A, Raj SS. Clinical and autopsy analysis of delayed diagnosis and missed injuries in trauma patients. *Am Surg*. 2006;72:174–79.

11. Bhardwaj H, Porter A, Ishaq MK, Youness HA. Bilateral hemotympanum following diagnostic bronchoscopy. *J Bronchology Interv Pulmonol*. 2016;23,e5–6.

12. Newton K, Claudius I. Chapter 44: Neck. In: Marx J, Walls R, Hockberger R, eds. *Rosen's Emergency Medicine: Concepts and Clinical Practice*, 8th ed. Amsterdam, The Netherlands: Elsevier; 2014, pp. 421–30.

13. Kaji AH, Newton EJ, Hockberger RS. Chapter 43: Spinal injuries. In: Marx J, Walls R, Hockberger R, eds. *Rosen's Emergency Medicine: Concepts and Clinical Practice*, 8th ed. Amsterdam, The Netherlands: Elsevier; 2014, pp. 382–420.

14. Houshian S, Larsen MS, Holm C. Missed injuries in a level 1 trauma center. *J Trauma*. 2002;52:715–19.

15. Swaid F, Peleg K, Alfici R, et al. Concomitant hollow viscus injuries in patients with blunt hepatic and splenic injuries: an analysis of a National Trauma registry database. *Injury*. 2014;45:1409–12.

16. Miller PR, Croce MA, Bee TK, Malhotra AK, Fabian TC. Associated injuries in blunt solid organ trauma: Implications for missed injury in nonoperative management. *J Trauma*. 2002;53:238–44.

17. Mellnick V, Raptis C, Lonsford C, Lin M, Schuerer D. Traumatic lumbar hernias: do patient or hernia characteristics predict bowel or mesenteric injury? *Emerg Radiol*. 2014;21:239–43.

18. Mavrogenis AF, Panagopoulos GN, Kokkalis ZT, et al. Vascular injury in orthopedic trauma. *Orthopedics*. 2016;39:249–59.

19. Gruen RL, Jurkovich GJ, McIntyre LK, Foy HM, Maier RV. Patterns of errors contributing to trauma mortality: lessons learned from 2594 deaths. *Ann Surg*. 2006;244:37–46.

Index